Whiplash

A Patient-Centered Approach to Management

Whiplash

A Patient-Centered Approach to Management

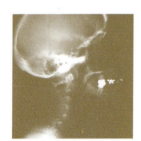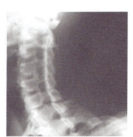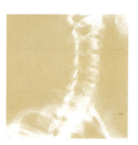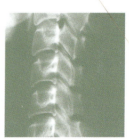

Meridel I. Gatterman

ELSEVIER
MOSBY

3251 Riverport Lane
St. Louis, Missouri 63043

WHIPLASH: A PATIENT-CENTERED APPROACH TO MANAGEMENT   ISBN: 978-0-323-04583-4
Copyright ©2012 by Mosby,Inc., an affiliate of Elsevier Inc.

Notices

Knowledge and best practice in this field are constantly changing. As new research and experience broaden our understanding, changes in research methods, professional practices, or medical treatment may become necessary.

Practitioners and researchers must always rely on their own experience and knowledge in evaluating and using any information, methods, compounds, or experiments described herein. In using such information or methods they should be mindful of their own safety and the safety of others, including parties for whom they have a professional responsibility.

With respect to any drug or pharmaceutical products identified, readers are advised to check the most current information provided (i) on procedures featured or (ii) by the manufacturer of each product to be administered, to verify the recommended dose or formula, the method and duration of administration, and contraindications. It is the responsibility of practitioners, relying on their own experience and knowledge of their patients, to make diagnoses, to determine dosages and the best treatment for each individual patient, and to take all appropriate safety precautions.

To the fullest extent of the law, neither the Publisher nor the authors, contributors, or editors, assume any liability for any injury and/or damage to persons or property as a matter of products liability, negligence or otherwise, or from any use or operation of any methods, products, instructions, or ideas contained in the material herein.

International Standard Book Number: 978-0-323-04583-4

Executive Editor: Kellie White
Developmental Editors: Kelly Milford and Joseph Gramlich
Publishing Services Manager: Gayle May
Project Manager: Stephen Bancroft
Designer: Teresa McBryan

Working together to grow libraries in developing countries

www.elsevier.com | www.bookaid.org | www.sabre.org

ELSEVIER   BOOK AID International   Sabre Foundation

Printed in the United States of America

Last digit is the print number: 9 8 7 6 5 4 3 2 1

*To patients who have suffered whiplash-associated disorders
that they may receive the care necessary
to return them to pre-injury, functional status.*

Contributors

Michael Haneline, DC, MPH
Professor, Head of Chiropractic
Traditional and Complementary Medicine
International Medical University
Kuala Lumpur, Malaysia

Lisa Hoffman, DC, DACBR
Associate Professor
Diagnostic Imaging
University of Western States
Portland, Oregon

William J. Lauretti, DC
Associate Professor
Department of Chiropractic Clinical Sciences
New York Chiropractic College
Seneca Falls, New York

Sara Mathov, DC, DACBR, ATC
Assistant Professor
Diagnostic Imaging
University of Western States
Portland, Oregon

Bonnie McDowell, RPT, DC
Practicing Chiropractor
Ballad Towne Chiropractic Clinic
Forest Grove, Oregon

Christina Peterson, MD
Medical Director
The Oregon Headache Clinic
Clackamas, Oregon

Foreword

Whiplash, along with its frequent consequences in terms of pain and disability, is often considered only in physiological and biomechanical terms. It is not routinely addressed from a patient-centered, multifactorial and holistic point of view. However, perhaps even more than most conditions considered to be the result solely of musculoskeletal injury, whiplash and its sequellae are difficult to understand from a purely biomechanical/physiological perspective. Meridel Gatterman's book is therefore unique, and a welcome addition to the literature on this important topic.

Often "patient-centered care" is assumed to be most useful when dealing with patients with complaints that are not injury-related, or that are linked to lifestyle and behavior, since it emphasizes self healing, holism, and humanism. It also operates through a practitioner-patient partnership in which the patient's preferences and values are respected in the choice of treatment and management plans. This book shows that patient-centered care can readily be applied to an injury-related condition like whiplash.

It is important to note that when one reviews the current treatment of whiplash, as Dr. Gatterman states, "one can't help but feel unsatisfied and even frustrated with the overall results. The only definitive conclusion that can be drawn from the studies done to date is that the science supporting most clinical interventions for neck pain is incomplete and often conflicting, particularly when it comes to managing neck pain that is the result of whiplash." She goes on to say, further, that "the current state of evidence is almost completely silent on what to do with patients who don't recover in the acute stage and become chronic." The cost, in terms of suffering, lost work time and health care expenses, is considerable, for chronic neck pain.

Clearly we are missing something when dealing with such patients, and I suspect that it may be that we are failing to approach each patient as an individual, with his or her own story to tell—that is, that each individual's response to an injury to the highly complex structures of the neck can be quite different from that of other individuals. Thus, "one size fits all" management plans will not work for everyone, and large clinical studies which lump everyone together and focus on pain reduction exclusively, may not reflect the individual experience of the participants.

This book adds a much-needed new dimension to the management of whiplash, by emphasizing and detailing an approach that addresses, accepts and respects the patient not just as an injured neck, but as a whole and individual person in whom physiological, psychosocial, behavioral, and biomechanical factors interact and must be simultaneously addressed. It thoroughly describes the anatomy, physiology and biomechanics of whiplash, and also details how to conduct an appropriate examination. It comprehensively addresses management of this condition, emphasizing a conservative approach with the goal of restoring the patient to an active, high-functioning life. A great deal of attention is placed on the soft tissue structures involved in whiplash, which is a particularly important area for practitioners to thoroughly understand. All placed within the context of patient-centeredness, this comprehensive approach should go a long way toward finding ways to approach the treatment of whiplash-associated complaints in a more individualized manner, one that may much more effectively help those who suffer from them to regain optimal function.

Cheryl Hawk, DC, PhD, CHES

Preface

This book is designed to encourage clinicians to take a more patient-centered approach to those persons unfortunate enough to suffer whiplash trauma. It is increasingly evident that a strictly pathoanatomical diagnosis will not always restore patients to a preinjury status. Pathoanatomical causes of neck, head and upper extremity pain are not evident in up to 80% of patients following whiplash injury, yet dysfunction in these regions causes prolonged suffering when unrecognized. A patient-centered approach to the management of whiplash-associated disorders focuses on restoration of function in addition to management of pathoanatomical lesions. Technological advances have increased knowledge of functional causes of pain and advances in imaging while not always necessary can identify functional lesions in patients who do not respond to initial management programs.

The structures of the cervical spine are most vulnerable to trauma from motor vehicle crashes, and patients who experience whiplash injury often feel fragile, with loss of function beyond what is diagnosed as pathoanatomical states. Overlooked functional lesions can cause much unnecessary suffering and often expensive care if not recognized. This book explores both the traditional approaches to whiplash injuries but more importantly includes what is considered alternative therapies, including those designed to reduce pain from pain generators in strained muscles (Chapter 5) and improvement in function from manipulation of blocked joints (Chapter 8). The etiology of whiplash-associated headaches along with a more traditional approach to mechanism and management appears in chapter 7. The epidemiology of whiplash-associated disorders (Chapter 9) looks at data related to frequency, risk factors, economic issues and the cost to society. Chapter 10 focuses on patient safety comparing the safety and complications of therapeutic procedures. Factors related to a favorable prognosis and those responsible for chronic symptoms are discussed in Chapter 11.

This text presents a multimodal management approach to whiplash-associated disorders that puts the needs of patients ahead of doctors focused only on pathoanatomical lesions, and insurance providers who are profit motivated, neither of which is always in the patient's interest.

Meridel I Gatterman, MA, DC, MEd

Acknowledgments

Grateful appreciation is expressed to all of those who contributed to the completion of this of this book including Drs. Sara Mathov, Lisa Hoffman, Bonnie McDowell, Christina Peterson, Michael Haneline and William Lauretti. I wish to express thanks to Dr. Kim Humphreys for his constructive review and Dr. Anthony Rosner for the further development of evidence tables. I appreciate the many hours of discussion provided by Dr. Christina Peterson whose ongoing contribution greatly enhanced this work. I wish to thank librarians Marcia Thomas and Carol Lynn Webb who provided assistance in obtaining valuable reference material.

Gratitude is expressed to Drs. George Goodman, President and Elizabeth Goodman, Dean of University Programs, Logan College Chiropractic who provided use of the Purser Center at Logan University, and Emily Ratliff, Purser Center Event Planner for organizing props and crews and Chris LaRose, Technical Manager for ensuring that there were no technical problems during the video shoot.

I especially wish to thank Dr. Donna Mannello for graciously participating in the figure and video productions and models Dr. Robin Waterbury and Alison Leonard. Also gratitude is expressed to Carolyn Kruse for providing voice over comments.

Great appreciation is expressed to Kellie White and the hard working staff at Elsevier including Emily Thompson, editorial assistant, Stephen Bancroft, Project Manager and especially Kelly Milford, Developmental Editor who patiently worked with me to bring the book to completion. I am also grateful for the inclusion of figures from Elsevier books by Drs. Gregory Cramer, Susan Darby, Ronald Evans, and Joseph Muscolino.

Lastly, my love and appreciation go to my husband Mike for his continued support, understanding and patience.

Table of Contents

Whiplash

A Patient-Centered Approach to Management

Chapter 1

Introduction

Meridel I. Gatterman

Perhaps there are no other conditions that beg more for a patient-centered approach to management than whiplash injuries. Individual variability to the whip-like action associated primarily with motor vehicle accidents continues to generate controversy, much needless suffering, and in many cases unnecessary legal action. The range of works on the subject includes those whose authors are clearly patient advocates, including one with a foreword by a noted claimant's attorney,[1] and on the other end of the spectrum, a study funded by an insurance society.[2] Patients with injuries from whiplash have often been maligned as malingerers who are seeking a large settlement from a third party.[3] Unusual symptoms such as blurred vision, tinnitus, dizziness, nausea, paresthesias, numbness, and back pain are often suspect when added to the more common symptoms of neck and head pain.[4] Acknowledging patients' symptoms with medically unexplained disorders becomes easier with a patient-centered approach.[5] There is an enormous difference between getting patients the care they need to prevent needless disability and helping them to get a monetary settlement based on disability that can be prevented. Clinicians have an ethical responsibility to provide care that returns the patient as close to pre-injury status as possible.

WHIPLASH AS AN ENTITY

In 1923 an American orthopedist, H.E. Crowe, applied the label "whiplash" to the effects upon the neck and upper trunk from a sudden acceleration/deceleration force.[6] Injury from whiplash associated with the rear-end collision was recognized by the mid 1930s as more patients with neck injuries were seen.[7] In 1945 Davis[8] described the mechanism of head-on collisions where a sudden forceful flexion of the neck is followed by recoil in extension. By the 1950s traumatic injuries associated with whiplash were increasingly diagnosed by the medical profession. In a published report in 1953, Gay and Abbott[9] used the term "whiplash injuries of the neck." By 1974 Hohl[10] reported on a longitudinal study on the factors influencing prognosis of soft tissue injuries of the neck in automobile accidents.

Despite a steady effort on the part of automobile manufacturers to make motor vehicles safer when involved in crashes, people continue to suffer injuries. Safety initiatives include introduction of headrests and higher seat backs, first lap and then also shoulder restraints, energy-absorbing car structures, and air bags. Nonetheless, occupants of motor vehicles continue to be injured and experience a variety of symptoms not always accompanied by objective signs.

1

WHIPLASH: WHAT IS IT?

"Whiplash" is a term used to describe a mechanism whereby the neck is whipped in one direction and recoils in the opposite direction. It is not a diagnostic term and it does not give an indication of the structures injured from this action. There has been an effort to replace the term "whiplash injuries" with other terms, including "acceleration/deceleration syndrome,"[11] yet the term persists. Other terms used to describe these injuries include cervical strain or sprain,[7] whiplash-associated disorders (WADs),[2] and soft tissue injuries of the neck.[10] For consistency in this book "whiplash" will be used to refer to the mechanism of injury and not a diagnosis, while the structures and tissues injured will be specifically named. Abandonment of the term "whiplash" will not change the issues surrounding the term; only addressing the issues directly will address the many controversies that surround injuries caused by this mechanism.

THE EPIDEMIOLOGY OF WHIPLASH INJURIES

The epidemiological characteristics of whiplash injuries have not been adequately studied, and there is much controversy surrounding the studies to date. (See Chapter 9.) To better understand the epidemiology of whiplash, good population-based research is needed both for incidence rates and risk factors and for clinical presentation and prognosis.[4] Population rates of whiplash injury, determined from automobile claims, vary from country to country and region to region. This variability may be due to accident rates, population characteristics, vehicle size, traffic density, and distances driven. Variability is also caused by automobile structures and administrative rules governing claims and compensation and differences in jurisdictional tort systems. Studies that rely on emergency room departments generally underrepresent the incidence of whiplash injury because the signs and symptoms of these injuries may not develop for some time after the event.[4] Emergency room data from rural and small town hospitals may be overrepresented when a major route for long-distance travel passes through the area. Personal risk factors for whiplash injury include age and gender. The late teens and early 20s have the highest risk of whiplash injury. Men have greater neck musculature for a given head size than women; consequently, they may have lower actual injury rates.

PATIENT-CENTERED CARE

Health care has been evolving away from a "disease or condition-centered" model toward a patient-centered model.[12] Patient-centered care can be traced back to the humanistic psychology and the client-centered therapy developed by the psychotherapist Carl Rogers.[13] Based on philosophical and ethical considerations, patient-centered care became the family practice model for the Department of Family Medicine at the University of Western Ontario in London, Ontario, Canada, in the 1980s.[14] Similarly, a patient-centered paradigm based on traditional chiropractic practice was identified as the optimal paradigm for chiropractic education and research in 1995.[15] By 2001 a report by the Committee on the Quality of Health Care of the Institute of Medicine included patient-centered care as one of the aims for the 21st-century health care system.[16]

Patient-centered care is not found in any single country,[3,17-19] nor is it the purview of any one discipline or specialty.[14-15] There are remarkable similarities in the characteristics of a patient-centered paradigm identified as the optimal paradigm for chiropractic education and research[14] and a model of patient centeredness found in the British literature[19] (Table 1-1). This similarity occurs across disciplines and in a number of countries. An interdisciplinary approach to the management of whiplash-associated disorders based on patient-centered care can prevent needless suffering and disability as well as lower health care costs.[20]

THE CHARACTERISTICS OF PATIENT-CENTERED CARE

Patient-centered care emphasizes self healing, a holistic approach to the patient, and a humanistic attitude with regard to the patient-practitioner relationship. Patient-centered practitioners work with patients as partners, both preferring minimally invasive procedures and therapies when appropriate. They provide care that is respectful of and responsive to individual patient preferences and needs, ensuring that patient values guide all clinical decisions.[15] Clinician expertise, scope of practice, and supporting evidence are all determining factors in patient-centered care.

EMPHASIS ON SELF-HEALING

It is important that patient-centered practitioners emphasize to patients that their body has the innate

TABLE 1-1

Characteristics of Patient-Centered Care

Characteristics of Patient-Centered Care*	Domains of Patient Centeredness Model†	Characteristics of Integrative Medicine‡
Recognition and facilitation of the inherent healing capacity of the person, with a preference for minimally invasive care	Less reliance on drugs; only 25% wanted a prescription	Understanding of the body's innate mechanisms of healing and CAM strategies
Recognition that care should ideally focus on the total person	Understanding the whole person	Refocus on the patient as a whole
Acknowledgment and respect for the patient's values, beliefs, expectations, and health care needs	Exploring the experience of disease and illness and the patient's feelings and ideas about the problem	Practitioner acts with compassion and pays attention to patient's spiritual and emotional needs
Health promotion and a proactive approach that encourages patients to take responsibility for their health	Health promotion, health enhancement, risk reduction, and early detection of disease	Care that promotes health by teaching patients the best way to improve their health
The patient and patient-centered practitioner act as partners in decision making	Finding common ground (partnership), sharing power, and establishing priorities and treatment goals	Involves patients as active partners in their care

*Gatterman MI: A patient-centered paradigm: a model for chiropractic education and research *J Altern Complement Med* 1995; 1:371-386.
†Little P, et al: Preferences of patients for patient centred approach to consultation in primary care: observational study, *BMJ* 2001; 322:1-7, 2001.
‡Snyderman R, Weil AT: Integrative medicine: bringing medicine back to its roots, *Arch Intern Med 2002*; 162:395-397, 2002.
CAM: complementary and alternative medicine.

ability to heal based on knowledge of the mechanisms that regulate and repair the human body.[15] Patients with whiplash injuries commonly fear that they will not return to pre-injury status. Whereas a small percentage of patients will have residual problems, the vast majority can return to pre-injury status with appropriate care. Reassurance and understanding are intrinsic and important components of patient management.[18] Emotional support is essential to allaying fear and anxiety. Suffering is not just physical pain and other distressing symptoms; it also encompasses significant emotional and spiritual dimensions.[16] Patient-centered care attends to the anxiety that accompanies injury whether due to uncertainty, fear of pain, disability, or disfigurement.[16] Patients with whiplash-associated injuries commonly feel vulnerable. They may be overly

concerned that they have suffered an injury to their neck which they associate with permanent disability. It is important that patients understand that the body is endowed with a basic vitality and adaptability giving it the ability to heal.[21] Patient-centered care that embraces self-healing strategies promotes compliance when life habits and environmental factors are addressed.[17]

HOLISTIC APPROACH TO THE PATIENT

Humans are complex organisms, and whiplash-associated injuries often are more than just simple neck strains or sprains. A holistic approach to patient care recognizes that there is a relationship among the component parts of the body, and an injured or dysfunctional body part should not be seen as separate from the body as a whole. Dysfunction in one area can extend beyond a localized area. Patient-centered practitioners focus on the whole patient both directly and through collaboration. Patient-centered care has moved away from the narrow vision of treating a single body part only. Specialists are not immune from the responsibility of treating the patient as a whole person. A specialty license does not mean that the clinician is excused from treating the patient in the context of how his or her life has been affected by his or her condition.[17]

Focusing on the whole person helps the clinician understand incongruity between the patient's distress related to the seemingly minor nature of his or her symptoms and the patient's failure to recover in the expected time from his or her injuries.[15] Care of the total person requires a willingness to address the full range of difficulties that patients bring to their doctors related to their condition, including psychological and social problems in addition to the customary physical dysfunction. Involvement of family and friends is the dimension of patient-centered care that focuses on the contribution that they make to the recovery and well-being of the patient.[14]

A HUMANIST ATTITUDE

It is important that health care practitioners acknowledge and respect patients' values, beliefs, and expectations. Physical contact with patients helps to allay fears, provide comfort, and establish a therapeutic bond. It is important that there is a connection in a meaningful and helpful way.[15] Patient-centered care encompasses qualities of compassion, empathy, and responsiveness to each patient's wants, expressed needs, and preferences.[14] It is highly customized and incorporates cultural competence[14] given that the patient's perspective of his or her condition is usually part of a much wider conceptual model. The conceptual model is the cultural lens through which the patient views his or her situation.[21] It is important, however, that symptoms or behavior not be ascribed to the person's "culture" when they are really due to an underlying physical or mental problem.[22]

Patient-centered practitioners approach patients with unconditional positive regard, empathy, and genuineness.[15] Acceptance of the patient's feelings relative to the patient's condition helps to validate the experience and makes the patient feel safe and acknowledged.[2,23] Cassell questions why scientific-

technological thinking should be in competition with (and in fact over) the humanist mode of thought.[24] He makes the point that one should not exclude the other.[24]

WORKING WITH PATIENTS AS PARTNERS

The patient-practitioner relationship is the most emphasized component of patient-centered care. The relationship that is the foundation for patient-centered care, compared with the traditional relationship, demands a sharing of power and control between the practitioner and the patient.[17] Patients should be given the opportunity to exercise the degree of control they choose over health care decisions that affect them. Rather than needing to "take charge," patient-centered practitioners are able to accommodate differences in patient preference and to encourage shared decision making.[17] This requires listening and imparting information in a nonjudgmental way. Patients want to know what is wrong with them (diagnosis), how it will affect them (prognosis), and what can be done to manage their condition.[16] They need answers that are accurate and in a language that they understand.[24] The explanatory model must be technically correct and in the context of the patients' experience of their injury.[24]

Ethically, patients have the right to receive information from practitioners and to discuss the benefits, risks, and cost of appropriate treatment alternatives.[25] Patient-centered communication is not merely an ethical imperative but can lead to better health outcomes[25,26] and lower health care costs.[20] Finding common ground and enhancing the patient-practitioner relationship sets priorities and goals of treatment and promotes a caring and healing relationship.[27]

SHARED DECISION MAKING

The goal of patient-centered care is to customize care to the specific needs and circumstances of each individual, modifying the care to respond to the person, not the person to the care.[16] Involvement of patients in decisions about the management of their condition can foster compliance and increase patient satisfaction. Patient-centered practitioners prefer conservative measures in the management of whiplash injuries.[15] Not all patients want prescriptions,[19] and although early use of nonsteroidal anti-inflammatory drugs (NSAIDs) has been demonstrated to have a beneficial effect on pain and neck function in the acute phase of whiplash injuries,[28] adverse side effects may make alternative manual methods preferable.[29] Early mobilization[30] and manipulation[2,31] in acute whiplash injuries have been demonstrated to be effective, and the risks versus benefits must be considered. Regardless of how mobility is obtained following whiplash injury, early return to functional movement with the least risk of side effects is in the best interest of the patient. Patient-centered management of whiplash injuries focuses on safe, effective, economical, and evidence-based methods of treatment.

INTEGRATIVE CARE

Integrative care has emerged as a new model for health care. It is often used to refer to a blending of the best of conventional (allopathic) and complementary and alternative medicine (CAM).[32] It is healing-oriented care that emphasizes the relationship between patient and practitioner.[33] The dictionary definition of *integrate* is "to unite with something else," while *integration* means "the incorporation of equals into society."[34] Yet, implicit in the merger process for mainstream medicine is an inequality in power and worthiness between conventional and CAM approaches. That is, the politically dominant "larger unit" (i.e., conventional medicine in the Western world) carries the values, culture, and conceptual framework into which it expects the smaller unit (i.e., CAM) to assimilate. It operates under the assumption that each CAM intervention once tested and proven effective (through the biomedical paradigm) can be incorporated into conventional care as now practiced.[32] The prevailing conventional care that relies on pharmaceutical medicine cannot assimilate CAM therapies that are based on a different paradigm.

THE PARADIGM CONCEPT

Science is conducted within a paradigm that provides a disciplinary matrix, the glue that holds the discipline together.[35] Paradigm is as important to solving puzzles in the practice of a discipline as it is to researching a discipline. It provides a framework or way of looking at the results of empirical inquiry. A paradigm provides a lens for viewing the world based on habits of mind and webs of belief.

CLASHING PARADIGMS

The current ferment within health care stems largely from a clash between the reductionistic and holistic paradigms.[15] This conflict can be traced to ancient Greece, where the Coans led by Hippocrates adhered to a holistic worldview in which the patient was viewed as a whole. In contrast, the Cnidian School focused on diseases of parts located in organs or organ systems.[36] The Coan School held that disease had a natural basis that was the result of an imbalance within the person. Coan decision making was person oriented, emphasizing the structure-function relationship. Promotion of health included diet, exercise, and a balanced life. The Cnidian tradition saw diseases as real entities with an existence distinct from the person.[36] The current biomedical model dominated by specialists is a legacy of the Cnidian School.[37] A patient-centered paradigm that follows the Coan tradition of Hippocrates is the most useful paradigm to manage patients with whiplash injuries.

The power of the dominant paradigm is enormous, and health conceptions are related to existing worldviews. Health care research and treatment practices today are directed by the prevailing reductionistic paradigm, thereby limiting the understanding and advancement of holistic models. The dominant reductionistic medical worldview cannot accommodate the holistic perspective characteristic of the patient-centered paradigm.

Each paradigm provides a set of scientific and metaphysical beliefs, a theoretical framework in which scientific theories can be tested, evaluated, and applied.

WHAT IS INTEGRATIVE CARE?

Integrative care represents a higher-order system of care that emphasizes wellness and healing of the entire person (bio-psycho-socio-spiritual dimensions). The integrative care model described by Snyderman and Weil is based on the same characteristics as patient-centered care and the domains of patient centeredness.[38] (See Table 1-1.) They emphasize that the practitioner of integrative care is not only trained in scientifically based medicine but is also open minded and knowledgeable about the body's innate mechanisms of healing. They identify the need to refocus on the patient as a whole and the primacy of meaningful patient-physician relationships. They stress the need to involve patients as active partners in their care, noting the insufficiency of science and technology alone to shape the ideal practice of medicine.

Patient-centered integrative care puts the patient's needs and preferences first, ensuring that patient values guide all clinical decisions.[15] It is nonhierarchical, bringing together alternative and complementary therapies with conventional medicine. Patient-centered care relies on active participation of the patient in developing and carrying out the treatment plan. Patients receiving functionally integrated care have a supportive therapeutic alliance with at least one member of the health care team to reduce time spent by other members of the team so as to deliver a more efficient and effective treatment regime.

Ethical integrated care accomplishes the following:

- Seeks reliable evidence-based information about the safety and effectiveness of those therapies provided
- Applies common sense when balancing risks and benefits in making therapeutic decisions
- Emphasizes weighing risks and benefits in considering situation-specific variables, including the patient's beliefs, cultural values and practices, therapeutic goals, and the type and severity of the patient's injuries
- Applies the ethical principles of autonomy (empowerment), nonmaleficence (not causing harm), beneficence (promoting patient welfare), and justice (fair and equitable care)
- Provides patients with any information that is pertinent to treatment decisions

When surveyed, patients strongly prefer patient-centered care[18] that is integrated to serve their interests.

EVIDENCE-BASED CARE

The reductionistic paradigm that drives the research into the pathophysiological basis of disease is not adequate for studying a patient-centered approach to whiplash injuries.[15] Where methodological issues are being co-opted by paradigmatic issues, methods that acknowledge a different worldview must be applied.[39] Observational study designs inherently accommodate the multifactorial nature of patient-centered practice and the development and adaptation of multidimensional outcome measures that capture mental-emotional-physical changes during treatment. Complementary and alternative medicine whole systems research goes beyond the limitations and inadequacies of the randomized controlled trial.[40] Whole systems are complex, and therefore no one method can adequately capture the meaning, process, and outcomes of these interventions.[40] Evidence-based medicine that accepts only randomized controlled trials tends to devalue the individuality of patients, shifts the focus of clinical practice away from care of the individual toward the care of populations, with the complex nature of sound clinical judgments not fully appreciated.[41] Whereas randomized controlled trials may establish strong causality through the enhancement of internal validity, generalizability is sacrificed.[32] Outcome design that evaluates integrative care should include at least one arm in the design that tests the effect of the total sum of the interventions under consideration.[32] The worldviews and roles of persons within the health care system influence the selection of outcome goals and their relative weighting.

Implicit in the worldview of integrative medicine and consistent with the patient-centered approach, is the belief that the patient is the most important stakeholder. Higher priority must be given to the patient's needs and values than is common within the conventional health care system.[32] As Sackett has noted, evidence-based care is the conscientious, explicit, and judicious use of the current best evidence in making decisions about the care of individual patients. He notes that it integrates individual clinical expertise with the best available external evidence from systematic research.[42] Patient-centered care evaluates the individual patient's clinical state, predicament, and preferences, and applies the most efficacious interventions to maximize the quality and quantity of life for that person.[42] There is no clash between the patient-centered worldview and evidence-based practice when Sackett's original concept of what constitutes evidence is applied. When evidence is interpreted in the strictest sense, relying solely on randomized controlled trials, then the patient-centered paradigm and evidence-based paradigms clash. Evidence-based care based on a patient-centered paradigm makes this book the appropriate approach to treating whiplash in the patient's interest.

REFERENCES

1. Frigard LT: *847.0: The whiplash injury*, Richmond Hill, NY, 1970, Richmond Hall.
2. Spitzer WO, et al: Scientific monograph of the Quebec Task Force on Whiplash-Associated

Disorders: redefining "whiplash" and its management, *Spine* 20(8S):1S-73S, 1995.

3. Ferrari R: *The whiplash encyclopedia: the facts and myths of whiplash*, Gaithersburg, MA, 1999, Aspen Pub.

4. Skovron ML: Epidemiology of whiplash. In Gunzburg R, Szpalski M, editors: *Whiplash injuries: current concepts in prevention, diagnosis, and treatment of the cervical whiplash syndrome*, Baltimore, 1998, Lippincott Williams & Wilkins, pp 175-181.

5. Malterud K: Understanding the patient with medically unexplained disorders—a patient-centered approach, *New Zealand Fam Pract* 29(06):374-379, 2002.

6. Crowe H: *Injuries to the cervical spine.* Paper presented at the meeting of the Western Orthopaedic Association, San Francisco, 1928.

7. Jackson R: *The cervical syndrome*, ed 4, Springfield, IL, 1977, Charles C Thomas.

8. Davis AG: Injuries of the cervical spine, *JAMA* 127:149-156, 936, 1945.

9. Gay JR, Abbott KH: Common whiplash injuries of the neck, *J Am Med Assoc* 152:1698-1704, 1953.

10. Hohl M: Soft-tissue injuries of the neck in automobile accidents: factors influencing prognosis, *J Bone Joint Surg Am* 56A:1675-1682, 1974.

11. Foreman SM, Croft AC: *Whiplash injuries: the cervical acceleration/deceleration syndrome*, ed 3, Baltimore, 2002, Lippincott Williams & Wilkins.

12. Expanding Patient-centered care to empower patients and assist providers, AHRQ Publication No. 02-0024, May, 2002, U.S. Department of Health and Human Services. http://www.ahrq.gov/qual/ptcareie.htm

13. Meador B, Rogers CR: Person-centered therapy. In Corsini RJ, editor: *Current psychotherapies*, ed 2, Itasca, IL, 1979, FE Peacock Pub, pp 131-184.

14. McCracken EC, et al: Patient-centred care: the family practice model, *Can Fam Physician* 29: 2313-2316, 1983.

15. Gatterman MI: A patient-centered paradigm: a model for chiropractic education and research, *J Altern Complement Med* 1:371-386, 1995.

16. Committee on Quality of Health Care, Institute of Medicine: *Crossing the quality chasm: a new health system for the 21st century*, Washington, DC, 2001, National Academy Press.

17. Stewart M, et al: *Patient-centered medicine: transforming the clinical method*, London, 1995, Sage.

18. Meland E: *Patient centered method and self directed behaviour change*, Universitetet i Bergen Institiutt for samfunnsmedisinske fag. http://www.uib.no/isf/people/paticent.htm. Accessed March 26, 2006.

19. Little P, et al: Preferences of patients for patient centred approach to consultation in primary care: observational study, *BMJ* 322:1-7, 2001.

20. Epstein RM, et al: Patient-centered communication and diagnostic testing, *Ann Fam Med* 3:415-421, 2005.

21. Fulder S: The impact of non-orthodox medicine on our concepts of health. In Lafaille R, Fulder S, editors: *Towards a new science of health*, London, 1993, Routledge, pp 105-117.

22. Helman CG: *Culture, health and illness*, ed 3, Oxford, 1997, Butterworth-Heinemann.

23. Coulehan J: Chiropractic and the clinical art, *Social Sci Med* 21:383-390, 1985.

24. Cassell EJ: *The healer's art*, Cambridge, MA, 1995, RMIT Press, pp 98-99.

25. Council on Ethical and Judicial Affairs: *Code of medical ethics*, 1998-1999, American Medical Association.

26. Ethical Force Program: *Patient-centered communication*, 2005, American Medical Association.

27. Stewart M, et al: The impact of patient-centered care on outcomes, *J Fam Pract* 49:805-807, 2000.

28. Szpalski M, et al: Pharmocologic interventions in whiplash-associated disorders. In Gunzburg R, Szpalski M, editors: *Whiplash injuries: current concepts in prevention, diagnosis, and treatment of the cervical whiplash syndrome*, Baltimore, 1998, Lippincott Williams & Wilkins, pp 175-181.

29. Dabbs V, Lauretti WJ: A risk assessment of cervical manipulation vs. NSAIDs for the treatment of neck pain, *J Manipulative Physiol Ther* 18(8):530-536, 1995.

30. Mealy K, Brennen H, Fenelen GCG: Early mobilisation of acute whiplash injuries, *Br Med J* 8:656-657, 1986.

31. Cassidy JD, Lopes AA, Yong-Hing K: The immediate effect of manipulation versus mobilization on pain and range of motion in the cervical spine: a randomized controlled trial, *J Manipulative Physiol Ther* 15:570-575, 1992.

32. Bell I, et al: Integrative medicine and systemic outcomes research: issues in the emergence of a new model for primary health care, *Arch Intern Med* 162:133-140, 2002.

33. Maizes V, et al: Integrative medical education: development and implementation of a comprehensive curriculum at the University of Arizona, *Acad Med* 77(9):851-852, 2002.

34. Mish FC, editor: *Merriam-Webster Collegiate Dictionary*, ed 10, Springfield, MA, 1993, Merriam-Webster Inc.

35. Kuhn TS: *The structure of scientific revolutions*, ed 2, Chicago, 1970, University of Chicago Press.

36. Phillips TJ: Disciplines, specialties and paradigms, *J Fam Pract* 27:139-141, 1988.

37. Jamison JR: Chiropractic philosophy versus a philosophy of chiropractic: the sociological implications of differing perspectives, *Chiro J Austral* 21:153-159, 1991.

38. Snyderman RS, Weil AT: Integrative medicine: bringing medicine back to its roots, *Arch Intern Med* 162:395-397, 2002.

39. Cassidy CM: Unraveling the ball of string: reality, paradigms, and the study of alternative medicine, *Advances: J Mind-Body Health* 10:5-31, 1994.

40. Verhoef MJ, et al: Complementary and alternative medicine whole systems research: beyond identification of inadequacies of the RCT, *Complement Ther Med* 13:206-212, 2005.

41. Tonelli MR: The philosophical limits of evidence-based medicine, *Acad Med* 73:1234-1240, 1998.

42. Sackett DL: Evidence-based medicine, *Spine* 10:1085-1086, 1998.

Chapter 2

Functional Anatomy of the Cervical Spine

Meridel I. Gatterman

The spine is a multilinked mechanical system that adapts to the complexity of motor functioning and kinetic demands.

In the cervical region, normal movement, as in all regions of the spine, is dependent on spinal motion segments[1] (Table 2-1). In the lower cervical spine, the motion segments are typical of the spine in general, whereas the three upper cervical motion segments are atypical.[2] The typical motion segment is made up of two vertebral bodies, the intervening intervertebral disc, two posterior spinal joints, neurological elements confined within the two lateral recesses and intervertebral foramina, plus all the connective and muscular tissues supporting and limiting intersegmental movement (Figure 2-1, Table 2-2). The upper two cervical motion segments provide for a wide range of movement (Figures 2-2, 2-3, 2-4) even though no intervertebral discs separate the anterior portions of these segments. The occipito-atlantal articulation (C0-C1) has the two paired condyles of the occiput, which fit into the concave articular surfaces of the atlas (Figure 2-3A). The body of the atlas in the atlantoaxial (C1-C2) segment is replaced anteriorly with the peg-like odontoid process of the axis. (See Figures 2-3B, 2-3C, 2-4.) This process is bounded anteriorly by the anterior arch of the atlas and posteriorly by the transverse cruciate ligament. Despite the lack of intervertebral discs that allow six degrees of freedom of movement in the typical motion segment, the two atypical upper spinal motion segments contribute to a considerable amount of movement in the upper cervical region. (See Table 2-1.) The C0-C1 articulation allows for cervical flexion and extension, while the C1-C2 motion segment accounts for 50% of the total cervical rotation. However, the increased demand for motion in the cervical spine affects its strength properties. In comparison to the lumbar spine, the cervical spine has approximately 20% of its bending strength and 45% of its compressive strength, making it more vulnerable to bending injuries.[3] The joints of Luschka (uncovertebral joints) and the transverse foramen through which the vertebral arteries pass are peculiar to the cervical spine.

EMBRYOLOGICAL DEVELOPMENT OF THE SPINAL MOTION SEGMENTS

The vertebrae of the spinal column are derived from mesenchyme, which subsequently undergoes chondrification and ossification.[4] Before reaching its final condition, the spinal column passes through four major stages: the nonsegmental axis, the segmented mesoderm, chondrification, and ossification (Box 2-1). The major embryological stages leading to the development of the spinal column and associated structures involve a recombination

TABLE 2-1

Range of Movement (in Degrees) of Cervical Motion Segments

	C0-C1	C1-C2	C2-C3	C3-C4	C5-C6	C6-C7	C7-T1
Flexion and extension*	15§	15	12	17	21	23	21
Lateral bending†	3§	—	14	14	14	14	14
Axial rotation‡	—	83	6	13	13	14	11

Modified from Adams M: Biomechanics of the cervical spine. In Gunzburg R, Szpalski M, editors: *Whiplash injuries: current concepts in prevention, diagnosis, and treatment of the cervical whiplash syndrome.* Baltimore, 1998, Lippincott Williams & Wilkins, pp. 13-20.
§Data from Kapandji IA: The physiology of the joints, vol 3, The trunk and the vertebral column, London 1974, Churchill Livingstone.
*Data from Dvorak J, et al: Spine 13:748-755, 1988.
†Data from Penning L: Normal movement of the cervical spine, Am J Roentgenol 130:317-326, 1978.
‡Data from Dvorak J, et al: Spine 12:197-205, 1987.

TABLE 2-2

Primary Function of the Components of the Lower Cervical Spinal Motion Segments

Vertebrae	Support spinal column and protect spinal cord
Intervertebral discs	Unite vertebrae and provide shock absorption
Zygapophyseal joints	Guide and restrict motion
Anterior and posterior longitudinal ligaments	Connect vertebrae and support spinal column
Ligamentum nuchae	Connects laminae and protects spinal cord
Z joint capsules	Reinforces the zygapophyseal joints
Intertransverse, supraspinous, and interspinous ligaments	Add stability to the spinal column
Transversospinalis muscles	Segmental position sensors
Short segmental muscles	Segmental position sensors
Uncovertebral joints	Restricts lateral flexion

BOX 2-1 Four Stages of Skeletal Axis Development

Nonsegmental axis (notochord)
Segmented mesoderm (somites, sclerotomes)
Chondrified vertebral elements
Ossified vertebral column

of the somites that allows for segmental spinal motion (Figure 2-5A-D).

The first stage is the formation of the nonsegmented notochord, a flexible rod of mesenchymal cells enclosed in a thick, membranous sheath. The notochord forms the axis around which the vertebral column develops. A condensation is the first cellular product of epithelial/mesenchymal

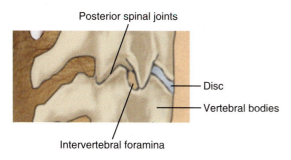

Posterior spinal joints

Disc

Vertebral bodies

Intervertebral foramina

Figure 2-1   The typical motion segment is made up of two vertebral bodies, the intervening intervertebral disc, two posterior spinal joints, neurological elements confined within the two lateral recesses and intervertebral foramina, plus all the connective and muscular tissues supporting and limiting intersegmental movement.

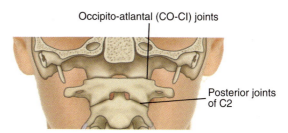

Occipito-atlantal (CO-CI) joints

Posterior joints of C2

Figure 2-2   The upper two cervical motion segments provide for a wide range of movement even though no intervertebral discs separate the anterior portions of these segments.

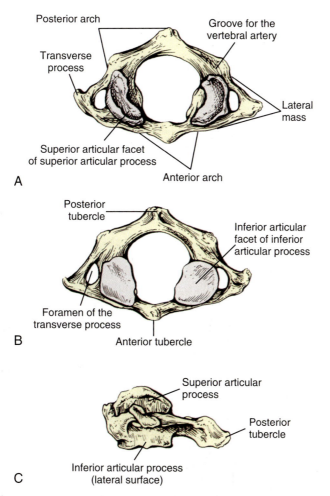

Posterior arch

Groove for the vertebral artery

Transverse process

Lateral mass

Superior articular facet of superior articular process

Anterior arch

A

Posterior tubercle

Inferior articular facet of inferior articular process

Foramen of the transverse process

Anterior tubercle

B

Superior articular process

Posterior tubercle

Inferior articular process (lateral surface)

C

Figure 2-3   **A,** Superior. **B,** Inferior. **C,** Lateral views of the first cervical vertebra, the atlas.

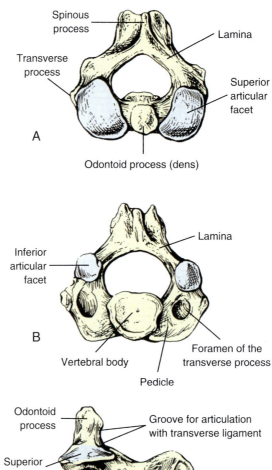

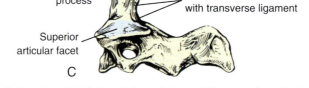

Figure 2-4   **A,** Superior. **B,** Inferior. **C,** Lateral views of the second cervical vertebra, the axis.

interactions. These condensations are the basic units from which morphology is constructed during development. Five developmental criteria identify a condensation:

- Number of stem cells
- Time of condensation initiation
- Mitotically active fraction
- Rate of cell division
- Rate of cell death[4]

Somatogenesis

Somites begin formation as discrete clusters of mesenchymal cells that undergo segmentation in a cranial to caudal progression beginning around the third week of intrauterine life; this stage is termed "compaction." A single somite can be described as having six faces, like a cube, with each facet having

a slightly different fate. Further, the position along the embryo can alter the developmental fate of the somite. During this stage, mesenchymal cells multiply rapidly, enclosing the notochord ventromedially as segmented sclerotomes. (See Figure 2-4A.) These will give rise to the bones, joints, and ligaments of the spinal column. Sclerotomal cells later migrate dorsally around the spinal cord, forming the neural arches. The mesenchymatous models in the third stage produce a cartilaginous vertebral column. Single mesenchyme cells will differentiate into chondroblasts when they are maintained in a rounded configuration. In the fourth stage of spinal development, ossification of the cartilaginous vertebral column occurs.[4]

The segmental nature of the mature vertebral column reflects its origin from the mesenchymal somites of the early embryo. During the fourth

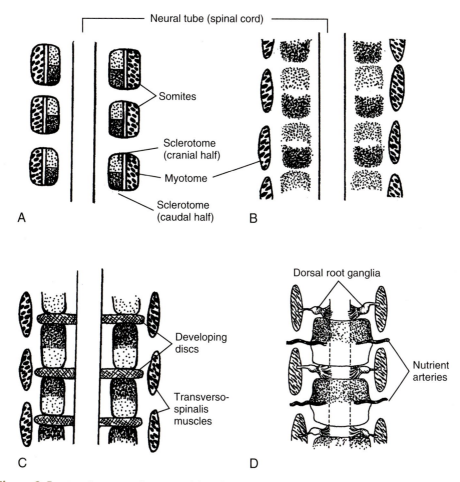

Figure 2-5   **A and B,** Recombination of the sclerotome occurs around a transverse split that forms the sclerotomic fissure. **C,** The denser caudal section of the sclerotome unites with the looser cranial half of the adjacent caudal sclerotome. The space between the recombined sclerotomal is filled with mesenchymal cells that become the precursors of the intervertebral discs. **D,** The adjacent myotomes do not split with the sclerotome; thus, the segmental muscles bridge the developing vertebrae. This bridging provides the mechanical relationship for the transversospinalis muscles to move and stabilize the individual motion segments.

week, the ventromedial wall of each somite separates into a mass of diffuse cells, forming the sclerotomes from which the vertebrae originate.[4] The cells of the dorsolateral part of the somite make up the dermomyotome. The dermatome or skin plate lays the foundation for the dermis, and the myotome or muscle plate is the forerunner of striated muscle. This differentiation becomes clinically significant to sclerotomal and dermatomal pain patterns and their origin, corresponding to the development of the spinal nerves directly opposite their respective somites.

The sclerotomal cells from each somite pair are densely packed in the caudal region and loosely packed in the cranial region. (See Figure 2-4A.) As development proceeds, a sclerotomic fissure separates these areas (see Figure 2-4B), and the component halves of adjacent sclerotomes reunite in new combinations. (See Figure 2-4B.) The denser caudal section of each original sclerotome joins the looser cranial half of the adjacent caudal sclerotome. (See Figure 2-4C.) These recombinations then become the primordia of the vertebrae. Their fusion around the notochord produces the vertebral centrum (body). The cranial portion of the condensed caudal mass, which is farthest from the nutrition provided by the artery, increases in density, forming the precursor of the intervertebral disc. The poor vascularity of the early intervertebral disc is lost in adult life, and the nutritional demands are met by diffusion from lymph.

The mesenchymal cells located between the cephalic and caudal portions of the original sclerotome segments fill the space between the two precartilaginous vertebral bodies as precursors of the intervertebral discs.[4] Whereas the sclerotomal mesenchyme forming the body of the vertebrae replaces the notochordal tissue that it surrounds, the notochord expands as localized aggregates of cells and matrix, thus forming the nucleus pulposus of the intervertebral disc where it persists until the second decade. The notochord then undergoes mucoid degeneration that forms the noncellular matrix of the nucleus pulposus. The nuclear material after 10 embryonic weeks is surrounded by the circular fibers of the annulus fibrosis, which is formed into a laminated fibrous zone from fibroblastic cells. These two structures form the intervertebral disc, giving it a double origin: the central nucleus pulposus from the notochord, and the annulus from the fibroblastic extension of the vertebral bodies.

The skeletal muscles develop from the dorsolateral or myotomal portion of the somite. When the vertebral bodies recombine, the adjacent myotomes that do not split now span the intervertebral fissure. Thus, the myotome-derived muscles are in a position to move, monitor, or stabilize adjacent vertebrae relative to each other. (See Figure 2-5.) This mechanical relationship establishes the elements of the spinal motion segments defined as *two adjacent vertebrae and the connecting tissue binding them to each other.*[5] With recombination of the sclerotomal portions, the intersegmental arteries originally located between the sclerotomes eventually pass into the middle of the vertebral bodies. (See Figure 2-5.)

The fibers of the ventral roots grow out from neuroblasts in the anterior and lateral parts of neural gray horn to supply the myotomes of the mesodermal somites. These fibers form the somatic and visceral motor efferents of the ventral nerve roots. The fibers of the dorsal roots are developed from the neural crest cells that form the spinal ganglia just medial to each primitive mesodermal somite and dorsolateral to the spinal cord. The spinal nerves eventually enter and exit through the intervertebral foramina.

Dorsal and lateral to the developing centra (body of the vertebra), the less dense portions of the sclerotomes form the precartilaginous neural arches and transverse processes, while denser portions give rise to the intervertebral ligaments.[4] Segmentation seems to be induced by the pull of the notochord, which acts as an organizer in effecting the centrum. The neural crest cells that develop into the dorsal root ganglia appear to act as organizers for vertebral arch segmentation.

COMPONENTS OF THE LOWER SPINAL MOTION SEGMENTS

Vertebrae

The lower cervical vertebrae have three parts that are associated with movement: the anterior (ventral) body, the medial (neural) arch, and the lateral transverse and posterior (dorsal) spinous processes (Figures 2-6A, 2-6B). All three parts have a predominant function in addition to sharing common functions. The anterior portion serves mainly as a load distributor. The medial portion serves to guide and restrict motion that is dependent on the geometry, size, and spatial orientation of the articular facets (articular processes). The combined anterior and medial portions provide necessary protection

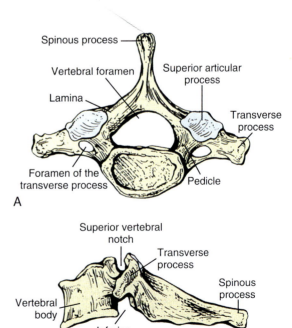

Figure 2-6   **A,** Superior and **B,** Lateral views of the seventh cervical vertebra, the vertebral prominens.

to the spinal cord, meninges, and their vessels. The lateral transverse and posterior spinous processes function as lever-like extensions for the attachment of muscles and the stabilizing ligaments. The foramen of the transverse processes provides openings through which the vertebral arteries pass upward through the transverse processes.

All three parts of the vertebrae interact for normal vertebral movement to occur.

The complete column of bodies and discs forms a strong but flexible central axis. The intervertebral discs provide for stability and movement, as connectors between vertebrae, and as separators that function as deformable spacers that allow for movement. The intervertebral foramen between adjoining neural arches near their junctions with the vertebral bodies allows passage of mixed spinal nerves, smaller recurrent nerves, and blood and lymphatic vessels.[6]

The vertebral bodies are convex anteriorly and concave posteriorly where they complete the vertebral foramen. The vertebral arch has on each side a vertically narrow ventral part, the pedicle, and dorsally a broader lamina. Adjacent vertebral notches contribute to the intervertebral foramen when the three-joint complex (disc and two zygapophyseal joints) articulates.[6] The side-to-side diameter of the cervical vertebrae increases from C2 to C7 to allow the lower vertebrae to support the greater weight that they are required to carry. The anterior surfaces of the vertebral bodies can develop osteophytes (bony spurs). Asymptomatic osteophytes that occur in 20% to 30% of the population can become clinically significant with injury to the cervical spine. Swelling that causes pressure on the more anteriorly located esophagus or trachea may lead to difficulty swallowing (dysphagia) and difficulty with speech (dysphonia). The superior and inferior surfaces of the vertebral bodies are described as being sellar or saddle shaped. The superior surface is concave from left to right as a result of the raised lateral lip. The superior surface is convex from front to back because of the beveling of the anterior surface.

Intervertebral Discs

The intervertebral discs of the cervical spine make up more than 20% of the superior-inferior length of the cervical spine. These structures allow the large amount of movement that occurs in the cervical region. Intervertebral discs are situated between adjacent surfaces of vertebral bodies between C2 (axis) and C3 through C7 and T1. The discs provide

almost 40% of the height of the cervical spine from C2 to C7. The C2-C3 interbody joint is the most superior disc capable of affecting a spinal nerve (C3 spinal nerve).[7]

Each intervertebral disc is a fibrocartilaginous coupling that forms an articulation between the bodies of the vertebrae. It serves both to unite the adjacent vertebral bodies and to hold them apart by means of the hydrostatic pressure of the centrally located nucleus pulposus. The nucleus exhibits considerable elastic rebound that allows the disc to assume its original physical state upon release of pressure. Recently, elastin content in the disc has been studied. Approximately 2% of the disc is made up of elastin, with the outer annulus fibrosus, inner annulus fibrosus, and nucleus pulposus having similar levels of elastin. Although the exact function of elastin in the healthy disc is unknown, degenerated discs exhibited a significant increase in elastin content, particularly in the inner annulus fibrosus. The increase in elastin content is thought to be in response to the deformation of the lamellar structure during radially applied loads, thereby resisting delamination.[8]

From the time of appearance of the epiphyseal ring, at puberty, the outer lamellae of the annulus fibrosis are anchored in this bony ring. The inner lamellae of the young adult annulus fibrosis remain continuous with the lamellar structure of the cartilage plates, forming a complete cartilaginous envelope around the nucleus pulposus. The outer fibrous lamellae of the annulus are almost indistinguishable in structure from the fibrous longitudinal ligaments that bridge many segments. Some inner fibers of the longitudinal ligaments attach to the vertebral rims at each level. The fibers of the annulus fibrosis only bridge one segment. Sections of the annulus show alternating directions of the collagen fibers in adjacent lamellae. They are arranged such that the alternating spiral arrangement of the fibers in successive layers gives great strength, limiting movements, especially rotation.

Mercer and Bogduk[9] demonstrated that the annulus fibrosus of the cervical disc is different than that of the lumbar spine. Instead of a ring of concentric lamella, the annulus fibrosus is arranged in a crescent-shaped mass of collagen that is thick anteriorly and tapers toward the uncinate processes laterally (Figure 2-7). The annulus fibrosus is deficient posterolaterally and posteriorly; only a thin vertical layer of annular fibers is present. (See Figure 2-7.) Mercer and Bogduk[9] concluded that the annulus fibrosus was more like an interosseous

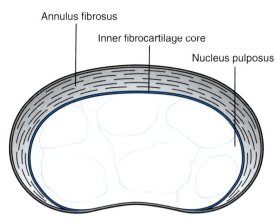

Figure 2-7   Superior view of a cervical intervertebral disc illustrating the crescent-shaped annulus fibrosus.

ligament than a ring of annular fibers around the nucleus pulposus. The difference in morphology of the cervical disc may help to explain some of the difference in biomechanics of the cervical spine related to the lumbar or thoracic spine.

The epiphyseal cartilage plates form a hard bony ring with a large central part of hyaline cartilage that persists in the adult as part of the envelope of the nucleus. In the cartilage plate, the lamellae of the annulus intimately lock with persisting parts of the cartilage model of the fetal vertebral body. Spaces in the bony end plates permit 10% of the vascular spaces of the vertebral marrow to come in contact with the cartilaginous plates, important pathways for diffusion of nutrients from the vascular spongiosa into the central parts of the disc.

In the adult nucleus pulposus there is a progressive increase in the collagen content with a corresponding decrease in the cell population. The sparser cell population associated with reduced vascularity continues to produce proteoglycans. The peripheral annulus contains a few small blood vessels. Normal adult discs have a high level of hydration and can absorb water readily, particularly in the nucleus. Disc turgor is created by the high water content that is maintained by the enveloping cartilaginous envelope. The nucleus pulposus is separated from the central parts of the vertebral bodies by only thin cartilaginous plates. At the centers of these, where the notochord originally penetrated the cartilage plates, there are weak areas where sudden axial loading of the spine may cause herniation of the young turgid nucleus into the vertebral spongiosa. These depressions in the vertebral end plates are called Schmorl's nodes and are found

commonly in children and over a third of all adults. They apparently produce little if any adverse effect on the functioning of the intervertebral disc.[10]

The intervertebral disc has been found to have both vasomotor and sensory innervation.[11] The vasomotor fibers are associated with the small vessels located along the superficial aspect of the annulus fibrosis. The sensory fibers are thought to be both nociceptive (pain sensitive) and proprioceptive. Mendel et al[12] found sensory fibers throughout the annulus fibrosis in cervical intervertebral discs. They were most numerous in the middle third of the disc (superior to inferior) and were consistent with those that transmit pain. In addition, pacinian corpuscles and Golgi tendon organs were found in the posterolateral aspect of the disc. The posterior aspect of the disc receives its innervation from the recurrent meningeal (sinuvertebral) nerve. The posterolateral aspect of the annulus receives both direct branches from the anterior primary division and also branches from the gray communicating rami of the sympathetic chain. The lateral and anterior aspects of the disc primarily receive their innervation from branches of the gray communicating rami and also from branches from the sympathetic chain. It does not appear that nerve fibers are present in the nucleus pulposus.[12]

The intervertebral disc, while serving both to unite and to separate the vertebral bodies, also allows the universal movements characteristic of the typical spinal motion segment. In addition, this anterior component of the functional unit of the spine, normally the primary weight-bearing part of the spinal column, is as such subjected to enormous compressive forces. The harmful effects of axial compression are magnified by the stress of motion, which adds shearing and torsional forces to the disc.

Disc degeneration occurs with aging and is manifested by a complex process of changes. The disappearance of notochordal cells in the first decade of life from the nucleus pulposus is followed by loss of its gel-like structure from a decrease in cells, water, and proteoglycans from the extracellular matrix. The annulus fibrosus also loses its shape, which provides mechanical strength.[13]

It is little wonder that the pathomechanical states resulting from disc degeneration that occurs with the aging process have such a devastating effect on spinal motion. The vicious cycle is established because the nutrition of the disc is dependent on imbibition from surrounding tissues that in turn are affected by spinal motion for normal distribution of tissue fluid. Restricted joint motion can

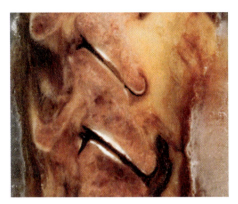

Figure 2-8 Lateral view of the lower cervical posterior (zygapophyseal) joints.

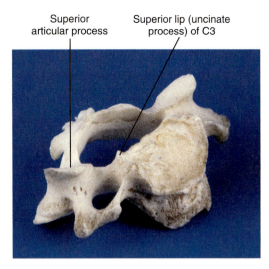

Superior articular process   Superior lip (uncinate process) of C3

Figure 2-9 The uncovertebral joints (joints of Luschka) are formed when the uncinate process of the lower vertebra articulate with small indentations found on the inferior surface of the upper vertebra.

therefore have a detrimental effect on the health of the disc and be a contributing factor to disc degeneration.

Posterior Spinal (Zygapophyseal) Articulations

The posterior spinal articulations, commonly referred to as the zygapophyseal joints, are true diarthrodial joints with characteristics similar to those of peripheral diarthrodial joints (Figure 2-8). They have articular cartilage, a loose capsule lined with synovial membrane, reinforcing ligaments, and related muscles. They appear on both sides of the posterior aspect of the lower cervical motion segments, guiding and restricting movement. The shape and the orientation of these small joints vary according to their location. The articulating surface of each superior and inferior articular process is known as the articular facet. The junction between the superior and inferior articular facets on one side of two adjacent vertebrae is known as a zygapophyseal joint (Z joint). Thus, there is a left and right Z joint between each pair of vertebrae.[14] The planar joint surfaces are covered with hyaline cartilage approximately 1 mm to 3 mm in thickness that thins with age.[14] Depending on their orientation, which varies along the length of the spine, the Z joints contribute to weight bearing. Axial load-sharing between anterior and posterior elements appears controversial with weight bearing by the Z joints dependent on spinal location and posture.

Uncovertebral Joints (Joints of Luschka)

When viewed from the lateral or anterior aspect, raised lips at the superior aspect of the typical cervical vertebral bodies become apparent. These structures arise as elevations of the lateral and posterior rims on the top surface of the vertebral bodies (uncinate processes) (Figure 2-9). Normally the uncinate processes allow for flexion and extension of the cervical spine and help to limit lateral flexion. In addition, the uncinate processes serve as barriers to posterior and lateral intervertebral disc protrusion. When the uncinate processes of one vertebra articulate with the small indentation found on the inferior surface of the vertebra above, the articulations are referred to as uncovertebral joints or joints of Luschka. These small synovial joints are limited medially by the intervertebral discs and laterally by the capsular ligaments. The uncovertebral joints frequently undergo degeneration with resulting bony outgrowth. The degree of uncovertebral joint arthrosis parallels the loss of disc height. Osteophytes from the uncovertebral joint can potentially impinge upon the adjacent exiting cervical spinal nerve root and can deflect the course of the vertebral artery.[7] Hall, in 1965, described three stages of degeneration of the joints of Luschka.[15]

Spinal Ligaments

The Articular Capsules
The articular capsules of the Z joints are thin and loose and attached peripherally to the articular facets of adjacent zygapophyses[7] (Figure 2-10). The capsules are longer and looser in the cervical region than in the lumbar and thoracic regions to

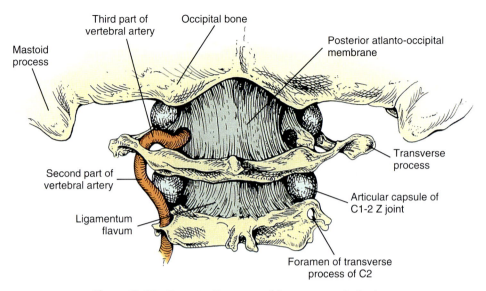

Figure 2-10   Posterior ligaments of the upper cervical spine.

accommodate for the greater amount of movement in the cervical region. The capsule consists of an outer layer of dense fibroelastic connective tissue, a vascular central layer made up of areolar tissue and loose connective tissue, and an inner layer made up of a synovial membrane.[7] The anterior and medial aspect of the Z joint capsule is made up of the ligamentum flavum. The synovial membrane lines the articular capsule including the portion made up by the ligamentum flavum.[7]

Synovial folds are synovial lined extensions of the capsule that protrude into the joint space covering part of the articular cartilage.[16,17] These intracapsular structures have been identified as synovial fold projections into the Z joint at all levels of the cervical spine.[18] Yu et al[18] identified four distinct types of cervical Z joint menisci on magnetic resonance imaging. These menisci ranged from thin rims to thick protruding folds (Figure 2-11).

The ligaments of the spine are arranged so as to provide postural support between vertebrae, with a minimum expenditure of energy, while at the same time allowing for adequate spinal motion.[2] They must also restrict motion within physiological limits so as to protect the neural elements of the spine. The spinal ligaments are designed to resist tensile forces acting parallel to the direction in which the fibers run. They also contribute to the maintenance of natural spinal curvature. Vertebral ligaments may be classified as long spinal ligaments and short intersegmental ligaments. The long spinal ligaments are continuous supporting bands running

the entire length of the spine, while the intersegmental bands connect adjacent vertebrae.

Long Spinal Ligaments

The long spinal ligaments include the anterior and posterior longitudinal ligaments and the supraspinous ligament. The anterior longitudinal ligament is a broad fibrous network attached to the anterior surfaces of the vertebral bodies. It forms a strong bond that runs from the anterior upper sacrum to the cervical spine where it attaches to the front of the body C2, the anterior tubercle of C1, and to the basilar occipital bone. The width of the anterior longitudinal ligament is diminished at the level of each intervertebral disc where it attaches to the annular fibers. It has several layers, the most superficial fibers being longest and extending over three to four vertebrae. The intermediate fibers extend between two and three vertebrae, while the deepest fibers run from one body to the next. Laterally short fibers connect adjacent vertebrae.[6] The anterior longitudinal ligament narrows considerably between the atlas and occipital bone and blends with the atlanto-occipital membrane (Figure 2-12). Functionally, the anterior longitudinal ligament limits extension and excessive lordosis in the cervical region. It is frequently damaged in extension injuries to the cervical[19] and lumbar areas.[7]

The posterior longitudinal ligament, unlike the anterior longitudinal ligament, is wider at the level of the intervertebral discs where it is interwoven

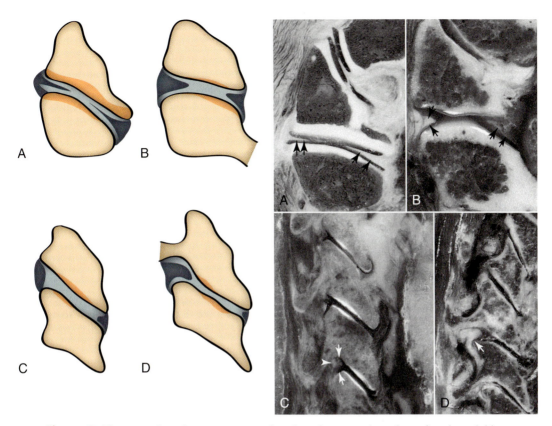

Figure 2-11 Examples of menisci. **A,** Washer-shaped menisci have been found in children. **B,** Menisci that extend into the joint spaces have been noted in the lateral atlanto-axial joints of adults. **C,** Menisci that do not extend into the joint spaces are found in C2-3 to C6-7 in adults. **D,** Menisci composed of collagen, fat, and cartilage that may extend into degenerated Z joints have also been reported.

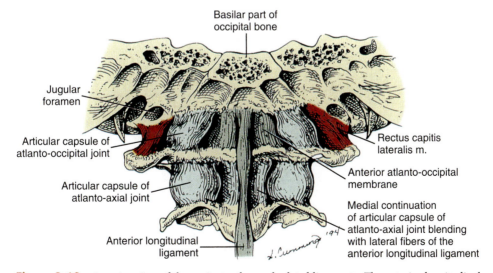

Figure 2-12 Anterior view of the occiput, atlas, and related ligaments. The anterior longitudinal ligament narrows considerably between the atlas and occipital bone and blends with the anterior atlanto-occipital membrane. The articular capsules of the atlanto-occipital and lateral atlantoaxial joints are also seen clearly in this figure.

into the annular fibers (Figure 2-13). It runs inside the spinal canal from the sacrum to the body of the axis. It attaches to the posterior superior and posterior inferior margins of the vertebral bodies. The upward extension of the posterior longitudinal ligament is the tectoral membrane, which continues

cephalad as a strong broad band also attached to the basilar part of the occiput[6] (Figure 2-14). The ligament is wide band in the cervical spine attaching to the intervertebral discs and adjacent vertebral bodies, narrowing and becoming more denticulate as it descends toward the lumbar region where it limits the ability to restrain posterior bulging of the intervertebral discs.[20] Its superficial fibers bridge three or four vertebrae, while deeper fibers extend between adjacent vertebrae as perivertebral ligaments close to and fused with the intervertebral disc.[6] A perivertebral membrane anterior to the deepest layer and attaching to the pedicles has also been found.[20] The posterior longitudinal ligament adds stability to the vertebral column.

The supraspinous ligament extends from the sacrum, along the tips of the spinous processes, to C7 where it becomes the ligamentum nuchae in the cervical spine (Figure 2-15). From C7 to the occiput the ligamentum nuchae is a flat, membranous structure, the most superficial fibers extending over three to four vertebrae, the intermediate fibers extending between two and three vertebrae, while the deepest fibers connect adjacent spines. It is the first structure to rupture in extreme flexion.[7] Mechanically, the ligaments deform in response to the separation between vertebrae. In addition, the posterior and anterior longitudinal ligaments can be stretched by bulging of the disc. Excessive

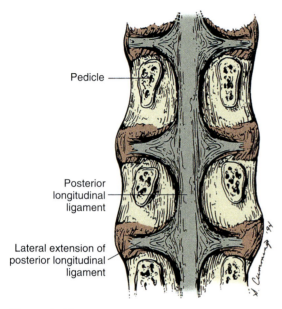

Figure 2-13   Posterior longitudinal ligament is shown coursing along the anterior aspect of the lumbar vertebral canal.

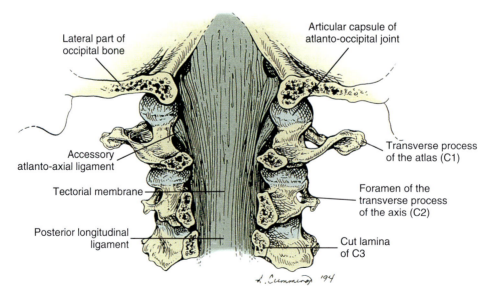

Figure 2-14   Posterior aspect of the occiput, posterior arch of the atlas, laminae and spinous processes of C2 and C3, neural elements, and meninges have all been removed to show the ligaments of the anterior aspect of the upper cervical vertebral canal and foramen magnum.

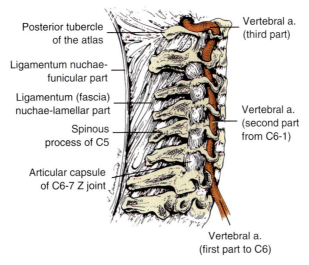

Figure 2-15 The supraspinous ligament becomes the ligamentum nuchae in the cervical spine.

traction at the attachment points of these two ligaments causes spur formation, which can be visualized radiographically.

Intersegmental Ligaments

The intersegmental ligaments that connect adjacent vertebrae include the ligamenta flava, the interspinous, intertransverse, and capsular ligaments.

The ligamenta flava extend from the anterior superior borders of the laminae to the anterior inferior borders of the laminae above (Figure 2-16). They connect adjacent vertebrae from the sacrum to the axis bridging the posterior elements of the spinal canal.[6] Their attachments extend from zygapophyseal capsules to where the laminae fuse to form spines. Where their posterior margins meet, they are partially united, with intervals for veins connecting internal to posterior external vertebral venous plexuses.[6] These fibroelastic structures permit separation of the lamina in flexion and at the same time brake the movement so that its limit is not reached abruptly.[6]

The elastic property of these ligaments assists in the restoration of the vertebral column to the neutral position following flexion. Additionally it protects the spinal cord from impingement by folding, which would occur with a nonelastic structure. A ligament made of collagen would just as well resist flexion but would not shorten without buckling. It may also protect the discs from injury.[6] The ligamenta flava form the medial and anterior aspects of the capsular ligaments. Because of the elastic nature of these ligaments' anterior

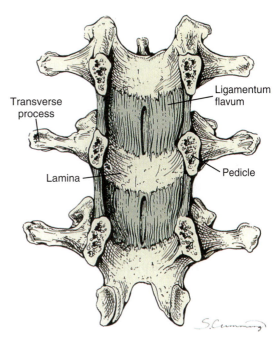

Figure 2-16 The ligamentum flavum (an elastic ligament) that forms the medial and anterior aspects of the capsular ligaments.

movement, the posterior joints of the spine may be less restricted, predisposing the joints to movement disorders. It has also been suggested that the shortening and lengthening of the ligamenta flava with spinal motion results in small, frequent, repetitive movements that assist in the nutrition of the posterior joint cartilage, the nucleus pulposus, and the cartilage plates of the disc, a function that would be expected to be absent or impaired by joint fixation.

The interspinous ligaments are thin and almost membranous. They connect adjacent spinous processes, and their attachments extend from the root to the apex of each process, meeting the supraspinous ligament at the back and the ligamenta flava in front. In the cervical region they are only slightly developed as part of the ligamentum nuchae.[6] The interspinous ligaments add stability to the spine by checking excessive flexion.[6] Along with the supraspinous ligament the interspinous ligaments are typically the first structures to rupture in extreme flexion.[7]

The intertransverse ligaments connect the ipsilateral transverse processes of adjacent vertebrae. They are largely replaced by intertransverse muscles in the cervical region and consist of a few scattered fibers in this area. The intertransverse ligaments become taut in contralateral lateral flexion.[21]

The capsular ligaments are attached immediately peripheral to the lateral margins of the articular facets joining adjacent articular processes. (See Figure 2-12.) As stated previously, medially and anteriorly the joint capsule is formed by a lateral continuation of the ligamentum flavum. Posteriorly the capsule is much thinner and loosely attached. Laxity of the capsule posteriorly and inferiorly, in addition to the elastic properties of the medial and anterior fibers, allows considerable range of movement in different directions. Disc degeneration leads to telescoping or imbrication of the facets, with destruction of the articular cartilage as the posterior joints increasingly bear weight.

Ligaments of the Upper Cervical Spine

The upper cervical ligaments are those associated with the occiput, atlas, and the anterior and lateral aspects of the axis.

Posterior Atlanto-Occipital Membrane

The posterior atlanto-occipital ligament is a thin membrane that attaches to the posterior arch of the atlas and posterior rim of the foramen magnum, spanning the distance from between the left and right lateral masses. Laterally this broad ligament arches over the right and left grooves for the vertebral artery. This allows for the passage of the vertebral artery, vertebral veins, and the suboccipital nerve. (See Figure 2-10.) When this ligament ossifies, it is known as a posterior ponticle, creating the arcuate foramen found in one third of subjects studied.[6] Compromise of the structures passing

through the bony opening as opposed to a membranous ligament needs further study.

Tectoral Membrane

The tectoral membrane is the superior extension of the posterior longitudinal ligament. It attaches to the posterior aspect of the body of C2, crossing over the odontoid process and inserting onto the anterior rim of the foramen magnum. (See Figure 2-14.) This ligament limits both flexion and extension of the atlas and occiput.[7] Recent research suggests that due to the presence of many elastic fibers, the tectoral membrane assists the alar and transverse ligaments in limiting extension and particularly flexion movements. The elastic fibers in the middle portion of the tectoral membrane allow it to stretch over the odontoid process during flexion (similar to a "hammock"), thereby inhibiting the odontoid process from impinging posteriorly into the cervical canal. The tectoral membrane does not have an effect on lateral flexion movement.[22]

Accessory Atlantoaxial Ligaments

The paired atlantoaxial ligaments (left and right) course from the base of the odontoid process to the inferior medial surface of the lateral mass of the atlas on the same side (Figure 2-17). They strengthen the posterior medial aspect of the capsule of the lateral atlantoaxial joints.[7]

Cruciform Ligament

The cruciform ligament is made up of transverse and longitudinal components that form a strong ligamentous protection of the spinal cord. The transverse portion runs from one lateral mass of the atlas to the opposite lateral mass. The anterior portion is lined with a thin layer of cartilage that forms a diarthrodial joint with the odontoid process that passes posterior to this ligament. The transverse portion of this ligament holds the atlas in its proper position, thereby preventing compression of the spinal cord during flexion of the head and neck. (See Figure 2-17.) Functionally it allows the atlas to pivot on the axis. The transverse ligament is stronger than the dens, which usually fractures before rupture of the ligament.[6] The superior longitudinal band of the cruciform ligament runs from the transverse ligament to the anterior lip of the foramen magnum. It is interspersed between the apical ligament anteriorly and the tectoral membrane posteriorly. The inferior longitudinal band attaches the transverse portion to the ligament to the body of C2. The longitudinal bands of the

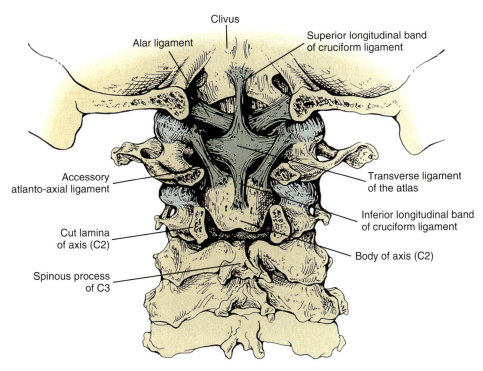

Figure 2-17 Anterior aspect of the vertebral canal and foramen magnum as seen from behind. The tectoral membrane has been removed, and many of the upper cervical ligaments can be seen. Notice the centrally located cruciform ligament with its narrow superior and inferior longitudinal bands and its stout transverse ligament. The alar and accessory atlanto ligaments can also be seen.

cruciform ligament hold the transverse portion in its proper position, assisting in holding the atlas against the odontoid process.[7]

Alar Ligaments
The strong right and left alar ligaments run from the posterior and lateral aspect of the odontoid process to the occipital condyle on the same side. (See Figure 2-17.) Each alar ligament limits contralateral atlantoaxial rotation. The left alar ligament becomes taut on rotation to the right and vice versa. The slight upward movement of the axis during rotation permits a wider range of movement by reducing tension in the alar ligaments, the capsules, and accessory ligaments of the lateral atlanto-occipital joint.[6] The alar ligaments also help to check lateral flexion as well as rotation and are also known as the check ligaments.[7] If the tectoral membrane and cruciform ligaments become torn, the alar ligaments also limit flexion of the upper cervical spine. The alar ligaments are most vulnerable to tearing during extreme movements of axial rotation and flexion. This combination of movement can occur during a rear-end motor vehicle

accident when the victim is looking in the rearview mirror.[23]

Apical Ligament of the Odontoid Process
The thin apical ligament is approximately 1 inch in length and fans out from the apex of the dens into the anterior margin of the foramen magnum between the alar ligaments (Figure 2-18). Its fibers blend with the deep fibers of the superior band of the cruciform ligament. The apical ligament is thought to prevent some vertical translation and anterior shear of the occiput.[24]

Anterior Atlanto-Occipital Membrane
The atlanto-occipital membrane runs from the superior aspect of the anterior arch of the atlas to the anterior margin of the foramen magnum in front of the apical ligament. (See Figure 2-12.) This broad membranous ligament blends laterally with the capsular ligaments of the atlanto-occipital articulation. It functions to limit extension of the occiput on C1. Fibers continuous with the anterior longitudinal ligament strengthen the anterior atlanto-occipital ligament medially and form a tough

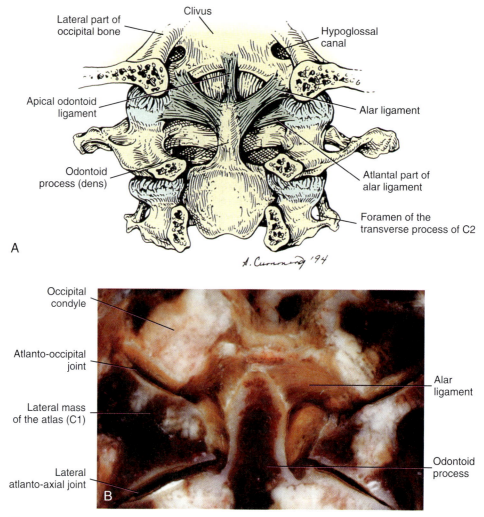

Figure 2-18 labels:

- Lateral part of occipital bone
- Clivus
- Hypoglossal canal
- Apical odontoid ligament
- Alar ligament
- Odontoid process (dens)
- Atlantal part of alar ligament
- Foramen of the transverse process of C2
- A
- A. Cumming '94
- Occipital condyle
- Atlanto-occipital joint
- Lateral mass of the atlas (C1)
- Alar ligament
- Odontoid process
- Lateral atlanto-axial joint
- B

Figure 2-18　The alar and apical odontoid ligaments. The tectoral membrane and cruciform ligaments have been removed.

central band between the anterior tubercle of the atlas and the occiput.[7]

Deep Spinal Muscles

Transversospinalis Muscles

The transversospinalis muscles run obliquely upward and medially from transverse processes to adjacent, and sometimes more distant, spinous processes. It is thought that these deep muscles function as postural stabilizers acting as dynamic ligaments that adjust small movements of the vertebral column, ensuring the efficient action of the long superficial muscles. Evidence suggests that these muscles are rich in muscle spindles, indicating that they act in response to position change,

thus serving as length transducers. These muscles are of such small physiological cross-sectional area that they generate only a few newtons of force, and because they work through a small moment arm, their contribution to rotational axial twisting and bending torque is probably minimal.[25] The vertebral column is made up of a series of small elements joined in series, and such a mechanical arrangement would buckle under compressive forces without a stabilizing mechanism.

The transversospinalis muscular group consists of the following: semispinalis thoracis, cervicis, and capitis; and multifidus and rotatores thoracis, cervicis, and lumborum. They are arranged such that from superficial to deep, the length of the muscles becomes progressively shorter.

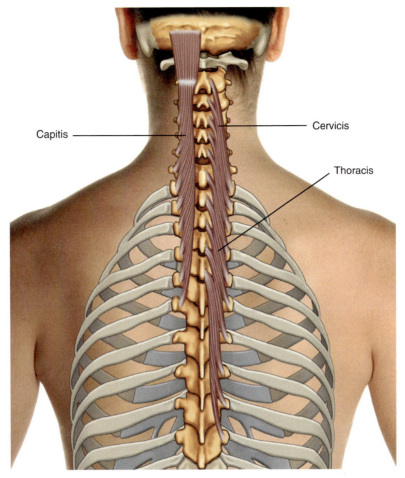

Capitis — — — — — Cervicis

— Thoracis

Figure 2-19 Posterior view of the semispinalis. The semispinalis thoracis and cervicis are seen on the right; the semispinalis capitis is seen on the left.

Semispinalis Thoracis

The semispinalis thoracis consists of thin, fleshy fasciculi interposed between long tendons. It arises below by a series of tendons that attach to the transverse processes of the sixth to the tenth thoracic vertebrae inserting above again by tendons into the spinous processes of upper four thoracic and lower two cervical vertebrae[21] (Figure 2-19).

Semispinalis Cervicis

The semispinalis cervicis is a thicker mass of muscle that arises below by a series of tendinous and fleshy fibers from the transverse processes of the upper five or six thoracic vertebrae, inserting above into the cervical spines from the fifth to the second (axis) cervical vertebrae. The insertion into the axis is the largest and is composed chiefly of muscle. (See Figure 2-19.)

Semispinalis Capitis

The semispinalis capitis is a thick powerful muscle that is the best developed of the semispinalis muscle group. It arises by a series of tendons from the tips of the spinous processes of the upper six or seven thoracic and seventh cervical vertebrae and from the articular processes of the fourth, fifth, and sixth cervical vertebrae. It inserts into the medial part of the area between superior and inferior nuchal lines of the occiput. (See Figure 2-19.) Functionally the semispinalis thoracis, cervicis, and capitis extend the neck and head, laterally flex the neck and head, and contralaterally rotate the neck at the spinal joints.

Multifidus

Only the deepest fibers of the multifidus muscles are thought to span contiguous vertebrae. In the

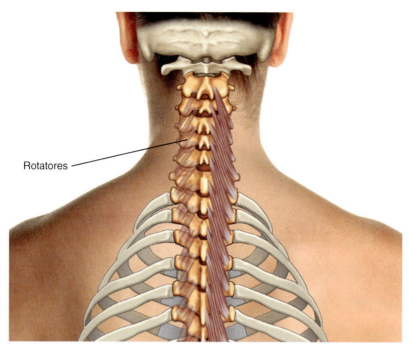

Rotatores

Figure 2-20 Posterior view of the right multifidus. The rotatores have been ghosted in on the left.

cervical region they arise from the articular processes. They run obliquely upward, attaching to the entire length of the spinous process of the vertebrae above (Figure 2-20). The fasciculi vary in length: the most superficial pass from one vertebra to the third or fourth above; those next in depth run from one vertebra to the second or third above; and the deepest connect contiguous vertebrae. They fill in the groove at the side of the spinous processes from the sacrum to the axis.[26]

Rotatores
The rotatores lay deep to the multifidus. They are best developed in the thoracic region, where they connect the upper and posterior part of the transverse process of the vertebrae to the lower border and lateral surface of the laminae of an adjacent superior vertebra (Figure 2-21). The first rotatores thoracis is found between the first and second thoracic vertebrae; the last between the eleventh and twelfth. In the lumbar and cervical regions, the rotatores lumborum and rotatores cervicis are irregular and variable, with attachments similar to those of the rotatores in the thoracic region.[26]

Interspinales
The interspinales are short, paired muscular fasciculi between the spines of adjacent vertebrae, one

on each side of the interspinous ligament.[6] They are present as small distinct bundles throughout the cervical region, beginning at the spinous process of C2 and continuing to the spinous process T1. Occasionally the cervical interspinales span more than two vertebrae[26] (Figure 2-22).

Intertransversarii
The intertransversarii are small muscles that run between the transverse processes of the vertebrae. They are best developed in the cervical region, where they consist of anterior and posterior slips separated by the ventral rami of the spinal nerves[21] (Figure 2-23). Theoretically the action of these muscles produces extension (multifidus and intertransversarii) and rotation (multifidus and rotatores), but it is likely that they function more as spinal stabilizers than prime movers.

Muscles That Move the Head and Neck

The muscles of the head and neck offer the first line of defense against whiplash injury.

Spinal motion segment immobility may be the result of primary muscle spasm in an otherwise normal segment or occur as a secondary compensatory mechanism in an attempt to stabilize a

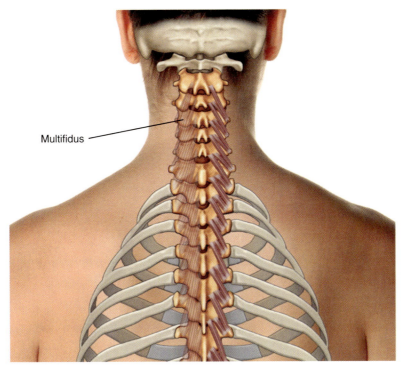

Figure 2-21   Posterior view of the right rotatores. The multifidi have been ghosted in on the left.

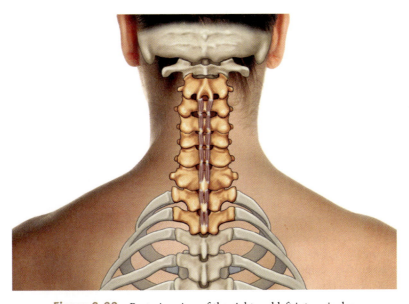

Figure 2-22   Posterior view of the right and left interspinales.

hypermobile segment. This muscle activity may be the variation in the pattern seen as paradoxical activity on electromyography of deep muscles. Clinical evaluation must await further studies of the complex arrangement of muscle bundles acting on the multitude of equally complex joints.[7]

Muscles Affecting the Cervical Spine

Superficial and Lateral Cervical Muscles

Trapezius. The trapezius muscle is a flat triangular muscle that extends over the back of the neck and upper thorax. The paired trapezius muscles form a diamond that attaches medially to the superior

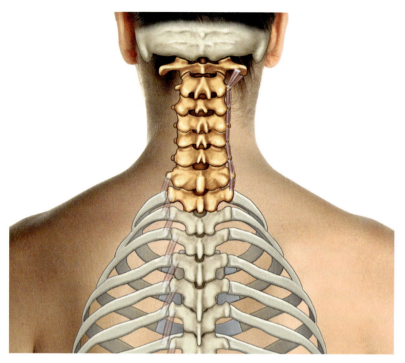

Figure 2-23   Posterior view of the right intertransversarii.

nuchal line of the occiput, the external occipital protuberance, ligamentum nuchae, and apices of the spinous processes and their supraspinous ligaments from C7 down to T12. Laterally it attaches to the lateral third of the clavicle, the acromion, and the spine of the scapula (Figure 2-24). The trapezius muscle is primarily a stabilizer of the scapula, but because of the upper attachment to the occiput and lower cervical vertebra, it can be affected in patients suffering from whiplash injury.[27] The upper trapezius acts synergistically with the sternocleidomastoid muscle in some head and neck movements.

Sternocleidomastoid. The sternocleidomastoid (SCM) muscle, as the name suggests, attaches inferiorly to the sternum and the clavicle and superiorly to the mastoid process of the occiput (Figure 2-25). Acting alone, one SCM will tilt the head toward the ipsilateral shoulder, simultaneously rotating the head so as to turn the face to the opposite side. Acting together from below, the muscles draw the head forward, assisting the longus coli to flex the cervical spine.[26] It is frequently injured in whiplash crashes.[27]

Intermediate Layers of Muscles Acting on the Cervical Spine
Splenius Capitis. The splenius capitis attach to the lower part of the ligamentum nuchae and

spinous processes of C7 through C3 or C4. The insertion is at the mastoid process, temporal bone, and occiput. The muscle passes upward and laterally under cover of the sternocleidomastoid muscle (Figure 2-26). Bilaterally they extend the head. Acting unilaterally they laterally flex and rotate the face toward the same side.[26]

Splenius Cervicis. The splenius cervicis originates from the spinous processes of T3 through T6 inserting on the transverse processes of C1 through C3 or C4 (Figure 2-27). Acting bilaterally they extend the neck. When they contract unilaterally they laterally flex and rotate the face toward the same side. Each is therefore synergistic with the contralateral sternocleidomastoid. Both the splenius capitis and the splenius cervicis are susceptible to the trauma of a rear-end collision, especially if the head and neck are somewhat rotated at the time of impact.[27]

Longissimus Muscles
The longissimus muscles are the longest of the erector spinae group. The entire longissimus group runs from the sacrum through to the mastoid process of the occiput (Figure 2-28). In the thoracic and cervical region, the longissimus capitis and longissimus cervicis are part of this group.

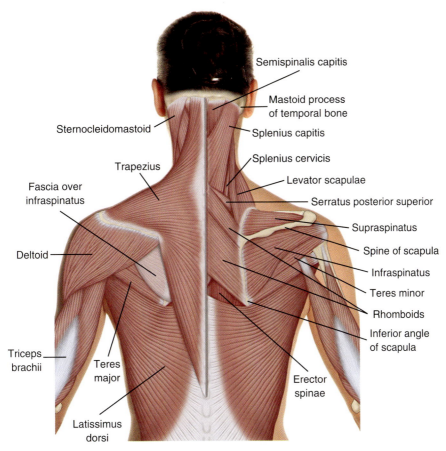

Figure 2-24 Posterior view of the cervical and thoracic muscles. The left side is superficial. The right side is deep. (The deltoids, trapezius, sternocleidomastoid, and infraspinatus fascia have been removed.)

Longissimus Capitis

The longissimus capitis muscle originates from the upper thoracic transverse process and articular processes of C4 through C7 and inserts onto the mastoid process. (See Figure 2-28.) Acting unilaterally it laterally flexes the head and rotates it to the same side. Acting together, the longissimus capitis muscles extend the head.[7]

Longissimus Cervicis

The longissimus cervicis muscle originates from the transverse processes of the upper five thoracic vertebrae and inserts into the transverse processes of C2 through C6. (See Figure 2-28.) Acting together the longissimus cervicis muscles extend the neck and head at the spinal joints.

Spinalis Capitis

The spinalis capitis (Figure 2-28) originates from the transverse processes of the C7 to the T6 or T7

vertebrae, the articular processes of C4 to C6, and sometimes from the spinous processes of C7 and T1. The fibers of this muscle blend with those of the semispinalis capitis and insert with it onto the occiput. When the right and left spinalis capitis contract, together they extend the head. Unilateral contraction results in lateral flexion of the head and neck and rotation of the head away from the side of contraction.[7]

Spinalis Cervicis

The spinalis cervicis muscle originates from the thoracic spinous processes and inserts onto the spinous processes of C2 and occasionally C3 and C4. (See Figure 2-28.) This small muscle functions to extend the cervical region.[7]

Semispinalis Cervicis

The semispinalis cervicis is a thick mass of muscle that originates from the transverse processes of the

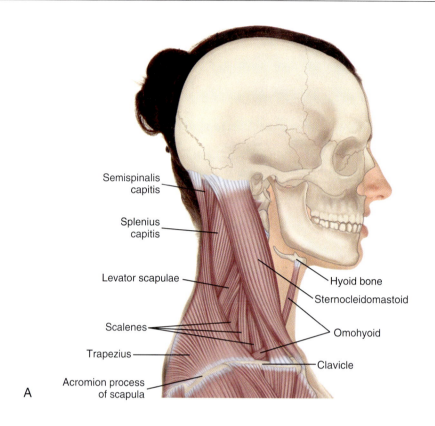

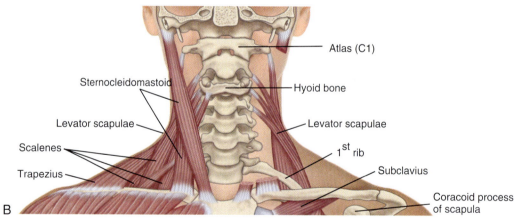

Figure 2-25   **A,** Lateral view of the superficial and lateral cervical muscles. **B,** Anterior view of the superficial and lateral cervical muscles.

upper five or six thoracic vertebrae and may also arise from the articular processes of the lower four cervical vertebrae. It inserts onto the spinous process of the axis and the spinous processes of C3 to C5 (Figure 2-29). The semispinalis cervicis extends the neck.[7]

Semispinalis Capitis

The semispinalis capitis is a thick powerful muscle that arises from the transverse processes of C7 to

T6 and the articular processes of C4 to C6 and inserts onto the occiput. (See Figure 2-29.) Acting together, the muscles extend the thoracic and cervical portions of the spine. Acting alone, the muscle rotates the vertebral bodies to the opposite side.[7]

Suboccipital Muscles

The suboccipital muscles are a group of four small muscles located inferior to the occiput in the most superior portion of the posterior neck. They are the

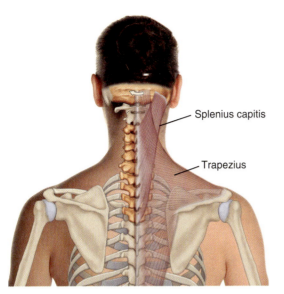

Figure 2-26   Posterior view of the right splenius capitis. The trapezius has been ghosted in.

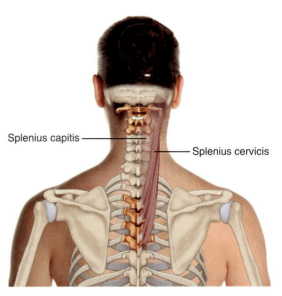

Figure 2-27   Posterior view of the right splenius cervicis. The splenius capitis has been ghosted in.

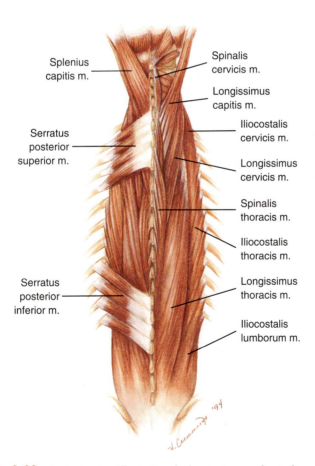

Figure 2-28   Posterior view illustrating the longissimus and spinalis muscles.

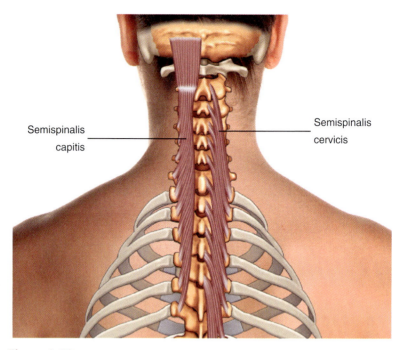

Figure 2-29   Posterior view of the semispinalis capitis and semispinalis cervicis.

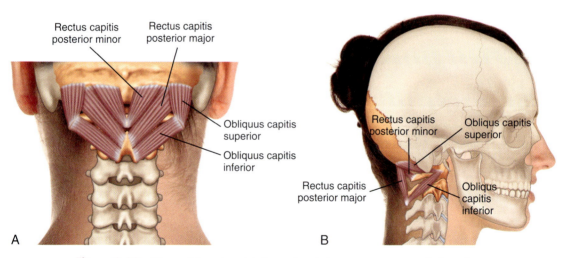

Figure 2-30   Views of the suboccipital muscles. **A,** Posterior view. **B,** Right lateral view.

deepest muscles in the region, located under the trapezius, splenius capitis, and semispinalis capitis.[7]

Rectus Capitis Posterior Major

The rectus capitis posterior major begins at the spinous process of C2, widens as it ascends, and attaches superiorly to the occiput (Figure 2-30). When acting bilaterally, the rectus capitis posterior muscles produce extension of the head. Unilateral

contraction turns the head so that the face rotates toward the side of the shortening muscle.[7]

Rectus Capitis Posterior Minor

The rectus capitis posterior minor (RCP minor) muscle is located medial to and partly under the rectus capitis posterior major. It attaches inferiorly to the posterior tubercle of the atlas, becoming broader as it ascends. It inserts on the occiput and is made up of a medial and deep part.[28] (See Figure 2-30.) It has been found that the rectus capitis posterior minor attaches to the posteriorly spinal dura in the posterior atlanto-occipital space.[29] In particular, the deep and medial parts of the RCP minor travel in an anteroinferior direction and attach to the spinal dura via their fascia and tendinous fibers.[28] Contraction of this muscle produces extension of the head.[7]

Obliquus Capitis Superior

The obliquus capitis superior arises from the transverse process of the atlas. It widens as it runs superiorly and posteriorly, inserting onto the occiput lateral to the attachment of the semispinalis capitis, overlapping the insertion of the rectus capitis posterior major. (See Figure 2-30.) Bilateral contraction produces head extension. Unilateral contraction produces lateral flexion of the head to the same side. It is probable that the obliquus capitis superior muscles, with the two rectus muscles, act as postural stabilizers rather than prime movers.[7]

Obliquus Capitis Inferior

The obliquus capitis inferior muscle is the larger of the two obliquus muscles. It originates on the spinous process of C2, passes laterally and lightly superiorly to insert onto the transverse process of C1. (See Figure 2-30.) The obliquus capitis inferior rotates the atlas such that the face is turned to the same side of contraction.[7] The length of the transverse processes of the atlas gives this muscle a considerable mechanical advantage.

Recently, Elliott et al[30] have shown that whiplash patients (WAD II) demonstrated on MRI quantifiably different amounts of fatty infiltration of posterior cervical muscles (suboccipital and other spinal extensors) compared to control participants. Fatty infiltration was found to be the greatest in the RCP major and minor as well as multifidi and at the C3 level. It is not currently known whether the fatty infiltration pattern is due to structural damage, nerve injury, or generalized disuse atrophy. However, future work may help to identify the underlying mechanism as well as indications for treatment and management approaches to address these problems.

Anterior Cervical Muscles

The anterior muscles of the cervical vertebrae are responsible for flexing the neck and occiput. They may be injured during extension injuries of the cervical region.

Longus Colli

The right and left longus colli are located along the anterior aspect of the cervical vertebral bodies. The vertical portion originates from C5 to T4 and inserts onto the vertebral bodies of C2 to C4. The inferior oblique portion originates from the vertebral bodies of T1 to T3, passing superiorly and laterally to insert onto the anterior tubercles of the transverse processes of C5 and C6. The superior oblique portion of the longus colli muscle originates from the anterior tubercles of the transverse processes of C3 to C5. It courses superiorly to insert onto the anterior tubercle of the atlas by means of a narrow tendon (Figure 2-31). This tendinous insertion can be ruptured during an extension injury of the neck. Together the three parts of this muscle flex the neck. The superior and inferior oblique parts may also aid with lateral flexion. The inferior oblique part also rotates the neck to the opposite side.[7]

Longus Capitis Muscle

The longus capitis muscle is located anterior and slightly lateral to the longus colli muscle. It originates as thin tendons from the anterior tubercles of the transverse processes of C3 to C6. The tendinous origins unite to form a muscular band that courses superiorly to insert onto the occiput anterior to the foramen magnum (Figure 2-32). The longus capitis muscle acts to flex the head.[7]

Recent research has shown that patients with neck pain, particularly from whiplash trauma, exhibit impaired function of the deep neck flexors (longus colli and longus capitus). The impaired muscle function includes weakness, fatigue, and abnormal activation patterns, and results in greater activation of larger superficial muscles such as the SCM to compensate.[31-35] Management of neck pain and whiplash patients needs to incorporate muscle strength, endurance, and coordinated activation exercises to address deep neck flexor muscle dysfunction.

Rectus Capitis Anterior

The rectus capitis anterior muscle is a small muscle located deep to the inserting fibers of the longus capitis muscle. It originates from the anterior aspect of the lateral mass and the most medial part of the transverse process of the atlas. This muscle inserts onto the occiput in front of the occipital condyle (Figure 2-33). The rectus capitis anterior flexes the head.[7]

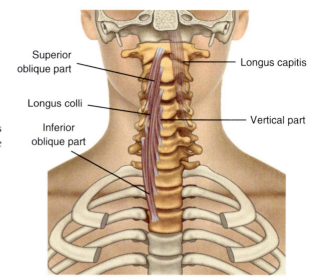

Figure 2-31 Anterior view of the right longus colli. The longus capitis has been ghosted in on the right.

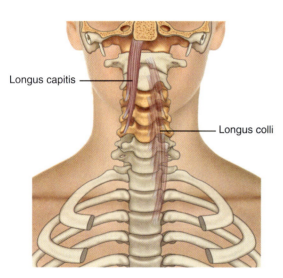

Figure 2-32 Anterior view of the right longus capitis. The longus colli has been ghosted in on the right.

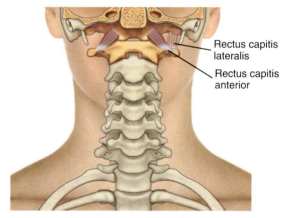

Figure 2-33 Anterior view of the rectus capitis anterior. The rectus capitis lateralis has been ghosted in on the right.

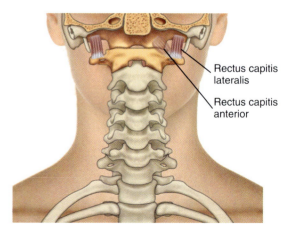

Figure 2-34 Anterior view of the rectus capitis lateralis bilaterally. The rectus capitis anterior has been ghosted in on the right.

Rectus Capitis Lateralis

The rectus capitis lateralis is a small muscle that originates from the anterior aspect of the transverse process of the atlas. It courses superiorly to insert into the jugular process of the occiput (Figure 2-34). The rectus capitis lateralis laterally flexes the occiput on the atlas.[7]

Lateral Cervical Muscles

The lateral cervical muscles (the scalene-anterior, medius, and posterior) extend obliquely between the upper two ribs and the cervical transverse

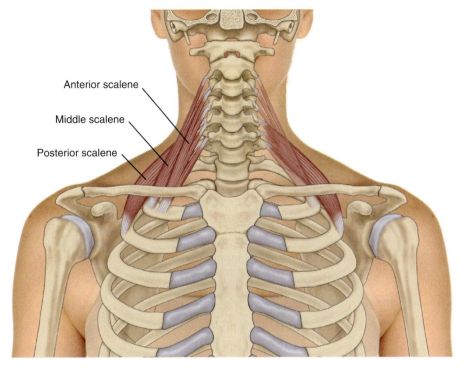

Figure 2-35   Anterior view of the anterior scalene muscles. The posterior scalenes are ghosted in the middle on the left.

processes. Because the lateral cervical muscles are frequently injured during whiplash trauma, the proximity of the anterior scalene to the lower brachial plexus, subclavian artery, and vein can give rise to compression syndromes affecting the ipsilateral upper extremity.[7]

Scalenus Anterior
The scalenus anterior lies at the side of the neck deep to the sternocleidomastoid. It is attached above to the anterior tubercles of the transverse processes of C3 through C6. The slips descend almost vertically to attach by a narrow tendon to the first rib (Figure 2-35). Acting from below, the scalenus flexes the neck and laterally flexes and rotates it to the opposite side.[26]

Scalenus Medius
The scalenus medius is the largest and longest of the scalene muscles. It is attached above to the transverse process of the axis and the lower five cervical vertebrae. Below it attaches to the upper surface of the first rib. (See Figure 2-35.) Acting from below, the scalenus medius flexes the cervical vertebral column to the same side.[26]

Scalenus Posterior
The scalenus posterior is the smallest and most deeply situated of the scalene muscles. It courses between the transverse processes of the fourth, fifth, and sixth cervical vertebrae to the outer surface of the second rib. (See Figure 2-35.) The scalenus posterior bend the lower end of the cervical part of the vertebral column to the same side.[26]

Intervertebral Foramen
The intervertebral foramen (IVF) is a short, elliptical canal forming an aperture for the exit of the segmental spinal nerves and the entrance of blood vessels and nerve branches that supply the structures of the vertebral canal (Figure 2-36). It is bounded superiorly and inferiorly by the respective pedicles of the adjacent vertebrae. The anterior portion is formed by the dorsum of the intervertebral disc covered by the posterior longitudinal ligament. The articular capsules of the posterior joints and the ligamenta flava contribute to the posterior aspect of the foramen. This opening provides a margin of safety in the healthy spine with the caliber of the canal larger than the collective size of the structures that pass through it. The remaining space

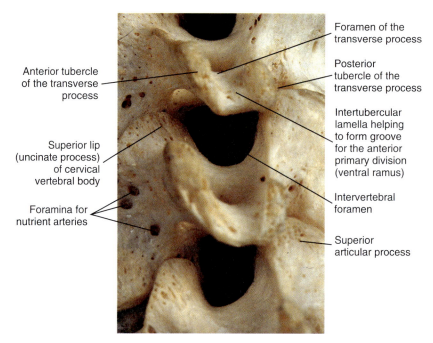

Anterior tubercle of the transverse process

Superior lip (uncinate process) of cervical vertebral body

Foramina for nutrient arteries

Foramen of the transverse process

Posterior tubercle of the transverse process

Intertubercular lamella helping to form groove for the anterior primary division (ventral ramus)

Intervertebral foramen

Superior articular process

Figure 2-36   Obliquely oriented view of the cervical intervertebral foramina. Note that the superior uncinate process of a typical cervical vertebral body forms a portion of the anterior border of the IVF.

is occupied by loose areolar tissue and fat, to accommodate the relative motions of the canal contents.

However adequate the canal size may appear, the bore is readily affected by anomalies and pathological and pathomechanical changes. Anomalous development may take the form of lateral recess stenosis or the presence of transforaminal ligaments. Pathological changes affecting foraminal size can include degenerative disc disease, the most serious form of which is frank disc herniation and osteoarthritic outgrowths from the posterior joints. Pathomechanical changes may be secondary to loss of disc height with the possibility of facet imbrication and subluxation[36,37] or displacement due to joint jamming.

Any of these conditions have the potential to diminish the size of the IVF and may be a source of interference with normal neurological function. Problems related to specific areas of the spine are further discussed, along with the unique characteristics of regional spinal dynamics.

Neurological Components

One of the most basic and important functions of the spinal column is protection of the spinal cord. The vertebral canal affords this protection and is occupied by the spinal cord, the meninges, and associated vessels. The combined vertebral motion segments form a hollow, flexible pillar comprised of the vertebral bodies anteriorly and the posterior vertebral arches made up of the pedicles and laminae. Passing through this canal from the brain stem to the conus medullaris is the spinal cord, housed in a bony, protective casing. Covering the spinal cord are the meninges (dura mater, arachnoid mater, and pia mater) that lie beneath the epidural adipose tissue and venous plexus.

The discovery by Hack et al in 1995[29] that the rectus capitis posterior minor muscle attaches to the posterior spinal dura in the posterior atlanto-occipital space, opened up the possibility of another mechanism for cervicogenic headaches. In 1998 Mitchell, Humphreys, and O'Sullivan[38] identified another connective tissue attachment to the spinal dura in the posterior atlantoaxial space between C1 and C2. In 2003 Humphreys et al[39] demonstrated that the rectus capitis posterior minor and C1-C2 connective tissue attachments to the spinal dura are linked in a connective tissue complex.

Further research by Nash et al in 2005[28] has demonstrated dural attachments in the posterior atlanto-occipital space. It is now thought that the medial and deep fibers of the rectus capitis posterior minor attach to the spinal dura by fascia and tendinous fibers and that the posterior atlanto-occipital membrane is part of the rectus capitis posterior minor fascia and tendon.

It is hypothesized that the posterior dural connections play a biomechanical role in protecting the spinal cord from pinching or bucking during physiological motions and that trauma, particularly the flexion and posterior translation of the head during the early phases of rear impact whiplash trauma, may abnormally traction the spinal dura. Clinically this may result in cervicogenic headaches and neck pain.

Beneath the transparent pia mater, dorsal and ventral rootlets can be discerned attaching to the spinal cord. These rootlets divide the spinal cord into spinal cord segments. The dorsal and ventral rootlets unite to form a single mixed spinal nerve containing both sensory and motor fibers.[7] The rootlets are exceedingly delicate and vulnerable. When subjected to adhesions, they undergo irreversible changes.[7] Once inside the IVF, the spinal nerve thickens as a result of the merging of the motor and sensory neurons and the presence of the

dorsal root ganglion (DRG). The sensory sources of neural innervation to spinal structures that have their cell bodies in the DRG include the following: (1) the anterior primary division (ventral ramus), (2) the posterior primary division (dorsal ramus), (3) the recurrent meningeal nerve, and (4) sensory fibers that course with the sympathetic nervous system (including fibers that run with the sympathetic trunk and also the gray communicating rami).[6] The spinal nerves formed by the union of the dorsal and ventral roots exit through the respective intervertebral foramina of each spinal motion segment protected by the dural root sleeve. As the mixed spinal nerve exits the IVF, it divides into two parts: a posterior primary division (dorsal ramus) and an anterior primary division (ventral ramus) (Figure 2-37). The posterior primary division further divides into a medial branch, which supplies the zygapophyseal joints and the transversospinalis group of deep back muscles, and a lateral branch, which supplies the sacrospinalis group of deep back muscles.[6] The anterior primary division innervates the ventrolateral aspect of the trunk and extremities. Passing back through the IVF are the tiny sinuvertebral nerves formed by the union of a

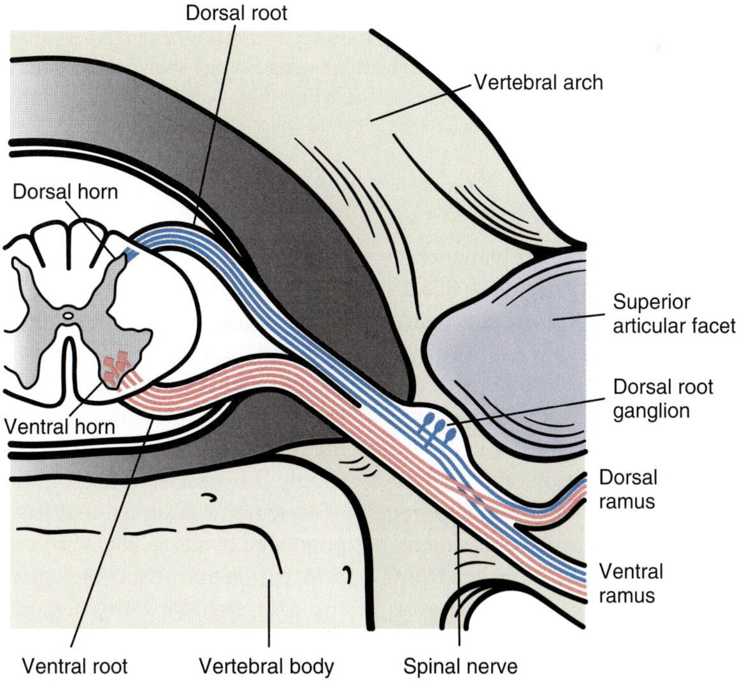

Figure 2-37   Components and somatic branches of a typical spinal nerve. The dorsal and ventral roots unite within the intervertebral foramen to form a spinal nerve. The spinal nerve branches into a dorsal ramus and ventral ramus. Each ramus contains motor and sensory fibers. Note: Sympathetic fibers are not shown.

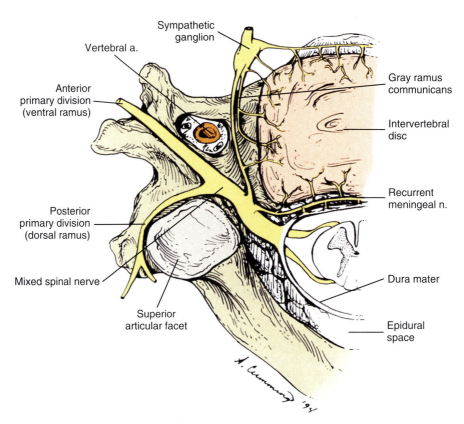

Figure 2-38   Superior view of a typical cervical segment showing the neural elements. Notice the dorsal and ventral roots, spinal nerve, and posterior and anterior primary divisions (dorsal and ventral rami). The posterior primary division can be seen dividing into a medial and lateral branch. The recurrent meningeal nerve is shown entering the intervertebral foramen. Fibers arising from the middle cervical ganglion and the gray communicating ramus also are shown. Notice that these fibers supply the anterior and lateral aspects of the intervertebral disc, vertebral body, and anterior longitudinal ligament.

spinal afferent and a sympathetic postganglionic root. This recurrent branch innervates the articular connective tissues of the vertebral canal (Figure 2-38). The sinuvertebral nerve originates just distal to the dorsal root ganglion, where it unites with the autonomic fibers from the gray ramus communicans. It curves upward around the base of the pedicle and divides into a superior and inferior branch. Numerous filaments are distributed to the periosteum, the posterior longitudinal ligament, the dura, and the epidural vessels. Branches from each level anastomose with an overlapping consistent with the mutual overlapping of the segmental sensory nerve distribution, suggesting that discogenic pain from a single level may involve more than one recurrent branch of the spinal nerves.

In addition to innervation of the posterior articulations and muscles derived from the posterior rami of the spinal nerves (see Figure 2-38) branches supply the articular capsules of the facets, the ligamenta flava, and the interspinous ligaments. Each intervertebral joint is innervated by two spinal nerves, a consequence of its embryonic origin from two vertebral (sclerotomal) segments, and in agreement with Hilton's law, as these are the nerves that supply the muscles acting on the joint.

Research has shown that facet joint capsules are populated by nerve fibers involved in pain and proprioception and that these sensory fibers are sensitive to stretch. McLain[40] demonstrated that Type I, II, and III mechanoreceptors are present in human cervical facet joints. More recently, Chen et al[41] have shown that A-delta and C-fiber receptors are present in the cervical facet joint capsules. A-delta fibers are thin, myelinated fibers that convey fast pain while C-fibers are larger unmyelinated fibers involved in chronic or dull pain. The presence of mechanoreceptors and pain fibers indicates that the central nervous system monitors activity within facet joints and that sensory input is important to the function of the cervical spine.

Sensory nerves containing the neuropeptide substance P and calcitonin gene-related peptide have also been found in facet joints, further supporting their role in pain generation and proprioceptive function.[42]

Several facet joint injury mechanisms have been proposed, including facet joint impingement, synovial fold pinching, and facet joint capsular strain.[43] In support of the facet joint capsular strain model, work by Lu et al[42] and Cavanaugh et al[43] demonstrated a relationship between capsular stretch and sensory fiber discharge such that higher capsular strains resulted in nociceptive discharge while low stretch levels activated proprioceptive mechanoreceptors.

Cervical Spinal Nerves

The dorsal ramus of the C1 spinal nerve is unique, passing above the posterior arch of the atlas after exiting the spinal canal. It abruptly divides into a ventral and dorsal ramus. The dorsal ramus (suboccipital nerve) runs between the posterior arch of the atlas and the vertebral artery, providing motor innervation to the suboccipital muscles. The C2 spinal nerve branches into a dorsal and ventral ramus, posterior to the lateral atlantoaxial joint. The dorsal ramus loops superiorly around the inferior border of the obliquus capitis inferior muscle and then divides into medial, lateral, superior communicating and inferior communicating, and a branch to the obliquus capitis inferior. The lateral branch of the dorsal ramus of C2 helps to supply motor innervation to the longissimus capitis, splenius capitis, and semispinalis capitis muscles. The medial branch of the dorsal ramus of C2 is large and is known as the greater occipital nerve that courses superiorly to provide a broad area of sensory innervation to the scalp. Disorders of the upper cervical spine, including irritation of the greater occipital nerve or the C2 ganglion, have been demonstrated to cause headaches.[37,44-46] Causes of irritation to the nerve or ganglion include direct trauma to the posterior occiput and entrapment between traumatized and or hypertonic cervical muscles, particularly the semispinalis capitis.[7]

The C3 spinal nerve is the most superior nerve to pass through an IVF. It branches into a dorsal and ventral ramus within the lateral aspect of the IVF. The dorsal ramus of C3 passes posteriorly between the C2 and C3 transverse processes, where it divides into deep and superficial medial branches, a lateral branch, and a communicating branch with the C2 dorsal ramus. The superficial medial branch of the dorsal ramus is known as the third occipital nerve. Because of its close relationships with the bony elements of the C2-C3 IVF, the third occipital nerve has been implicated as a cause of headaches that frequently accompany generalized osteoarthritis of the cervical spine.[47] Local anesthetic block of the third occipital nerve has provided relief of occipital and suboccipital headaches in 10 consecutive patients with suspected cervicogenic headaches.[48]

The spinal nerves of C4 through C8 exit through respective IVF. Structures of the cervical region innervated by the nerves of the dorsal rami can produce pain in the cervical region. The ventral rami of cervical spinal nerves form the cervical and brachial plexuses, which innervate the anterior neck and upper extremities. Injury to these structures can lead to a variety of signs and symptoms.

THE AUTONOMIC NERVOUS SYSTEM

The autonomic nervous system has been described as that part of the nervous system concerned with regulation of the internal environment of the body. It is divided into the sympathetic and parasympathetic systems. The autonomic nervous system in not a separate system but is an integral part of the somatic and visceral peripheral nervous systems and of the central nervous system. The parasympathetic system is connected with the central nervous system in the cervical area through the oculomotor, facial, glossopharyngeal, and vagus cranial nerves. Clinically, patients with neck pain from whiplash trauma have demonstrated altered control of oculomotor function. Treleaven, Jull, and LowChoy in 2005 and 2006[49,50] showed that chronic whiplash patients with or without dizziness had altered control of eye movement during gaze as measured by the smooth pursuit neck torsion test. It is now thought that neck trauma from whiplash causes dysfunction of normal eye movements, likely due to disturbed cervical afferentation.

The sympathetic system originates in mediolateral gray matter of the base of the anterior horns of the spinal cord from C4 through C8 in the cervical region. The cervical sympathetic chain lies anterior to the longus capitis muscle. It is composed of three ganglia: superior, middle, and inferior

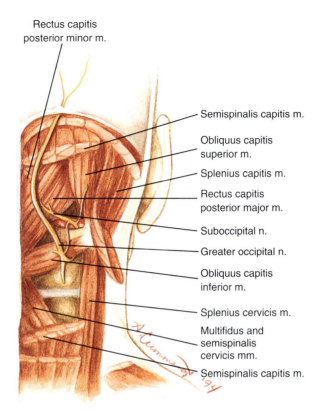

Rectus capitis
posterior minor m.

Semispinalis capitis m.

Obliquus capitis
superior m.

Splenius capitis m.

Rectus capitis
posterior major m.

Suboccipital n.

Greater occipital n.

Obliquus capitis
inferior m.

Splenius cervicis m.

Multifidus and
semispinalis
cervicis mm.

Semispinalis capitis m.

Figure 2-39 Illustration of the suboccipital region demonstrating the greater and suboccipital nerves in relation to the surrounding muscles.

(Figure 2-39). The superior ganglion is the largest, lying inferior to the occiput and anterior to the transverse processes of C2 and C3. Hyperextension injuries to the neck, especially during rotation, can compress the C2 ganglion between the posterior arch of the atlas and the lamina of the axis.[7]

The middle cervical ganglion is not always present. When present it lies anterior to the transverse processes of C6. The inferior ganglion usually unites with the first thoracic ganglion to form the cervicothoracic (stellate) ganglion located just inferior to the transverse process of C7. Swelling in the anterior strap muscles in the cervical region can cause irritation of the cervical ganglion trapped between the transverse processes and muscle.

Vascular Components

External Vertebral Venous Plexus

The external vertebral venous plexus is a network of veins surrounding the external aspect of the vertebral column. It is associated with both posterior and anterior elements of the vertebral column and can be divided into an anterior plexus surrounding the vertebral bodies and a posterior plexus

associated with the neural arches. These plexuses communicate with segmental veins throughout the spine, including deep cervical veins, intercostal veins, lumbar veins, and ascending lumbar veins in addition to the internal vertebral venous plexus that lies within the vertebral canal. The external and internal vertebral plexuses communicate through the IVF and also directly though the vertebral bodies. The veins that run through the IVF, connecting the two plexuses, surround the exiting spinal nerve and form a vascular cuff around the nerve.[7]

Internal Vertebral Venous Plexus

The internal vertebral venous plexus is located beneath the bony elements of the vertebral foramina (laminae, spinous processes, pedicles, and vertebral body). It is embedded in a layer of loose areolar tissue know as the epidural (extradural) adipose tissue. The internal vertebral venous plexus is made up of many interconnected longitudinal channels, some that run along the posterior and anterior aspects of the vertebral canal. They have no valves and therefore drainage is dependent on posture and respiration.

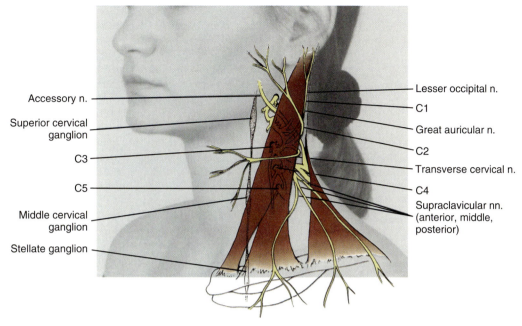

Figure 2-40   View of the neural elements with the vertebral artery and cervical ganglion.

Arterial Supply to the Spine

The external aspect of the vertebral column receives its arterial supply from branches of regional deep arteries. The internal aspect of the vertebral canal receives its arterial supply from segmental arteries that send branches into the IVF. The spinal segmental artery divides into three branches on entering the IVF. One branch courses posteriorly, supplying the posterior arches of neighboring vertebrae; an anterior branch supplies the posterior longitudinal ligament, the posterior aspect of the vertebral body, and the surrounding tissues; and a third branch, the neural branch, runs to the mixed spinal nerve.

A close relationship exists between the extensive and abundant blood supply of arterial branches that form the anterior lateral and posterior spinal arteries of the spinal cord.[7]

The Vertebral Arteries

The vertebral arteries are significant because of their close relationship to the cervical nerves, the cervical vertebrae, and the nerve plexus derived from the sympathetic chain. In the cervical region, vertebral arteries extend upward through the transverse foramina from the sixth cervical vertebra along the uncovertebral joints, a common site of degenerative arthritic changes. These arteries loop over the posterior arch of the atlas and continue

through the foramen magnum (Figure 2-40). The relationship of the sympathetic plexus surrounding the vertebral artery is complex and sometimes referred to as the vertebral plexus of nerves or vertebral nerve. (See Figure 2-39.) This deep plexus is derived from small branches of the vertebral nerve, the stellate, the middle cervical ganglia, and the cervical ventral rami. (See Figure 2-39.) These fibers form vascular branches that create a dense neural plexus around the vertebral arteries. The vertebral arteries have been found to produce pain. The afferents for their nociceptive sensation run with the autonomic fibers. Spur formation of the upper cervical zygapophyseal or uncovertebral joints can cause headaches.[7]

CONCLUSION

The functional approach to disorders of spinal movement requires a thorough understanding of the concept and components of the vertebral motion segment.[1] The interaction and movement between spinal motion segments are of great importance to spinal function. The upper cervical motion segments are atypical, and although they do not have discs, as do the motion segments of the lower cervical spine, they allow for considerable motion. (See Table 2-1.) Normal movement between adjacent vertebrae in the lower cervical spine is limited, but the cumulative effect over the whole column allows for considerable motion. (See Table 2-1.) The intervertebral discs provide both stability (by tying the vertebrae together) and motion (through their elastic deformability). The discs permit torsion and compressibility between vertebral bodies. The forces transmitted through the spinal column are smoothed out by the discs. Each motion segment exhibits an intrinsic equilibrium that is dependent on healthy discs. Aberrant motion of one element of the motion segment can affect other elements of the same motion segment, as well as adjacent segments. This must be considered along with the soft tissue pathology that can accompany kinesiological dysfunction of the spine. Of great importance in whiplash injuries is restoration of normal motion in each segment of the cervical spine. (See Chapter 8.)

References

1. Schmorl G, Junghanns H: *The human spine in health and disease*, ed 2, translated by Beseman EF. New York, 1971, Grune & Stratton, p 35.
2. Gatterman MI: *Chiropractic management of spine related disorders*, ed 2, Baltimore, 2002, Lippincott Williams & Wilkins.
3. Przybyla AS, et al: Strength of the cervical spine in compression and bending, *Spine* 32(15):1612-1620, 2007.
4. Collins P: Embryology and development. In Williams PL, editor: *Gray's anatomy*, ed 38, British. Philadelphia, 1995, Churchill Livingstone, pp 264-270.
5. Gatterman MI, Hansen D: Development of chiropractic nomenclature through consensus, *J Manipulative Physiol Ther* 17:302-309, 1994.
6. Soames RW: Skeletal system. In Williams PL, editor: *Gray's anatomy*, ed 38, British. Philadelphia, 1995, Churchill Livingstone, pp 510-546.
7. Cramer GD, Darby SA: *Basic and clinical anatomy of the spine, spinal cord and ANS*, St Louis, 1995, Mosby.
8. Cloyd JM, Elliott DM: Elastin content correlates with human disc degeneration in the anulus fibrosus and nucleus pulposus, *Spine* 32(17):1826-1831, 2007.
9. Mercer S, Bogduk N: The ligaments and annulus fibrosus of human adult cervical intervertebral discs, *Spine* 24(7):619-626, 1999.
10. Taylor JR, Giles LGF: Lumbar intervertebral discs. In Giles LGF, Singer KP, editors: *The clinical anatomy and management of back pain series, vol 1, Clinical anatomy and management of low back pain*, Oxford, 1997, Butterworth-Heinemann, pp 49-71.
11. Bogduk N, Tynan W, Wilson A: The nerve supply to the human lumbar intervertebral discs, *J Anat* 132:39-56, 1981.
12. Mendel T, et al: Neural elements in human cervical intervertebral discs, *Spine* 17:132-135, 1992.
13. Hoogendoorn RJ, et al: Experimental intervertebral disc degeneration induced by chondroitinase ABC in the goat, *Spine* 32(17):1816-1818, 2007.
14. Cramer GD, Gudavalli R, Skogsbergh D: Functional anatomy of the cervical spine. In Herzog W, editor: *Clinical biomechanics of spinal manipulation*, New York, 2000, Mosby, pp 50-91.
15. Hall MC: *Luschka's joint*, Springfield, IL, 1965, Charles C Thomas.
16. Giles LG, Taylor JR: Human zygapophyseal joint capsule and synovial fold innervation, *Br J Reumatol* 26:93-98, 1987.
17. Xu G, et al: Normal variations of the lumbar facet joint capsules, *Clin Anat* 4:117-122, 1991.
18. Yu S, Sether L, Haughton VM: Facet joint menisci of the cervical spine: correlative MR imaging and cryomicrotomy study, *Radiology* 164:79-82, 1987.
19. Bogduk N: The anatomy and pathophysiology of whiplash, *Clin Biomech* 1:92-101, 1986.
20. Loughenbury PR, Wadhwani S, Soames RW: The posterior longitudinal ligament and peridural (epidural) membrane, *Clin Anat* 19(6):487-492, 2006.
21. Neumann DA: Axial skeleton: osteology and arthrology. In *Kinesiology of the musculoskeletal system: foundations for physical rehabilitation*, St Louis, 2010, Mosby, pp 251-310.
22. Tubbs RS, et al: The tectoral membrane: anatomical, biomechanical, and histological analysis, *Clin Anat* 20(4): 382-386, 2007.
23. Foreman SM, Croft AC: *Whiplash injuries: the cervical acceleration/deceleration syndrome*, ed 3, Baltimore, 2002, Lippincott Williams & Wilkins.
24. White AA, Panjabi MM: *Clinical biomechanics of the spine*, Philadelphia, 1990, JB Lippincott.
25. McGill SM: Functional anatomy of the lumbar and thoracic spine. In Herzog W, editor: *Clinical biomechanics of spinal manipulation*, New York, 2000, Churchill Livingstone, pp 26-49.
26. Salmons S: Muscle. In Williams, PL, editor: *Gray's anatomy*, ed 38, British. Philadelphia, 1995, Churchill Livingstone, pp 737-900.
27. Travell JG, Simons DG: *Myofascial pain and dysfunction: the trigger point manual, vol 1, Upper half of body*, Baltimore, 1983, Williams & Wilkins.
28. Nash L, et al: Configuration of the connective tissue in the posterior atlanto-occipital interspace: a sheet plastination and confocal microscopy study, *Spine* 30(12):1359-1366, 2005.
29. Hack GD, et al: Anatomic relation between the rectus capitis posterior minor muscle and the dura mater, *Spine* 20: 2484-2486, 1995.

30. Elliott J, et al: Fatty infiltration in the cervical extensor muscles in persistent whiplash-associated disorders, *Spine* 31(22):E847-E855, 2006.

31. Barton PM, Hayes KC: Neck flexor muscle strength, efficiency, and relaxation times in normal subjects and subjects with unilateral neck pain and headache, *Arch Phys Med Rehabil* 77:680-687 1996.

32. Falla D: Unraveling the complexity of muscle impairment in chronic neck pain, *Man Ther* 9:125-133, 2004.

33. Falla D, Jull G, Hodges PW: Feed forward activity of the cervical flexor muscles during voluntary arm movements is delayed in chronic neck pain, *Exp Brain Res* 157:43-48, 2004.

34. Falla D, et al: Neck flexor muscle fatigue is side specific in patients with unilateral neck pain, *Eur J Pain* 8:71-77, 2004.

35. Jull G, Kristjansson E, Dall'Alba P: Impairment in the cervical flexors: a comparison of whiplash and insidious onset neck pain patients, *Man Ther* 9:89-94, 2004.

36. Keim HA, Kirkaldy-Willis WH: Clinical symposia: low back pain, *Ciba-Geigy* 39:2-32, 1987.

37. Edmeads J: Headaches and head pains associated with diseases of the cervical spine, *Med Clin North Am* 62: 533-544, 1978.

38. Mitchell BS, Humphreys BK, O'Sullivan E: Attachments of the ligamentum nuchae to cervical posterior spinal dura and the lateral part of the occipital bone, *J Manipulative Physiol Ther* 21:145-148, 1998.

39. Humphreys BK, et al: Investigation of connective tissue attachments to the cervical spinal dura mater, *Clin Anat* 16:152-159, 2003.

40. McLain RF: Mechanoreceptor endings in human cervical facet joints, *Spine* 19:495-501, 1994.

41. Chen C, et al: Distribution of A-delta and C-fiber receptors in the cervical facet joint capsule and their response to stretch, *J Bone Joint Surg Am* 88(8):1807-1816, 2006.

42. Lu Y, et al: Neural response of cervical facet joint capsule to stretch: a study of whiplash pain mechanism, *Stapp Car Crash J* 49:49-65, 2005.

43. Cavanaugh JM, et al: Pain generation in lumbar and cervical facet joints, *J Bone Joint Surg Am* 88(Suppl 2):63-67, 2006.

44. Bogduk N, et al: Cervical headache, *Med J Aust* 143:202-207, 1985.

45. Bogduk N: An anatomical basis for the neck-tongue syndrome, *J Neurol Neurosurg Psychiatry* 44:202-208, 1989.

46. Boguk N: Headaches and the cervical spine (editorial), *Cephalalgia* 4:7-8, 1986.

47. Trevor-Jones R: Osteo-arthritis of the paravertebral joints of the second and third cervical vertebrae as a cause of occipital headaches, *S Afr Med J* 392-394, 1964; May.

48. Bogduk N, Marsland A: On the concept of third occipital headache, *J Neurol Neurosurg Psychiatry* 49:775-780, 1986.

49. Treleaven J, Jull G, LowChoy N: Smooth pursuit neck torsion test in whiplash-associated disorders: relationship to self-reports of neck pain and disability, dizziness and anxiety, *J Rehabil Med* 37(4):219-223, 2005.

50. Treleaven J, Jull G, LowChoy N: The relationship of cervical joint position error to balance and eye movement disturbances in persistent whiplash, *Man Ther* 11(2):99-106, 2006.

Chapter 3

Patient History and Mechanism of Injury

Meridel I. Gatterman

Identifying the mechanism of injury is crucial when taking an appropriate history of patients who have suffered whiplash trauma. The direction of force, patient's position, relationship of the head and spine, and state of tension in the neck muscles all help to determine the nature of the injuries suffered.[1] Most important is the position of the patient at the time of impact.[2] Patients who are unprepared for the impact have a tendency to suffer more severe injuries.[1] Passengers in the right front seat are injured more frequently because they are less prepared than the driver for a collision.[2] If the driver is turned looking in the rearview mirror at the time of impact, the nature of the injuries will be different than if facing forward. A head position that is rotated or inclined is more likely to produce more severe injury.[1]

It is important to evaluate the extent of sagittal plane forces, as well as forces in other planes. Asymmetrical rotational forces may be introduced by the shoulder harness that restrains one shoulder, allowing the other to be forced forward during the hyperflexion phase of the whiplash. The resultant shoulder girdle strain is a common clinical finding with motor vehicle accidents in which shoulder harnesses are worn. If severe torsion occurs, injury to the thoracolumbar region, lumbosacral junction, and the sacroiliac joint contralateral to the fixed shoulder may occur. Different structures will be injured if the victim is looking in the rearview mirror or stretching out the arm to protect others in the car at the time of impact. With the neck rotated 45 degrees, the physiological range of extension is half of this range, and the posterior joints can be pushed beyond this physiological range with possible sprain and joint locking. Serious injuries occur with the head forced into hyperextension. When the impact is from the side, a similar whiplash action occurs in the cervical spine, with the neck first snapped in the direction of the impact, followed by recoil in the opposite direction. Lateral flexion is limited, as the head strikes the shoulder or side of the vehicle.

MECHANICS OF WHIPLASH

Initially, in a rear-end impact, the torso of the victim translates backward while the head and neck remain stationary and the vehicle moves forward underneath. This is followed by the abrupt upward movement of the torso as the thoracic kyphotic curvature is straightened.[2] This sets the head into vertical acceleration that straightens and compresses the cervical spine. This is followed by a series of abnormal distortions of the neck. First there is an initial flexion of the upper cervical spine, followed by extension of the lower cervical segments.[2] This induces an S-shaped distortion in the entire

44

cervical spine.[3-6] This is then followed by extension of all levels of the cervical spine.[5] Yang and King[7] also found significant posterior shear deformation present with large facet capsular stretch. They considered this to be a major source of pain. Following the extension phase, the head is cantilevered forward into flexion with fanning of the spinous processes.[8]

STRUCTURES INJURED DURING THE FOUR PHASES OF WHIPLASH

When a vehicle is struck from behind, the occupant's torso is accelerated while the unrestrained head and neck lag behind.[8] As the head and neck are forced into extension, the anterior cervical muscles are stretched while contracting in an effort to prevent hyperextension. Most frequently injured by this phase are the "anterior strap muscles," including the sternocleidomastoid and scalene muscles.[2] The splenius capitus muscles are frequently injured, especially if the head and neck are rotated at the time of impact. Having the head turned at time of impact increases the risk of injury.[8]

Structures injured during the second phase of whiplash from a rear-end collision are those vulnerable to shear strain. Penning[9] speculates that the primary mechanism of injury in whiplash is actually hypertranslation of the head backward. He notes that it is the overstretching of the ligaments of the upper cervical spine, especially of the atlantoaxial segment (including the alar ligament), that leads to disorders of proprioceptive information. When ligaments and joint capsules are stretched, the axial traction permits the joints to separate and then subsequently compress with jamming and altered alignment. Ligamentous injury occurs when the cervical muscles become stretched to the point that the ligaments are called into play to stabilize the spine.[2] When the ligaments become stretched, further injury to the discs and articular capsules can ensue. Disc injury usually consists of a disruption of the annulus fibrosus viewed on radiographs as a widening of the posterior disc space, a narrowing of the anterior disc space, and often a concomitant anterior hypermobile subluxation caused by disruption of the posterior elements.[8] During phase 3, acceleration is diminished, with the head and torso thrown forward, straining the superficial posterior cervical muscles, including the upper trapezius. During phase 4, if the body is restrained by a seatbelt, the head will continue to move forward until it strikes the chest or an external object. This is the phase when the upper cervical posterior muscular and ligamentous elements of the cervical spine, including the suboccipital muscles, become injured. Croft[8] maintains that it is the upper cervical spine that sustains the greatest injury from whiplash because it tends to be the biomechanical pivot point sustaining the greatest whiplike action.

The biomechanical injuries seen clinically from the whiplash mechanism tend to follow a characteristic pattern. Ligamentous sprain at the C4-C5 to C5-C6 segments creates a hypermobility that may account for the degenerate changes commonly seen in the mid cervical region as a sequelae to whiplash injury. Hyperextension injuries caused by rear-end collisions frequently strain the anterior strap muscles (scalene and sternocleidomastoideus). If the head is rotated and tilted to one side, the torsional effect causes greater damage on one side than on the other. Forceful hyperextension injuries may produce traction on the anterior longitudinal ligament, which sprains the fibers attached to the intervertebral disc. An avulsion fracture may occur as a piece of bone is torn from the inferior margin of the vertebral body.[10] Rupture of the underlying annulus may occur, with displacement of nuclear material.[11] Compressive forces on the posterior structures may produce avulsions of the capsular ligaments, as infolding or creasing of the interlaminar ligaments and damage to the articular cartilage as the posterior joints are jammed together.[12] Extension with compression can produce a crushing of the posterior elements of the vertebra as in a roll over crash.

Hyperflexion injuries caused by head-on collisions may tear or stretch the nuchal ligaments, the capsular ligaments of the Luschka and posterior facet joints, the interspinous ligaments, and the other posterior ligaments of the neck.

Dislocation of the posterior facets with or without cord injury may occur, and in severe cases,[12] fracture of the posterior elements of the vertebrae as they are forced apart can occur. Compression fracture of the vertebral bodies can also occur and may not be visualized in early radiographs, becoming evident when more compression and healing have occurred.[6]

Whiplash injuries to neurological structures include contusion of the brain and spinal cord.[13] Damage to the cortex and cerebellum may occur from a contracoup as the brain hits the inner table of the skull on the opposite side, as well as from a direct blow to the skull. Damage to the spinal cord is produced by a combination of hyperextension and backward shearing forces. Trauma to the cord may also occur as the result of edema as well as transection. If the head is rotated at the time of impact, the shearing force may fracture a vertebral arch or posterior facet.[6] The lateral masses of the atlas and axis may suffer compression fractures, and a transverse process fracture may occur on the side of rotation. Ligaments on the contralateral side from rotation may be torn, causing dislocation of the atlas or axis.[6] More commonly seen are rotational subluxations of the atlas or the axis. Described by Jacobson and Adler[14] in 1956 as a pathological fixation in a position within the normal range of motion, this condition was described in detail by Coutts[15] in 1934. Wortzman and Dewar[16] report that rotational fixation is usually of a moderate nature, such as occurs in a flexion-extension injury in a rear-end collision. (See Chapter 8.) Current imaging using cervical roentgenography and conventional or computed tomography are used to show dislocations, subluxations, and fractures.[17] Magnetic resonance imaging (MRI) is more commonly used to assess different types of soft-tissue lesions related to whiplash injuries. Dynamic imaging may show functional disturbances. Flexion extension views, high resolution static MRI, and especially dynamic MRI warrant more widespread use.[18] (See Chapter 5.)

Injuries caused by side collision may produce strain of the lateral neck muscles and tearing of the alar and atlantoaxial ligaments and upper joint capsules. If severe, a wedging of the lateral aspect of a vertebral body and its associated lateral mass can occur.[19]

Direct traumatic insult to the nerve roots can produce neuropathy[20] in addition to inflammation in the dural sleeves and perineural tissues, which may result in fibrosis. Adhesions between the dural sleeves and the adjacent capsular structure may prevent normal motion of nerve roots. Irritation of the cervical sympathetics gives rise to a variety of symptoms.[21] Sympathetic ganglion damage as well as damage to sympathetic fibers in the spinal cord is thought to be responsible for these symptoms. Cervical sympathetic nerve irritation may occur by reflex stimulation as well as by direct trauma. Because of their close proximity to the vertebral arteries, the cervical sympathetics are particularly vulnerable to injury. The vertebral arteries and the encircling sympathetic nerves within the transverse foramen may be subjected to trauma as they are pulled backward against the posterior wall of their bony rings, or by subluxation or fracture of the adjacent bony structure, or injury to adjacent soft tissues.

Grieve[22] compares the mechanism of whiplash injury to multiple sprained ankles in the neck, with the added complications of nerve root and plexus traction injury, meningeal irritation, tearing of ligaments and muscle fibers, and trauma to blood vessels and lymphatics. He notes that the overall effect is an upset of sensitive structure and delicately balanced function.

HISTORY

The patient with whiplash most commonly gives a history of minor to moderately severe rear-end collisions[22] or other types of vehicular crashes, such as a head-on or side collision. Occasionally the patient suffering from whiplash presents with a history of a fall. A sideways fall on the outstretched arm can produce a lateral whiplash effect on the cervical spine. A blow such as from a swinging object may also produce whiplash. A severe form of whiplash-induced injury occurs with the "shaken baby" or "whiplash-shaken infant" syndrome. Injury occurs when an adult shakes an infant repeatedly in the fore and aft direction. This mechanism can cause severe injuries, including neurocognitive dysfunction, and can even be fatal.[8]

It is important to obtain as much information as possible about the mechanism of injury, particularly when a motor vehicle crash is the mechanism of injury. The direction of force, position and relationship of the head and spine, and state of tension of the neck muscles all help to determine the location of stress. The position of the patient at the time of impact should be noted. Was the patient looking straight ahead or positioned with the head or body turned? Was the patient driving? Was the arm outstretched? Did the head or another body part strike something? Did something loose in the vehicle strike the patient? Was the patient wearing a seat restraint (lap type or combined lap-shoulder harness), and what was the nature of the head support? Was there loss of consciousness or mental confusion? Was the patient thrown from the car? What were the relative sizes of the involved vehicles, make of the vehicles, and type of suspension in the injured party's vehicle? What was the approximate speed involved? Was the patient's foot down hard on the brake pedal or floor board? Was the seat torn loose? Did the backrest break away? Had there been a previous or old neck injury? The answers to these questions all aid in the assessment of the

---

| BOX **3-1** | **Questions Aiding in the Assessment of the Severity of Injury in Addition to Indicating Which Structures Are Involved** |

- Was the patient looking straight ahead or positioned with the head or body turned? Was the patient driving?
- Was the arm outstretched?
- Did the head or another body part strike something? Did something loose in the vehicle strike the patient?
- Was the patient wearing a seat restraint (lap type or combined lap-shoulder harness), and what was the nature of the head support?
- Was there loss of consciousness or mental confusion? Was the patient thrown from the car?
- What were the relative sizes of the involved vehicles, make of the vehicles, and type of suspension in the injured party's vehicle?
- What was the approximate speed involved? Was the patient's foot down hard on the brake pedal or floorboard?
- Was the seat torn loose? Did the backrest break away? Had there been a previous or old neck injury?

---

severity of injury in addition to indicating which structures are involved. (See Box 3-1.)

HISTORY RELATED TO CRASH SITE RECORDS

The Insurance Research Council provides data based on a sample of 42,000 auto injury claims that reports trends in injury claim patterns.[23] The police report typically indicates the party's position in the vehicle (driver or passenger) and whether there were visible or obvious injuries noted at the scene. Other information available will likely include loss of consciousness, seatbelt status, and whether there was ejection from the vehicle. If the patient was transported by ambulance, this will be noted, and ambulance medical records should include the physical and neurological status of the patient. Level of consciousness, bruising, fractures, lacerations, abrasions, and head, chest, or abdominal injuries will be included, and any spinal precautions, including collars splints or boards, will be noted.

EMERGENCY ROOM RECORDS

Anywhere from 43% to 50% of whiplash claimants are seen in emergency rooms without overnight admission to the hospital. The emergency room records will show assessment of vital signs, neurological status, and physical injuries. A radiological report will be available if x-rays were taken. If the patient is conscious, a report of pain rated by the patient at the time of admission will most likely be available. Simply stating a diagnosis as a whiplash injury or neck pain is not sufficient enough to describe the injury.

HISTORY RELATED TO SYMPTOMS

It is important to establish the patient's initial symptoms and note improvement, worsening, or return to pre-injury status. Activities that have been restricted because of pain or activities that increase the patient's symptoms should be recorded. Any time off from work or any work restriction should be determined and noted. It is important to establish whether there have been prior injuries to the same region of the body. This record should include when these injuries occurred, descriptions of pain, treatment extent, imaging and other test findings, and whether previous conditions had resolved. Any prior musculoskeletal conditions that made the patient more susceptible to injury should be assessed, including rheumatoid arthritis, other painful joint conditions, disc herniations, and spine or joint surgeries.

REFERENCES

1. Sturzenegger M, et al: Presenting symptoms and signs after whiplash injury: the influence of accident mechanisms, *Neurology* 44(4):688-693, 1994.
2. Gatterman MI, Hyland JK: Whiplash. In Gatterman MI, editor: *Foundations of chiropractic: subluxation*, 2nd ed, St Louis, 2005, Mosby, pp 429-447.
3. Grauer JN, et al: Whiplash produces an S-shaped curvature of the neck with hyperextension at the lower levels, *Spine* 22:2489-2494, 1997.
4. Kaneoka K, et al: Motion analysis of cervical vertebrae during whiplash loading, *Spine* 24:763-769, 1999.
5. Panjabi MM, et al: Mechanism of whiplash injury, *Clin Biomech* 13:29-49, 1998.

6. Eck J, Hodges SD, Humphreys SC: Whiplash: a review of a commonly misunderstood injury, *Am J Med* 110(8):651-656, 2001.

7. Yang KH, King AI: Neck kinematics in rear-end impacts, *Pain Res Manag* 8:9-85, 2003.

8. Foreman SM, Croft AC: *Whiplash injuries: the cervical acceleration/deceleration syndrome*, 3rd ed, Baltimore, 2002, Lippincott Williams & Wilkins.

9. Penning L: Backward hypertranslation of the head: participation in the whiplash injury mechanism of the cervical spine? *Orthopade* 23:268-274, 1994.

10. Hohl M: Soft tissue neck injuries. In Bailey RW, editor: *The cervical spine*, Philadelphia, 1983, JB Lippincott, pp 282-287.

11. Barnsley L, Bogduk N: The pathophysiology of whiplash, *Spine State Art Rev* 7:329-353, 1993.

12. Kirpalani D, Mitra R: Cervical facet joint dysfunction: a review, *Arch Phys Med Rehabil* 89(4):770-774, 2008.

13. Martin DH: The acute traumatic central cord syndrome. In Gunzburg R, Szpalaski M, editors: *Whiplash injuries: current concepts in prevention, diagnosis, and treatment of the cervical whiplash syndrome*, Philadelphia, 1998, Lippincott Williams and Wilkins, pp 129-134.

14. Jacobson G, Adler DC: Examination of the atlanto-axial joint following injuries with particular emphasis on rotational subluxation, *Am J Roentgenol* 76:1081-1094, 1956.

15. Coutts MB: Atlanto-epistropheal subluxations, *Arch Surg* 29:297-311, 1934.

16. Wortzman G, Dewar FP: Rotary fixation of the atlantoaxial subluxation, *Radiology* 90:479-487, 1968.

17. Bagley LJ: Imaging of spinal trauma, *Radiol Clin North Am* 44(1):1-2, 2006.

18. Van Goethem JWM, et al: Whiplash injuries: is there a role for imaging, *Eur J Radiol* 22:30-37, 1996.

19. Whitly JE, Forsyth HF: The classification of cervical spine injuries, *Am J Roentgenol* 83:633-644, 1960.

20. Davidson J, Larson IL, Risling M: Effects of pressure gradients on dorsal root ganglions—a possible whiplash injury mechanism, *J Biomech* 39(suppl 1):S148, 2006.

21. Fitz Ritson D: Cervicogenic sympathetic syndromes. In Gatterman MI, editor: *Foundations of chiropractic: subluxation*, St Louis, 2005, Mosby, pp 398-416.

22. Grieve GP: *Common vertebral joint problems*, New York, 1981, Churchill Livingstone.

23. Insurance Research Council: Auto injury insurance claims: countrywide patterns in treatment, cost, and compensation. ircweb.org/ircproducts/abstract.htm#20080213.

Chapter 4

Physical Examination

Meridel I. Gatterman

This chapter will outline the general physical examination and tests that aid in the differential diagnosis of the most common conditions that present in whiplash-injured patients. Succeeding chapters (5 through 8) cover a more detailed examination of specific whiplash-associated disorders. If imaging has been performed prior to the examination, such as in the emergency room, these views should be reviewed prior to beginning the exam. If clinical judgment suggests further imaging or if none has been performed, then it may be prudent for this to be ordered. It should be kept in mind with whiplash patients, as with other traumatic injuries, the symptoms are often worse the second day after the injury. In the case of fractures, these may not be clearly visualized on radiographs until a few days have passed; therefore, further imaging should be ordered and fractures should be ruled out if the patient's condition has worsened significantly. (See Chapter 5.) If instability is suspected, dynamic imaging should be ordered immediately.

Clinical assessment, including the physical examination, is a continuous process of evaluation, intervention, re-evaluation, and reflection.[1] Following the patient's story (Chapter 3), the subjective and objective examination is carried out. It is crucial in the initial stages of the examination to remember the fragility of the patient who may have suffered

both physical and mental trauma. Grieve[2] stresses the vulnerability of the whiplash patient to rough handling. He notes that these patients are quite different from those suffering from a single peripheral joint injury.

If the badly injured whiplash patient is handled vigorously with careless movement, the exacerbation can be severe, with headaches of hideous intensity, bizarre visual upset, psychic distress amounting to abject misery, and cervical pain of frightening viciousness.[2]

Patient-centered practitioners heed this caution.

LISTENING TO THE PATIENT

The patient's subjective complaints present a pattern that leads to a physical diagnosis. It is important to listen carefully to render a more precise diagnosis. It is not enough to simply use a muscle strain or ligamentous sprain as a diagnosis without identifying the structures involved. The physical diagnosis is formulated from the dysfunction presenting in the muscle injury and pain syndromes (Chapter 6), articular and ligamentous structures (Chapter 8), and the neurological system (Chapter 7). Skill in extracting the appropriate information requires care, patience, and an open mind. Gaining the patient's confidence is not only reassuring but encourages compliance with future therapeutic recommendations. Patient-centered care recognizes the individual differences in the general population that must be considered in the physical measurement and observation of patients with neck pain.

THE PAIN DRAWING

The pain drawing is a useful first step in formulating a diagnosis and can indicate both physical and psychological problems. Described by Ransford, Cairns, and Mooney as a psychological screen,[3] the pain drawing demonstrated better than 80% correlation with the hysteria and hypochondriasis levels of the Minnesota Multiphasic Personality Inventory. The pain drawing is also useful to guide the physical examination. When the pain drawing is consistent with anatomical referral patterns, no points are assessed for psychological disorders. When pain is indicated outside the boundaries of the body, in a nonanatomical pattern, over the entire body, in both the upper and lower extremities, or bilaterally in the absence of physical findings, then psychological assessment is indicated. One point for each abnormal physical pattern is assigned to the pain drawing. With a score higher than 3 points, there is less likelihood of a good outcome from treatment independent of psychological intervention.

It has been demonstrated that patients who are psychologically normal at the time of injury can develop abnormal psychological profiles if symptoms persist for 3 months.[4] If pain drawings are filled out each visit, later pain drawings may indicate psychological distress from ongoing pain. It must be kept in mind that patients exhibiting symptoms and signs of fibromyalgia will frequently indicate bilateral pain involving both upper and lower extremities. With careful palpation of the typical sites of exquisite tenderness on minimal pressure, a diagnosis of fibromyalgia can be differentiated. (See Chapter 6.)

The pain drawing can be an extremely useful first step to direct the examination to determine the structures injured. The patient can indicate not only the site of pain, but also different symbols can be used to indicate the type of pain (Figure 4-1). Travell and Simons[5] have mapped the referral patterns of trigger points found in muscles, and those with injury to the musculature from whiplash trauma can be readily identified through palpation using the pain diagram as a starting point. (See Chapter 6.)

CHIEF COMPLAINTS AND GENERAL ASSESSMENT

Recording the patient's chief complaints provides a starting point to guide treatment of the acute patient and suggests, if necessary, a prognosis for long-term management. Table 4-1 outlines the most common symptoms associated with whiplash trauma. Any medications being used should be noted, as heavy pain medication can affect physical findings. The physical examination is a general assessment that precedes focus on the chief complaints. This should include obtaining a blood pressure reading, temperature, heart rate, and vital signs. How the patient moves about, the patient's gait, and both standing and sitting posture should be observed. There is considerable variation in static posture between individuals, and the challenge is to determine the relevance of a patient's posture to the presenting signs and symptoms. A more dynamic analysis of posture generally provides more information. It is more useful to observe the patient's sitting posture to see if adequate mobility is present in the cervical region. If guarding is present, muscular control strategies should be noted. Assessment of shoulder girdle movement is necessary if upper extremity injury is suspected, and occasionally there will be low back and lower extremity problems that must be addressed.

ANALYSIS OF CERVICAL MOTION

Measurement and assessment of the active range of cervical motion, including pain response, is fundamental to examination of patients who have suffered whiplash trauma. Deficits in cervical range of motion have been shown to differentiate patients with neck disorders from asymptomatic subjects.[6-9] The use of an inclinometer provides a quantitative measurement of range of motion (Figures 4-2, 4-3, 4-4). Observation of the patient during range-of-motion testing gives a qualitative measure of the patient's pain response and pattern of control of movement.

SEGMENTAL CERVICAL MOVEMENT

The typical cervical vertebra is wider than it is high, with comparatively large vertebral foramina. Almost 40% of the height of the cervical spine from C2 to C7 is made up of intervertebral discs, so it is not surprising that it is the most mobile region of the spine. Stability is sacrificed, however, with this

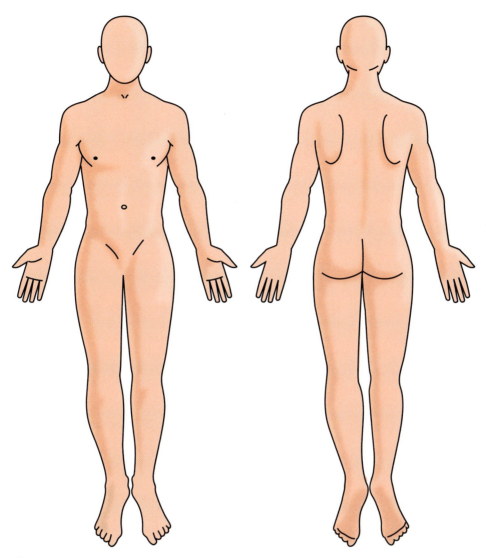

Figure 4-1 The pain drawing can indicate both physical and psychological problems. Different symbols are used to indicate different symptoms: numbness (.), pins and needles (o), burning (x), aching (*), stabbing (/).

mobility, making the cervical spine most vulnerable to injury. Each typical motion segment contributes 6 degrees of freedom of motion (Table 4-2). The movement of the C1 around the dens of C2 provides over 80 degrees of rotation. The condyles of the skull provide for slight flexion and extension with even less lateral flexion. (See Table 4-2.) Restriction of segmental motion, although it may contribute only slightly to overall cervical range of motion, can cause significant pain and dysfunction when not treated. (See Chapter 8.)

Assessment of segmental motion through hands-on examination should include static and motion palpation.[11] Following assessment of general cervical motion (see Figures 4-2, 4-3, 4-4), segmental symmetry and movement should be palpated. (See Chapter 8.) Tissue tone, texture, and temperature are also palpated.[11] This may require referral to a specialist such as a chiropractor if the practitioner is not trained and skilled in this procedure. A pulling away on palpation is an indication of localized tenderness. This may also be verbalized by the patient. Table 4-3 presents standardized grading for muscle strength, tenderness, frequency of spasm strain and sprain, in addition to a modified grading system for whiplash-associated disorders.

TABLE 4-1

Common Symptoms of Whiplash-Associated Injury

Symptom	Origin of the Symptom
Headache	Suboccipital muscles, zygapophyseal joints, myofascial trigger points, trigeminal nerve complex
Neck pain and stiffness	Cervical muscles, zygapophyseal joints, cervical nerve roots, cervical disc
Shoulder pain	Shoulder joint, rotator cuff, scapular muscles
Arm and hand numbness	Scalene muscles, zygapophyseal joints, cervical nerve roots, brachial plexus
Disorientation, irritability	Brain
Visual disturbances	Vertebral basilar artery network, brain stem, cervical spinal cord
Memory loss and difficulty concentrating	Brain
Vertigo	Cervical sympathetic nerves, vertebral artery, inner ear
Difficulty swallowing	Pharynx
Ringing in the ears	Temporomandibular joint, basilar arteries, cervical sympathetic chain, inner ear
Nausea	Vagus nerve
Dizziness, light-headedness	Cervical sympathetic nerves, brain, inner ear
Poor posture and balance	Paravertebral muscles, disturbed proprioceptors, zygapophyseal joints, cervical nerve roots

Modified from Evans RC: *Illustrated orthopedic physical assessment,* 3rd ed, St Louis, 2009 Mosby.

NEUROLOGICAL EVALUATION

The neurological evaluation challenges sensory, motor, and reflex functions.

Sensory function can be differentiated into pain and temperature, touch vibration, and position. Suspected peripheral lesions manifest locally: the more central the lesion is, the wider is the area of pain paresthesia or loss of motor function. Cerebral dysfunction is evaluated by noting the patient's mannerisms and orientation to time, space, and body parts. Further evaluation of cerebral function requires advanced imaging procedures and electro-diagnostic testing. Cerebellar lesions are characterized by repeated cogwheel-type muscle actions when the patient's eyes are open. The posterior columns of the spinal cord are the source of the dysfunction when repeated muscle actions are smooth and occur while the patient's eyes are open; however, when the eyes are closed these same muscular actions cannot be repeated as smoothly. Testing the cranial nerves determines brain stem dysfunction (Table 4-4).

Sensory Testing

Vibration sensation is carried by fibers in the dorsal or posterior columns of the spinal cord. It is tested by applying a vibrating tuning fork to bony prominences from distal to proximal. Most persons will be able to discern vibration or buzzing at the first joint of each digit. Occasionally the need to test the

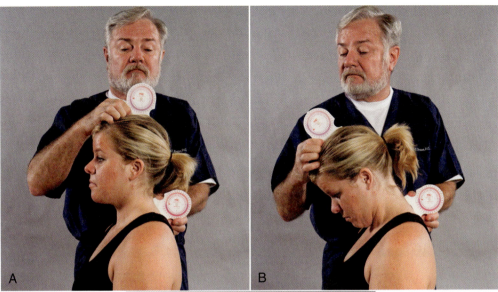

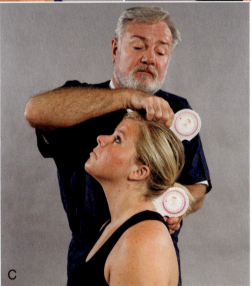

Figure 4-2 Cervical flexion and extension are measured with an inclinometer. The patient is seated with the cervical spine in the neutral position. **A,** The examiner places one inclinometer over the T1 spinous process in the sagittal plane. The second inclinometer is placed at the superior aspect of the occiput, or on top of the head also in the sagittal plane. Both inclinometers are zeroed in these positions. **B,** The patient flexes the head and neck forward. The examiner records both angles. The T1 inclination is subtracted from the cranial inclination to determine the cervical flexion angle. The expected amount of flexion is 60 degrees or greater from the neutral position. Cervical extension is measured from the neutral position as in A. **C,** The examiner places one inclinometer slightly lateral to the T1 spinous process in the sagittal plane. The second inclinometer is placed at the superior aspect of the occiput or on top of the head, in the sagittal plane. Both inclinometers are zeroed in these positions. The patient extends the head and neck, and the examiner records the angle of both inclinometers. The T1 inclination is subtracted from the occipital inclination to determine the cervical extension angle. The expected amount of extension is 75 degrees or greater from the neutral position.

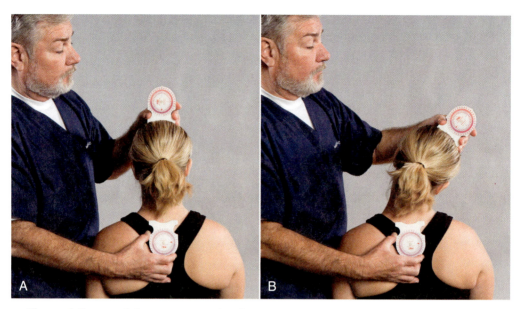

Figure 4-3   Lateral flexion is measured with an inclinometer and the patient seated with cervical spine in the neutral position. **A,** The examiner places one inclinometer on the T1 spinous process in the coronal plane. The second inclinometer is placed at the superior aspect of the occiput, or on top of the head also in the coronal plane. Both inclinometers are then zeroed. **B,** The patient laterally flexes the head and neck to one side. The examiner records the angles of both instruments. The T1 inclination is subtracted from the occipital inclination to determine the cervical lateral flexion angle. The expected amount of lateral flexion is 45 degrees from the neutral position. The procedure is then repeated for the opposite side.

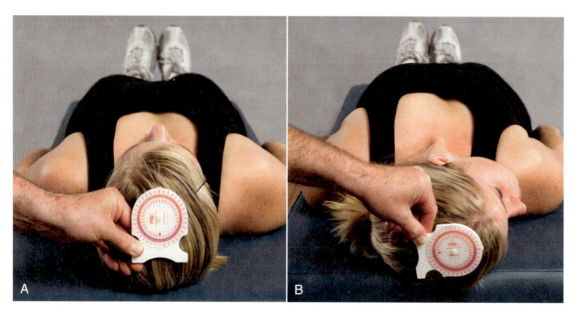

Figure 4-4   Rotation is measured with an inclinometer and the patient in a supine position. **A,** The examiner places the inclinometer at the crown of the head in the coronal plane. The instrument is zeroed. **B,** The patient rotates the head to one side, and the examiner records the angle of cervical rotation indicated on the inclinometer. The procedure is repeated on the opposite side. The expected range of cervical rotation is 80 degrees or greater from the neutral position.

TABLE 4-2

Range of Movement (in Degrees) of Cervical Motion Segments

	C0-C1	C1-C2	C2-C3	C3-C4	C5-C6	C6-C7	C7-T1
Flexion and extension*	15§	15	12	17	21	23	21
Lateral bending†	3§	—	14	14	14	14	14
Axial rotation‡	—	83	6	13	13	14	11

Modified from Adams M: Biomechanics of the cervical spine. In Gunzburg R, Szpalski M, editors: *Whiplash injuries: current concepts in prevention, diagnosis, and treatment of the cervical whiplash syndrome*, Baltimore, 1998, Lippincott Williams & Wilkins pp 13-20.
*Data from Dvořák J, et al: Functional radiographic diagnosis of the cervical spine: flexion/extension, *Spine* 13:748-755, 1988.
†Data from Penning L: Normal movements of the cervical spine, *Am J Roengenol* 130:317-326, 1978.
§Data from Kapandji IA: *The physiology of the joints, Vol 3, The trunk and vertebral column*, London, 1974, Churchill Livingstone.
‡Data from Dvořák J, et al: Functional radiographic diagnosis of the cervical spine: axial rotation, *Spine* 12:197-205, 1987.

next proximal major joint will arise, such as going to the ankle from the great toe. Various factors such as age, previous injury, or disease may explain a deterioration of distal sensation. Symmetry between the extremities is generally considered to be "normal" or clinically insignificant. Because fibers transmitting sensation cross at the level of the lower medulla and not in the spinal cord, unilateral alterations of sensation point to an ipsilateral peripheral or cord lesion. Position sense is carried by fibers in the dorsal column-medial lemniscal pathway. This sense is tested by firmly grasping a great toe or thumb and moving the digit in an up or down direction. The patient must have the eyes closed to remove visual clues, and inform the examiner of the onset and direction of movement. Symmetry between the tested parts is the critical finding. Because fibers cross at the level of the lower medulla, unilateral findings suggest an ipsilateral cord lesion. Bilateral losses are associated with ataxia (a loss of muscular coordination and impairment of gait).

Pain sensation is easily tested with a pin or paper clip. By tapping the patient's skin, the examiner can determine whether a lesion involves a peripheral nerve, dermatome, myotome, the cord, or brain. Pain and temperature information travels in the lateral spinothalamic tract. These fibers cross at the cord at the level of entry; therefore, a lesion in the cord will alter sensation on the contralateral side.

Reflexes

The biceps, triceps, and brachioradialis reflexes are most commonly tested in the upper extremities. In the lower extremities, the Achilles and patellar tendons are used for reflex testing. These reflexes are associated with segmental levels of the cord and occur when the tendon stretch activates the muscle spindles, sending a phasic, synchronous discharge to the cord. Testing involves identifying the tendon and then percussing it with a reflex hammer. Before concluding that a tendon reflex is absent or impaired, the patient should be distracted or the procedure reinforced by having the patient divert his or her gaze and in the lower extremities tightly pulling the hand apart while the tendon is percussed.

Testing for Muscle Strength

Loss of muscle strength has been associated with neck pain, most commonly in the neck flexors and extensors as well as the axioscapular muscles such as the upper trapezius. Early strength testing may aggravate symptoms, and pain inhibition can give false outcome measures when give way is because of a pain response rather than to a loss of muscle strength. Manual muscle testing of the sterno-cleidomastoid and trapezius muscle is performed

TABLE **4-3**

Standardized Charting Nomenclature

Grading Muscle Strength
5-Normal Complete range of motion against gravity with full resistance
4-Good   Complete range of motion against gravity with some resistance
3-Fair   Complete range of motion against gravity
2-Poor   Complete range of motion with gravity eliminated
1-Trace   Evidence of slight contractility; no joint motion
0-Zero   No evidence of contractility

Tenderness Grading Scale
Grade I   No tenderness
Grade II   Tenderness with no physical response
Grade III Tenderness with withdrawal (jump sign)
Grade IV   Withdrawal to nonnoxious stimuli (i.e., superficial palpation, pin prick, gentle percussion)

Frequency
Intermittent <25% of time (waking hours)
Occasional   25%-50%
Frequent   50%-75%
Constant   75%-100%

Grading Spasm
+1   Sustained contraction with mild resistance to passive motion
+2   Sustained contraction with moderate resistance to passive motion
+3   Muscle rigidity with complete resistance to motion in some direction
+4   Spasm triggered by movement, palpation, etc.
+5   Spasm present without external irritation, e.g., antalgic posture (splinting), contracture, etc.

Grading Muscle Strains
Grade I—Mild: Low grade inflammatory reaction, minimal swelling, no appreciable hemorrhage, some disruption of fibers
Grade II—Moderate: Laceration of fibers, appreciable swelling and edema, hemorrhaging into surrounding tissues (hematoma)
Grade III—Severe: Complete disruption of the muscle, tendon torn from the bone or pulled apart

Grading Sprains
Grade I—Mild: Few ligamentous fibers are torn
Grade II—Moderate: Ligamentous tearing without complete separation of the ligament
Grade III—Severe: Complete tearing of the ligament from its attachment or complete ligamentous separation
Grade IV—Sprain-fracture: Ligamentous attachment pulls loose with a fragment of bone (avulsion)

Modified Quebec Task Force Grading System for Whiplash Associated Disorders (WAD).

TABLE 4-4

Tests for Cranial Nerve Function

I	Smell (test each side independently)
II	Visual acuity (ability to read eye chart)
III	Light accommodation (papillary change to light)
III, IV, & VI	Eye movement (finger following)
V	Wink and ability to chew
VII	Facial muscle (smile and taste)
VIII	Auditory (hearing acuity and balance)
IX	Taste (gag reflex)
X	Voice (swallow)
XI	Shoulder shrug
XII	Tongue (motor)

with the patient seated (Figure 4-5). Posterolateral neck extensors are tested with the patient prone (Figure 4-6). The neck flexors are tested with the patient supine. (See Figure 4-6.) Posterolateral, anterolateral, and anterior neck flexors are tested with the patient supine (Figure 4-7). The prone and supine muscle tests may be conducted after the sitting provocation tests to prevent the patient from changing position unnecessarily.

PROVOCATION TESTS FOR CERVICAL SPINE DISORDERS

Provocation tests give valuable information by stressing specific tissues. When the test reproduces or exacerbates the patient's symptoms, the test is considered positive. In the cases of acute trauma from motor vehicle crashes, if fracture or instability is suspected, appropriate imaging is essential before provocation testing is begun (see Chapter 5). As the name suggests, provocation tests are designed to provoke or reproduce the patient's symptoms (pain and/or dysfunction), and extreme caution is necessary to prevent further injury to already damaged tissues. To avoid confusion, the tests will be described further according to the function they are testing rather than using eponyms to name the test. Depending on how acute and how much pain the patient is experiencing, the sitting tests may be conducted first to avoid painful changes in position.

Compression Tests

Compression tests may produce a cervical collapse sign (the neck will collapse or buckle during compression) in addition to producing localized and/or radicular complaints. The patient should be observed closely for a pain response and pressure should be released if the patient pulls away, buckles, or collapses. The patient is then questioned as to the exact location of the pain localized by one finger.

Foraminal Compression

In a healthy individual, approximately one fifth of the intervertebral foramen in the cervical region is filled by the dorsal and ventral nerve roots (medially) and the spinal nerve (laterally). In the neutral position, they are located in the inferior portion of the foramen, at or below the disc, with ample room for pain-free movement. Hypertrophy from degenerative changes (osteoarthritis) in the zygapophyseal joints may result in compression of the dorsal rootlets, dorsal roots, or dorsal root ganglion becoming symptomatic following injury to the cervical spine.[10] Inflammation with edema and swelling from whiplash trauma can compromise previously asymptomatic patients, causing neurogenic pain. Compression of the cervical spine can compress the foramen, eliciting lateralized and localized symptoms. Asking the patient to indicate the area of most intense pain using one finger to touch the area, as with any test, gives valuable information. Foraminal compression is tested with the patient seated (Figure 4-8).

Assessment of Cervical Nerve Function Through Compression

Acute disc herniation as well as zygapophyseal joint subluxation can produce nerve root compression. If the patient presents with the hand on top of the head for symptomatic relief, this suggests nerve root involvement since this position relieves radicular pain from nerve compression (Figure 4-9). Root pain may awaken the patient after several hours of sleep and may be relieved after 15 to 30

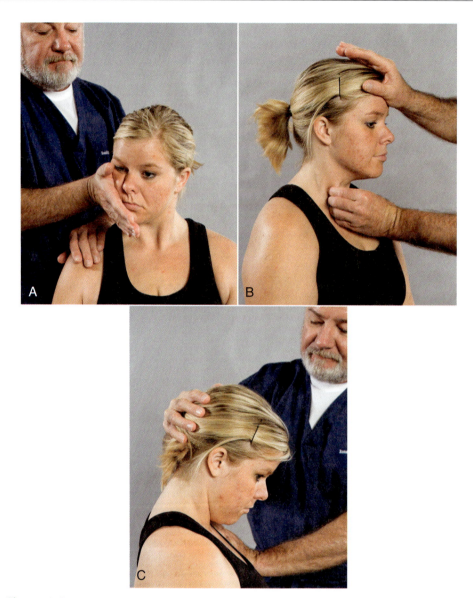

Figure 4-5   The strength of the sternocleidomastoid and trapezius muscles is assessed with the patient seated. **A,** Rotation against resistance. **B,** Flexion with palpation of the sternocleidomastoid muscle. **C,** Extension against resistance.

minutes upon sitting upright. Cervical compression is commonly performed by having the patient sit up and bend the head backward. If an exacerbation of radicular pain occurs when the head is laterally flexed in an attempt to approximate the ear to the shoulder as the examiner exerts downward pressure on the patient's head, then nerve root compression is suspected (Figure 4-10). Clinical findings associated with cervical nerve roots are outlined in Table 4-5.

Disc Herniation

Occasionally motor vehicle crashes result in disc herniation.[12] Although not a common occurrence, disc herniation is possible and should be explored when there has been significant impact or prior injury to the cervical spine. MRI can give a definitive diagnosis in these cases. (See Chapter 5.) A central posterior midline protrusion and spinal cord compression can produce a momentary sharp, radiating pain or paresthesia along the spine and into one or more of the extremities as the head and neck are passively flexed forward to the chest (Lhermitte's sign) (Figure 4-11).

Distraction

Distraction of the patient's cervical spine can offer relief from cervical nerve root compression, intervertebral foramen encroachment, and facet joint subluxation. A generalized increase in pain with cervical distraction can occur from muscle spasm as the neck is tractioned. The signs and symptoms of nerve root compression may be relieved when the intervertebral foramen is opened. Pressure on the joint capsules of the zygapophyseal joints is also decreased by distraction. With the patient seated, the examiner exerts upward pressure on the patient's head (Figure 4-12).

DIFFERENTIATION OF STRAIN FROM SPRAIN

To differentiate a strain from a sprain, the cervical spine is moved through an active range of motion

---

TABLE **4-5**

Clinical Findings Associated with Cervical Nerve Roots

Root	Disc	Muscle	Reflex	Sensation
C5	C4-C5	Deltoid/biceps	Biceps	Lateral arm
C6	C5-C6	Biceps/wrist extensors	Brachioradialis	Thumb, ring and index fingers, lateral forearm
C7	C6-C7	Triceps/wrist flexors/finger extensors	Triceps	Middle finger, ring finger
C8	C7-T1	Hand intrinsic/finger flexors		Ring and fifth fingers, medial forearm

Adapted from Watkins RG: *The spine in sports*, St Louis, 1996, Mosby.

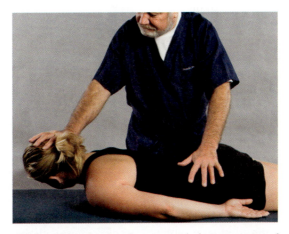

Figure 4-6   The posterolateral head and neck extensors (splenius capitis and cervicis, and cervical erector spinae) are tested with the patient prone. The patient resists posterolateral extension with the face turned toward the side tested. The upper trapezius, also a posterolateral neck extensor, is tested in a similar manner with the face turned away from the side examined. The examiner applies pressure in, and anterior direction against, the posterolateral aspect of the head.

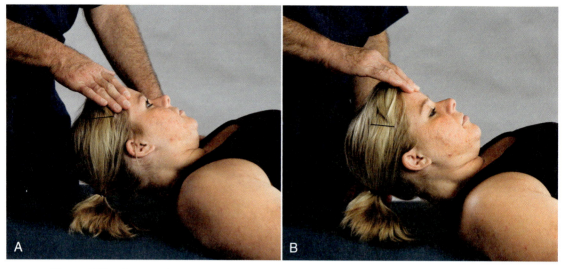

Figure 4-7 The anterolateral and anterior head and neck flexors are tested with the patient supine. **A,** The sternocleidomastoid and scalene muscles are tested when the patient attempts anterolateral neck flexion. The examiner applies pressure to the temporal region of the head in an obliquely posterior direction. If the neck muscles are strong enough to hold the head but not strong enough to flex completely, the patient may try to lift the head from the table by raising the shoulder. This movement occurs especially in the tests for right and left neck flexors because the patient attempts to aid the maneuver by taking some weight on the elbow or hand, allowing the shoulder to rise from the table. To prevent this movement, the examiner holds the patient's shoulder flat on the table. **B,** The bilateral contraction of the neck flexors is tested as the patient tries to flex the cervical spine by lifting the head from the table toward the sternum while keeping the mouth closed and the chin depressed. The examiner applies pressure to the forehead in a posterior direction. Pressure is applied over the thorax if the patient has weak abdominal muscles and in children under 5 years old.

and then through a passive range of motion (Figure 4-13). Pain during resisted range of motion (isometric contraction) signifies muscle strain. Pain during passive range of motion signifies ligamentous sprain. This maneuver can be used to determine ligamentous sprain or muscular strain of any joint or series of joints. Occasionally the patient has both a muscle strain and ligamentous sprain. Whiplash trauma can produce injury to multiple structures that must be differentiated if the clinician is to provide optimal management of the patient's condition.

If the patient holds the weight of the head with both hands and exhibits a markedly splinted cervical spine, then instability is suspected. If removal of this support is not tolerated or the patient cannot rise from the supine position without lifting the head with the hands, then further imaging to rule out severe sprain or fracture is necessary (Figure 4-14) (see Chapter 5).

ASSESSMENT OF VERTEBRAL ARTERY FUNCTION

The vertebral arteries are vulnerable to injury in the foramina of the cervical spine. Vertebral arterial damage with abnormalities in blood flow can occur with a whiplash injury.[13] Vertebral artery insufficiency is a primary concern of clinicians managing patients with neck pain, especially if cervical manipulation is being considered.[14] The signs and symptoms of vertebral artery syndrome insufficiency (Table 4-6) may be provoked by placing the patient's neck in extension and rotation (Figure 4-15). This test must be performed with extreme caution and terminated at any point should the patient exhibit signs of vertebral artery insufficiency or discomfort with the test. If the patient exhibits a positive test, then further procedures, including manipulation in this position, are not recommended. This does not preclude other cervical manipulative procedures. (See Chapter 8.)

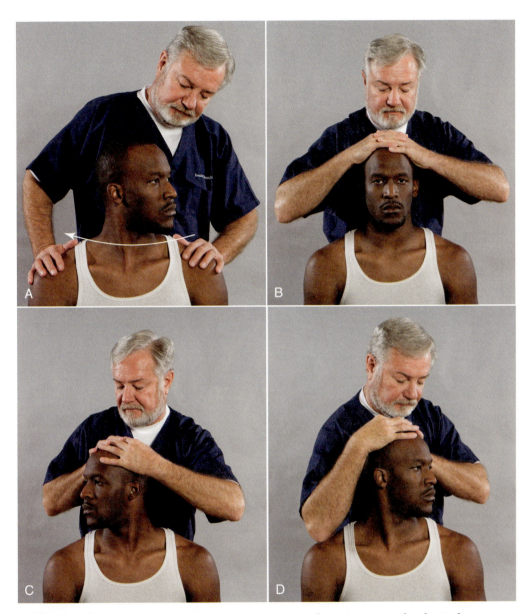

Figure 4-8 **A,** To begin foraminal compression testing, the patient is seated and actively rotates the head from side to side. Localization of any discomfort is noted. Alternatively, the examiner can passively rotate the patient's head from side to side while exerting strong downward pressure on the head. **B,** With the head and neck in a neutral position, the examiner progressively increases downward pressure (compression) on the head and neck. Symptoms may lateralize and localize at this point. **C,** From the neutral position, the head is rotated toward the side of complaint, and similar compression is applied. Reproduction of the complaint is a positive finding and suggests foraminal encroachment. **D,** The maneuver is repeated for the opposite side.

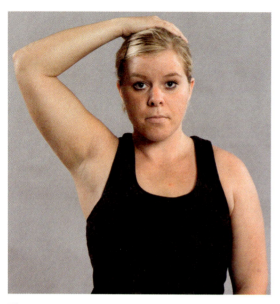

Figure 4-9 The patient presents with the hand on top of the head. If this position relieves radicular pain, this suggests nerve root syndrome.

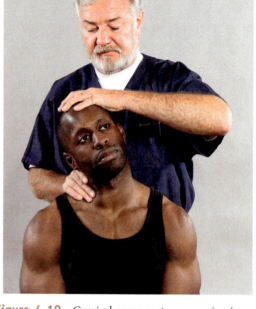

Figure 4-10 Cervical nerve root compression is performed by having the patient laterally flex the head in an attempt to approximate the ear to the shoulder. The examiner then exerts downward pressure on the patient's head. An exacerbation of radicular pain indicates a positive test.

TABLE **4-6**

Vertebral Artery Syndrome

Symptoms
Dizziness
Vertigo
Loss of consciousness
Blurred vision
Ataxia
Drop attack
Headache
Nausea
Tinnitus

Signs
Nystagmus
Blanching or cyanosis surrounding the mouth
Dysarthria
Dysphonia
Dysphagia

Tests
Extension and rotation
MRI/MRA

Modified from Gatterman MI: *Chiropractic management of spine related disorders*, 2nd ed, Baltimore, 2004, Lippincott Williams & Wilkins.

CERVICOBRACHIAL PAIN

Brachial plexus injuries are commonly traction injuries resulting from lateral neck flexion away from the involved side; however, compression of the brachial nerves can occur at several sites, including the compression from injured scalene muscles and other thoracic outlet syndromes. The main aim of clinical assessment of arm and hand pain following whiplash trauma is to differentiate nerve root compression from brachial plexus involvement. Somatic referred pain from trigger points in muscles is reproduced by pressure on the trigger point in the involved muscle. (See Chapter 6.) Motion palpation is used to determine whether exiting nerves are compromised by facet joint subluxation. (See Chapter 8.) The patient with referred pain may complain of a deep ache, whereas radicular pain is described as being sharp, shooting, or lancinating.[15] Table 4-5 outlines the clinical findings associated with the cervical nerve roots.

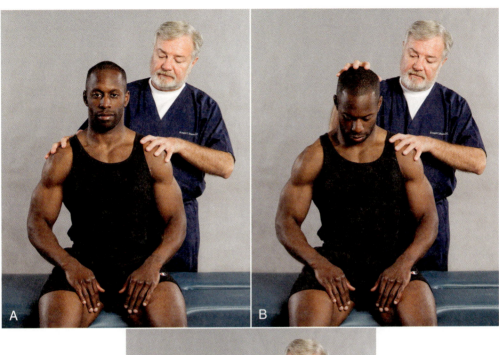

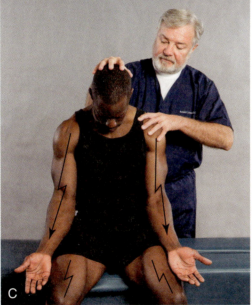

Figure 4-11   A, The patient sits comfortably but erect, with the head and neck in the neutral position. **B,** The head and neck are passively flexed toward the chest. **C,** The patient may experience a sharp, radiating pain or paresthesia along the spine and into one or more extremities. The presence of these symptoms suggests spinal cord compression or myelopathy.

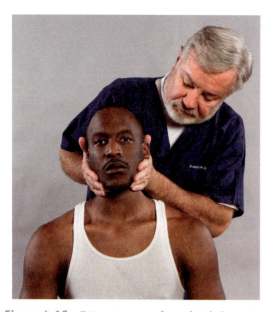

Figure 4-12   Distraction is performed with the patient seated, the spine erect, and the head and neck in neutral position. The examiner cups the patient's mandible and occiput and lifts the head. A positive finding is the relief of the patient's localized or radicular pain. The sign is confirmed if the symptoms return when the weight of the head is returned to the neck. Alternatively this test can be performed with the patient in the supine position.

Several provocation tests are employed to determine the genesis of arm/hand symptoms. Brachial plexus traction can be produced in both the sitting and supine positions. (See Figures 4-15, 4-16, 4-17.) In addition to the previously described tests for nerve root involvement (see Figures 4-9, 4-11), assessment for compromise of the cervical nerve root is tested (Figure 4-18). MRI and electro-diagnostic studies are used to confirm a diagnosis of nerve root compression. (See Chapter 5 and Table 4-4.)

It is important to note the frequent occurrence of cervicobrachial pain in chronic whiplash subjects.[16] In one study, 60% of chronic whiplash patients with symptoms that lasted longer than 3 months reported the presence of arm pain.[17] The origin of arm/hand symptoms is critical for appropriate management of these patients.

What underlies chronicity is failure to recognize patterns that can be confirmed by physical examination. Provocation tests are essential to test function and differentiate the patient's problems. Identification of specific loss of function and pattern recognition based on a careful examination

significantly impacts the clinician's diagnostic ability.

OUTCOME EVALUATION

Outcome evaluation is an ongoing process during the management of whiplash-associated disorders. Several outcomes can be monitored, including pain and functional status, both of which are important to patients. Assessment of patients' disability and their ability to perform their activities of daily living are important, not only to patients but also to the clinician who must have a rationale for ongoing management. Patient compliance with self-management programs and follow-up treatment is also enhanced by outcome evaluation.

Re-evaluation and modification of management programs are essential to patient-centered care, for each patient is an individual who may respond differently from others. There is no place for cookbook management in patient-centered care, even when the diagnosis is the same. Continuous assessment that monitors the patient's progress is of the utmost importance. Such re-evaluation informs the clinician in planning for any changes that may be needed for continuous progress in the patient's condition.

Treatment should cease once self-reported pain and disability scores are within normal limits, or when such scores have failed to change, indicating no further benefit from ongoing treatment. While this is appropriate for a cost-benefit analysis, disability scores may be challenged, especially if the purpose of rehabilitation is to prevent further reoccurrence of pain. Pain may be alleviated relatively quickly, but it would seem reasonable that a rehabilitation process would take 6 to 8 weeks for many and up to 12 weeks or longer for some. Management must be guided by changes in outcome measures of functional and physical impairment respecting cost.[14] Lack of change may suggest referral to a specialist in another field or another clinician of a different discipline. This is not to suggest that the patient continue on a medical merry-go-round with some patients medically stationary with some residual disability.[14]

NECK DISABILITY INDEX

The Neck Disability Index is a self-rated questionnaire that is the most widely used and most strongly validated instrument for assessing disability in patients with neck pain. Clinicians can confidently

Text continued on page 69.

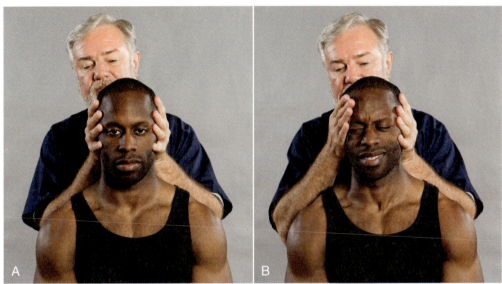

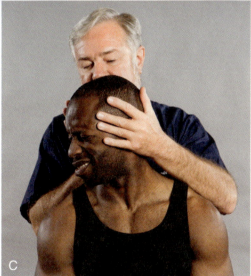

Figure 4-13   **A,** The patient is seated with the head and neck in the neutral position. The examiner grasps the patient's head with both hands. **B,** The patient actively attempts rotation of the head to one side against isometric resistance. Pain produced at this stage suggests muscle strain of the contracted musculature. The test is repeated with resistance on the opposite side. **C,** If isometric testing is negative for pain, the examiner passively rotates the patient's head and neck to one side to the limit of joint play. Pain produced on passive rotation suggests ligamentous injury. The maneuver is performed bilaterally.

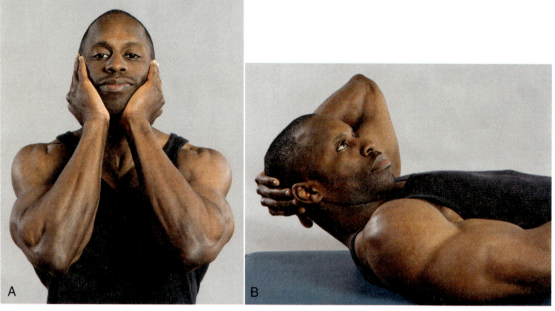

Figure 4-14 **A,** The patient holds the weight of the head with both hands and exhibits a markedly splinted cervical spine. If removal of this support is not tolerated or **B,** the patient cannot rise from the supine position without lifting the head manually, then further imaging to rule out severe sprain or fracture is suggested.

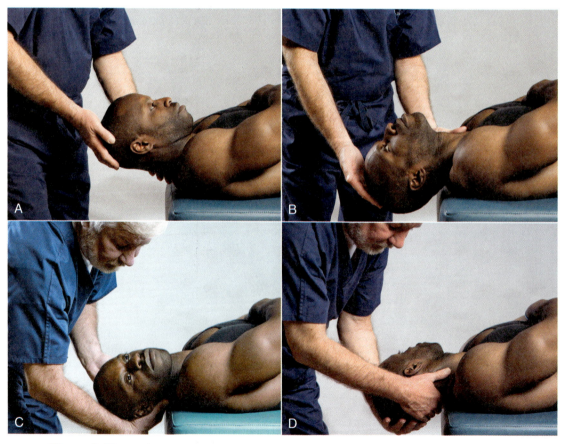

Figure 4-15 **A,** The patient is supine with the head extended off the end of the exam table. The examiner provides support for the weight of the skull. **B,** The examiner then brings the patient's head into extension. If no signs or symptoms are produced, the test proceeds. **C,** The examiner further brings the patient's head into extension and lateral flexion. The patient is instructed to keep the eyes open so the examiner may look for nystagmus and other neurovascular signs. **D,** The test is repeated on the opposite side. This test should be terminated immediately should discomfort arise or if signs of vertebral insufficiency are noted.

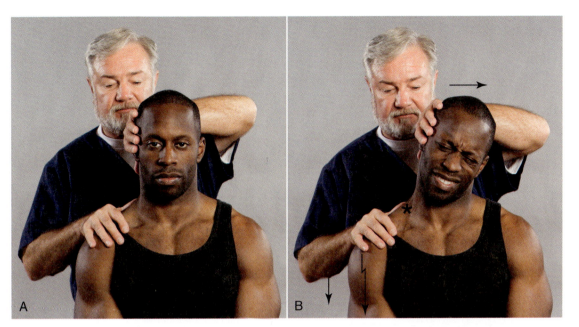

Figure 4-16 **A,** The patient is seated with the head and neck in the neutral position. The examiner contacts the lateral skull and superior aspect of the shoulder on the involved side. **B,** The examiner depresses the shoulder while flexing the head to the opposite shoulder in a slow, controlled fashion. Reproduction of symptoms suggests a brachial plexus irritation.

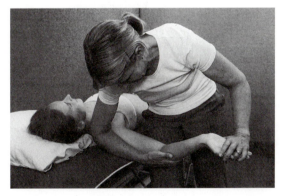

Figure 4-17 With the patient in the supine position, the shoulder is forcefully depressed while the wrist is extended. The shoulder is then externally rotated fully and the elbow is slowly extended. If the patient reports neurological symptoms in the hand within 10 degrees of full extension of the elbow, the test is considered positive for brachial plexus tension.

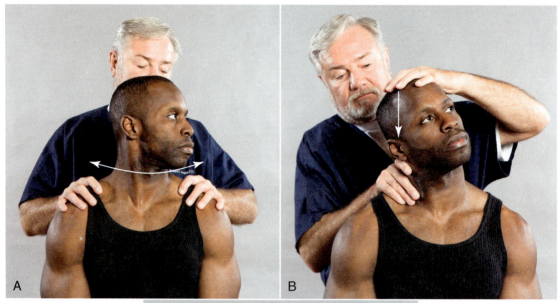

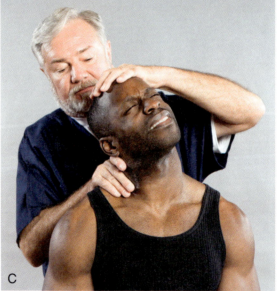

Figure 4-18 **A,** While seated comfortably with an erect posture, the patient actively rotates the head from side to side. Localization of pain is noted. **B,** The patient's head is laterally flexed to the side of complaint. The examiner gradually applies downward pressure to the head and neck. Reproduction of symptoms or collapse sign at this point constitutes a positive test and the remainder of the test is not completed. **C,** From the laterally flexed position, the neck is extended as far as the patient can tolerate. The examiner applies progressive downward pressure. Reproduction of radicular symptoms suggests nerve root compression. Localized spinal pain suggests facet involvement confirmed by motion palpation. (See Chapter 8.)

apply a "minimally clinically important change" value of 3 to 5 points in their practice settings. Patients can complete the questionnaire online and submit it for scoring. Used as part of the initial assessment, the Neck Disability Index provides a baseline for comparison of initial disability with periodic reassessment and final disability when the patient is assessed as medically stationary.

References

1. Maitland GD: *Maitland's vertebral manipulation*, 7th ed, London, 2005, Butterworth.
2. Grieve GP: *Common vertebral joint problems*, New York, 1981, Churchill Livingstone, pp 223.
3. Ransford AO, Cairns D, Mooney V: The pain drawing as an aid to the psychological evaluation of patients with low back pain, *Spine* 1:127-134, 1976.
4. Gargan MF, Bannister GC, Main CJ: *Behavioural response to whiplash injury.* Presented at the conference of the British Cervical Spine Society. Bowness-on-Windermere, UK November 7, 1992.
5. Travell J, Simons D: *Myofascial pain and dysfunction: the trigger point manual, vol 1, Upper half of body*, Baltimore, 1983, Williams and Wilkins.
6. Dumas JP, et al: Physical impairments in cervicogenic headache: traumatic vs. nontraumatic onset, *Cephalalgia* 21:884-893, 2001.
7. Dall'Alba P, et al: Cervical range of motion discriminates between asymptomatic and whiplash subjects, *Spine* 26:2090-2094, 2001.
8. Sterling M, et al: Characterisation of acute whiplash associated disorders, *Spine* 29:182-188, 2004.
9. Zwart JA: Neck mobility in different headache disorders, *Headache* 37:6-11, 1997.
10. Evans RC: *Illustrated physical assessment orthopedic assessment*, 3rd ed, St Louis, 2009, Mosby.
11. Barnsely L, Lord S, Bogduk N: The pathophysiology of whiplash, *Spine State Art Rev* 7:329-353, 1993.
12. Endo K, et al: Cervical vertigo and dizziness after whiplash injury, *Eur Spine J* 15:886-890, 2006.
13. Jull G, et al: Psychological and psychosocial factors in neck pain. In *Whiplash, headache, and neck pain: research-based directions for physical therapies*, New York, 2008, Churchill Livingstone, pp 87-99.
14. Bogduk N: The neck, *Bailliere's Clin Rheumatoid* 13:261-285, 1999.
15. Barnsley L, Lord S, Bogduk N: Clinical review. Whiplash injury, *Pain* 58:283-307, 1994.
16. Sterling M, Treleaven J, Jull G: Responses to a clinical test of mechanical provocation of nerve tissue in whiplash associated disorders, *Man Ther* 7:89-94, 2002.
17. Vernon H: The Neck Disability Index: state-of-the-art, 1991-2008, *J Manipulative Physiol Ther* 31:491-502, 2008.

Chapter 5

Imaging

Sara Mathov and Lisa Hoffman

INTRODUCTION

Imaging of the patient's cervical region following whiplash trauma, although not routine in mild cases, is necessary when moderate to severe trauma is associated with clinical findings indicating injury more severe than sprain or strain or when a patient's symptoms become chronic. An acceleration-deceleration mechanism of energy transfer to the neck, which may result from rear-end or side impact collisions or other mishaps, has been used to describe whiplash trauma and is included in the publication of the 1995 Quebec Task Force on Whiplash-Associated Disorders.[1] The energy transfer of this trauma can result in soft tissue injuries (whiplash injury), which may in turn lead to a wide variety of clinical manifestations (whiplash-associated disorders).[2] This description encompasses the diversity of the injuries occurring from this mechanism of trauma. Because of the wide range of impairment occurring from this injury, diagnosis and determination of the full extent of injury can be difficult, and the condition often creates a chronic problem that can last for years following the initial incident.[3]

The diagnosis of a whiplash-associated disorder (WAD) is often made clinically, after which the clinician may order imaging, such as radiographs, to further evaluate and determine the extent of the injury. Plain film radiographs are often the first step and are used to rule in (or rule out) more severe injury such as fracture or dislocation. Following a plain film evaluation, the clinician may choose to further investigate through the use of magnetic resonance imaging (MRI), computed tomography (CT), or other forms of advanced imaging. This chapter will cover the findings seen with these modalities and include the reasoning behind ordering advanced imaging for the evaluation of WAD. Although injuries to many areas of the body may occur, the scope of this chapter will be limited to injuries of the cervical spine, as this is the primary region of interest in the evaluation of whiplash injuries.

ACUTE INJURY

The role of imaging in the evaluation of acute whiplash injury is rather limited. Plain film radiographs are most commonly the first step in imaging evaluation. The goal of the x-ray examination is to determine whether there is more serious injury to the cervical spine, which would complicate the diagnosis of WAD.

Plain film radiographs of the cervical spine are routinely used to evaluate patients who have experienced significant trauma. In patients with a working diagnosis of WAD, the primary applications are to rule out fracture or dislocation and to detect evidence of instability.[4-6] Two notable clinical decision rules have been developed to predict the likelihood of significant spinal injury and provide an indicator of the need for cervical spine radiographs in alert and stable trauma patients. These are the National Emergency X-Radiography Utilization Study (NEXUS) criteria and the Canadian C-Spine Rule (CCR).[7,8] Both of these screening tools for significant cervical spine injury have been studied extensively, and comparative evaluations of the two sets of criteria have been done.[7-11] Both sets of criteria attempt to identify patients at low risk of significant cervical spine injury with the final goal of avoiding unneeded radiographs. The CCR is applied to alert (Glasgow Coma Scale score = 15) and stable blunt trauma patients and addresses three clinical or history factors:

1. The presence of any high-risk factor indicates a need for radiography. High-risk factors are identified as the following:
   - Age = 65 years or older
   - Dangerous mechanism of injury (Box 5-1)
   - Paresthesias in extremities
2. The absence of any of the low-risk factors that allow safe assessment of range of motion indicates a need for radiography. Low-risk factors are identified as the following:
   - Simple rear-end motor vehicle accident (MVA) (Box 5-2)
   - Sitting position in emergency department
   - Ambulatory at any time
   - Delayed onset of neck pain
   - Absence of midline cervical spine tenderness
3. Inability of the patient to actively rotate the neck 45 degrees to the right and left indicates a need for radiography.[7]

The NEXUS criteria also evaluate alert, blunt trauma patients. The rules identify a patient as being at virtually no risk of significant cervical spine injury if they meet four criteria[8]:

1. No neurological abnormality
2. No evidence of intoxication
3. No posterior cervical midline spine tenderness
4. No other distracting painful injury

Evaluation and comparison of these clinical decision criteria demonstrate a high level of sensitivity for both. In a study of over 8,000 patients presenting to emergency departments, the CCR would have missed one clinically significant fracture with sensitivity of 99.4%.[7] The NEXUS Low-Risk Criteria showed 99% sensitivity in a study of over 34,000 patients. It identified 810 of the 818 patients with cervical spine injury.[12] Application of the NEXUS rules appears to be applicable in geriatric patients, who have a somewhat higher rate of fracture as well.[13]

Although evaluation of these criteria outside the emergency department has not been studied, they could clearly be applied in a primary care setting. One concern for practitioners' considering manual therapies is the definition of "clinically important cervical spine injuries." The comparison study by Stiell et al[7] considered the following injuries to be "clinically unimportant fractures": osteophyte avulsion, a transverse process not involving a facet joint, a spinous process not involving lamina, or simple vertebral compression of less than 25% of body height. The overall incidence of significant fractures in the emergency department setting was about 2% of patients in the studies evaluating the CCR and NEXUS clinical guidelines.[7,8] In the primary care setting these criteria can be applied to stratify patients as high or low risk of significant cervical injury. The addition of criteria from the manual medicine guidelines for musculoskeletal injuries (Box 5-3) can aid the clinician in evaluating patient risk for other injuries that may contraindicate certain manual therapies. Though some of the specific criteria are debatable and not relevant to

BOX 5-1 High-Risk Mechanisms of Injury

Dangerous mechanism of injury:
- Fall from 1 m or 5 stairs
- Axial load to head
- High-speed MVA (>100 km/hr [>60 m/hr]); rollover; ejection
- Motorized recreational vehicle
- Bicycle collision

BOX 5-2 Complicated Mechanisms of Injury

MVA not considered simple rear-end:
- Pushed into oncoming traffic
- Hit by bus or large truck
- Rollover
- Hit by high-speed vehicle

General Clinical Indicators for Imaging

X-rays may be indicated within the first 30 days of injury if one of the following is present:

- Fever (>100° persisting longer than 48 hours)
- Unrelenting night pain or pain at rest
- Aberrant pain, paresthesia, or numbness
- Motor deficit
- Progressive neurological deficit
- Significant trauma
- Suspicion of fracture
- Suspicion of progressive disease
- Drug or alcohol abuse
- Chronic use of steroids
- Age over 50 years

the trauma patient, these criteria focus the practitioner on information that may indicate a higher risk of injury (e.g., a patient with ankylosing spondylitis is at greater risk of fracture than the general population). These guidelines also indicate that failure to respond to care in 4 weeks or a significant increase in symptoms or impairment warrants x-rays.[6]

Imaging information is applied in patient management plans to determine when conservative care, manipulation, and rehabilitation can be appropriately applied. In this scenario, plain film radiographs provide a diagnostic tool with good cost-benefit ratio. Radiographs are a readily available and relatively low cost imaging choice, but the potential significance of a missed fracture, dislocation, or instability is great. The minimal diagnostic series of anteroposterior, anteroposterior open-mouth, and neutral lateral views should be obtained in the primary care setting, although the lateral view typically provides the most information in cases of cervical trauma.

Radiographs are the initial imaging modality for ruling out fracture. The presence of fracture in the WAD patient may alter management by requiring surgical referral or by delaying or modifying rehabilitation plans. Clinical indicators of fractures may include increasing pain, pain unresponsive to care, and the development of neurological symptoms. Prior radiographs read as negative do not rule out fracture in the face of strong clinical evidence.[14-17] Evaluation of the major or unique forces involved in the injury may guide the clinician to higher levels of suspicion for certain types of fracture. Atlas (C1) fractures are associated with axial loading injuries whereas articular pillar fractures are associated with the combination of extension and rotation. Table 5-1 lists some common fractures with their associated force mechanism. Although the known forces may affect the level of suspicion of a given fracture, a lack of correlation should not rule out diagnoses with positive radiographic findings.

Fractures involving the vertebral bodies (compression/wedge or burst) are less likely to present with visible fracture lines. Stable compression fractures produce anterior wedging. The step defects and bands of condensation that indicate acute fracture may not be as prominent in the cervical spine as they typically are in the thoracic and lumbar vertebrae. MRI may be required to identify the edema associated with recent fracture. The clinician should be aware that C5 and C6 are common sites for developmental variation that results in a slightly decreased anterior body height. Anterior body height loss of more than 25% should be evaluated more thoroughly with MRI or CT to rule out significant involvement of the posterior elements. Burst fracture is indicated by posterior body height loss compared to the vertebrae above and below. Disruption of the posterior body margin is typically seen.[18] Burst fractures should be evaluated with MRI to identify canal stenosis or evidence of cord edema.

Fractures involving the posterior elements may be difficult to identify. The addition of oblique views may be helpful in better visualizing the posterior elements. Specific views of the articular pillars may be required. A variety of special views are intended to better visualize the odontoid process. Fracture of posterior elements should be evaluated with CT to determine stability and to identify any associated fractures.[5]

Careful attention should be paid to prevertebral soft tissues. Focal distention of soft tissues may be the only evidence of an otherwise occult fracture. As with most radiographic findings, the absence of prevertebral soft tissue distension does not rule out fracture or dislocation.[19,20]

Dislocation may occur with or without associated fracture. Assessment of vertebral landmarks on the lateral view (neutral, flexion and/or extension) can identify most dislocations. Initial radiographs may appear normal if spontaneous reduction has occurred. These cases may present later when the significant associated soft tissues damage allows the dislocation to recur. Some common patterns of

TABLE 5-1

Common Cervical Fractures/Dislocations with Mechanisms and Findings

Fracture Location/Type	Mechanism	Radiographic Findings
C1 burst (Jefferson)	Axial compression	Asymmetrical or widened paraodontoid spaces; lateral mass overhangs C2 by >2 mm; posterior arch fracture line
C1 posterior arch	Compressive hyperextension	Fracture lines may be difficult to detect
Odontoid	Complex and poorly understood; combinations of extreme flexion, extension, rotation, and shearing	Fracture line may be difficult to detect; angulation of odontoid
C2 traumatic pars (Hangman's)	Hyperextension; possibly flexion-distraction for Type II	Anterolisthesis of C2 possibly without alignment abnormality at spinolaminar junction line
Teardrop	Disruptive hyperextension or compressive hyperflexion	Triangular fragment at anteroinferior body corner
Vertebral body compression	Compressive hyperflexion; lateral hyperflexion	Anterior or lateral wedging of vertebral body
Burst, C3-C7	Axial compression with flexion	Loss of anterior and posterior body height
Articular pillar	Hyperextension and rotation	Oblique or pillar views may be required to visualize
Spinous process	Hyperextension or hyperflexion	Inferior displacement of fragment common
Transverse process	Lateral hyperflexion	Uncommon
Uncinate process fracture	Lateral hyperflexion	Uncommon

Taylor JAM, Resnick D: Skeletal imaging atlas of the spine and extremities, Philadelphia, PA, 2000, W.B. Saunders, pp 78-89.

dislocation are identified in Table 5-2. Cervical spine dislocations should be further evaluated with CT to detect associated fracture and determine effects on the neural foramina.[5] The forces associated with facet dislocation may lead to serious injury to the vertebral and other arteries as well. Clinical or radiographic findings suggesting vertebral artery injury warrant evaluation with magnetic resonance angiography.[5,21]

Ligamentous instability may present after acute symptoms have begun to resolve. Increased or new pain or neck symptoms, or the development of neurological symptoms in the absence of dislocation or fracture, may raise the suspicion of instability.[22] A Delphi survey of physical therapists listed the following symptoms of highest consensus for instability:

- Intolerance to prolonged static postures
- Fatigue and inability to hold head up
- Better with external support, including hands or collar
- Frequent need for self-manipulation
- Feeling of instability, shaking, or lack of control
- Frequent episodes of acute attacks
- Sharp pain, possibly with sudden movements

The following were identified as highest consensus for physical exam findings for instability:

TABLE **5-2**

Traumatic Dislocations

Dislocation	Mechanism or Tissue Injury	Radiographic Findings
C1-C2	Transverse ligament rupture	Increased atlantodental interval
Bilateral facet dislocation	Hyperflexion	"Perched facets"; anterolisthesis; interspinous widening
Unilateral facet dislocation	Hyperflexion with rotation	Abrupt, focal intersegmental rotation

---

- Poor coordination/neuromuscular control
- Abnormal joint play
- Motion that is not smooth throughout range of motion[23]

Instability (without associated fracture or dislocation) may not be evident on initial radiographs, as muscle spasm may obscure unstable segments.[22,24] Flexion-extension lateral radiographs should be performed after muscle spasm has subsided to allow adequate stress on joint structures (Figures 5-1, 5-2). Hwang determined in cadaveric studies that 60 degrees of cervical flexion-extension was needed to evaluate intersegmental motion.[25] Wilberger noted patients with initial flexion-extension films with small (1.5- to 3-mm) translations and angular displacements (5 to 10 degrees) showed radiographic evidence of instability (3.8- to 7-mm translation and 13 to 22 degrees angular displacement) 2 to 4 weeks later.[22] The Penning method has been widely used to evaluate intersegmental motion (Diagram from Penning, Dvorak.[26-28]). Henderson and Dorman also used an overlay tracing method to evaluate intersegmental motion. They used motion relative to vertebral body diameter to evaluate normal motion. They assigned a relative "rule of thumb" to designate excursion of less than 25% sagittal body diameter (SBD) as articular fixation and greater than 75% SBD as radiographic evidence of instability.[29] Using this method of tracings on an overlay is subject to error. Sagittal translation and rotation must be evaluated carefully, as landmarks may be difficult to consistently identify due to associated rotation or lateral flexion of segments. Digital radiographs with computer evaluation of intersegmental motion may provide the most accurate assessment. Frobin et al[30] report the accuracy of a computerized method of evaluating cervical spine intersegmental sagittal rotational (within 2 degrees) and translational motion (within 0.7 mm or 5% of vertebral depth). Their study employed corrections for radiographic distortion, variations in stature, and positioning errors (Figure 5-3). The center of a vertebra is determined by the intersection of diagonal lines from the four body corners. A midplane line is drawn through this center at the midpoints of the anterior and posterior body margins. The angle of the midplane lines between adjacent vertebrae is evaluated. The angle is recorded as positive if it opens anteriorly and negative if it opens posteriorly. The angle measured in extension minus the angle measured in flexion gives the rotational motion in degrees. A bisecting line is drawn between the two midplane lines. Perpendicular lines are drawn from the body midpoints to the bisecting line for both levels. Translational motion is measured by the change in distance between the two points on the bisecting line. To correct for magnification, the distance is expressed as a proportion of the anteroposterior body width (mean of superior and inferior body margins). Results were finally reported as "translational motion per degree of rotation" to take into account the wide range of rotational motion reported from studies of normal subjects. Adapted landmarks were used for C0-C2. This method appears to provide a reliable and reproducible measure of intersegmental motion. Kristjansson et al applied this method to compare women with chronic WAD grades 1 and 2 to women with chronic insidious neck pain and to a normal database. They found significant increases in sagittal rotational motion in the lower cervical spine of chronic WAD subjects compared to both normal and chronic insidious neck pain subjects.[30,31]

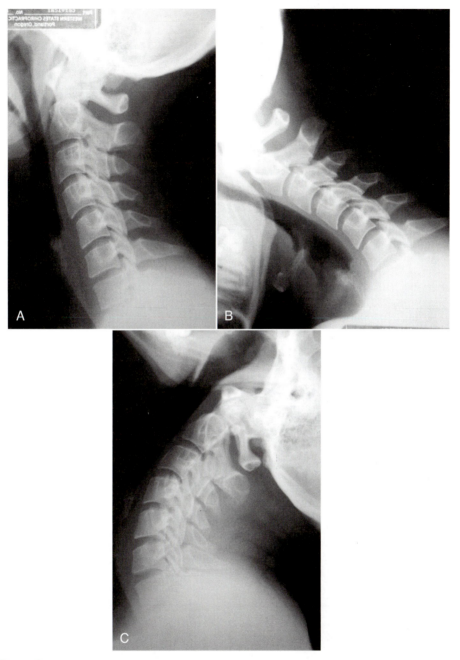

Figure 5-1 A 25-year-old male with no prior complaints, 5 days post-MVA. **A,** Neutral lateral shows straightening of the lower cervical curve though slight neck extension was present at the time of imaging. **B,** Flexion and **C,** extension views show essentially normal curves with no listhesis. (Incidentally noted is an oval soft tissue calcification or ossicle superimposed between the occiput and posterior arch of C1, which does not seem to affect motion.)

Whatever method is employed, sagittal translation alone is not adequate to evaluate for instability. Measurement of sagittal rotation should be performed as well. The most accepted standards for abnormal motion are for instability with the parameters set at 3.5-mm translation or 11-degree change in disc angle[33] (Figures 5-4, 5-5). Pediatric patients require caution in applying these parameters. In all cases, careful correlation with clinical presentation is required. The use of videofluoroscopy should be restricted to cases in which clinical suspicion of instability or aberrant motion is high and plain film

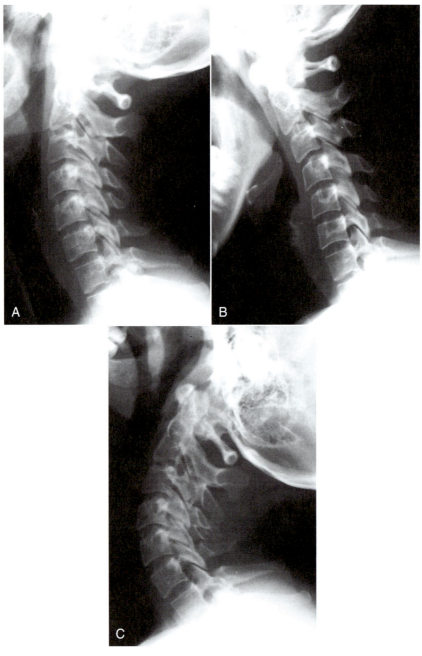

Figure 5-2 A 30-year-old female, 3 weeks post-MVA. **A,** Neutral radiograph is unremarkable. **B,** Flexion radiograph shows overall decrease in flexion. Most flexion occurs at C4-C5. **C,** Extension radiograph is unremarkable.

stress radiographs are normal or inconclusive. Much research remains to be done regarding what constitutes normal intersegmental motion of the cervical spine and what the clinical implications are of findings outside of these ranges.

The use of MRI in the evaluation of an acute WAD, in the absence of fracture or dislocation, is generally not necessary and has been examined in the literature. Ronnen et al[34] determined that there is "no indication for the use of MR imaging in the routine work-up in patients with acute whiplash injury in whom plain radiography of the cervical spine shows no signs of fracture or dislocation." Their evaluation of 100 whiplash patients found

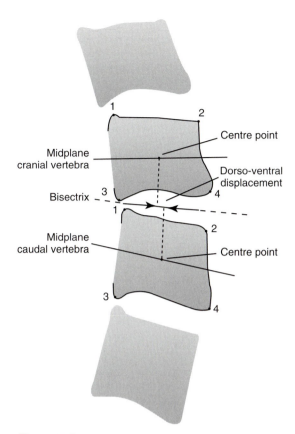

Figure 5-3 Changes in the cervical lordosis, particularly at C4-C5, have been noted in chronic WAD patients. The clinical significance of this observation and the presence of this finding in other conditions associated with neck pain are questionable.[32]

only one patient to have an abnormal finding that could be directly related to trauma (soft tissue edema in the region of the anterior longitudinal ligament from C3 to C7). The authors also indicated that those patients with kyphosis of the cervical spine did not have changes suggesting soft tissue injury and thus determined the source of kyphosis to be muscle spasm, which would negate the need for MRI evaluation. Another study,[35] which evaluated 178 whiplash patients using MRI in both the acute (within 3 weeks of the injury) and subacute (3 months post-injury) periods, did not find significant changes during those time frames. The most common finding among the patients at initial evaluation was mild disc degeneration, which was determined to be pre-existing and did not show change over the 3-month period of time. The authors concluded that MRI of the cervical spine is not necessary as a standard procedure following whiplash injury. Other studies found similar results,

supporting the idea that the use of MR imaging in the evaluation of acute whiplash injuries is not useful.[36-39]

CHRONIC INJURY

The use of advanced imaging with chronic WAD patients has been evaluated to a much greater extent in the literature. Recent studies have shown that an increased fatty signal on MR imaging in the cervical extensor musculature may be an indication of chronic WAD. These changes were seen especially in the rectus capitis posterior minor and major and deep cervical multifidus muscles.[40] The same authors also found an increase in the cross-sectional area of the cervical extensor musculature in patients suffering from chronic WAD.[41] These findings did not correlate to those seen in patients with chronic insidious neck pain, therefore suggesting that the cause is due to the chronic nature of the whiplash injury. In a separate study evaluating patients with chronic neck pain of an insidious onset, the cervical extensor musculature did not demonstrate quantifiable MRI changes in the fat content of the cervical extensor musculature and in fact were similar to the asymptomatic control group.[42] This study also reported a lack of sensory hypersensitivity and psychological distress in the insidious neck pain group which has been demonstrated in WAD patients.[42] All of these findings are significant in the way that they provide evidence of the chronicity of the injury (indicating that it is not just "in the patient's head"). However, it is not yet known whether these findings would affect treatment of the patient significantly, therefore necessitating the need for MRI evaluation.

There is also a body of evidence suggesting the necessity of evaluating the alar and transverse ligaments in chronic WAD patients. A 1987 study that examined by dissection 427 injured cervical spines (from high-speed MVAs) found 340 ligamentous injuries compared to 57 bony fractures.[43] This information would suggest that soft tissue injuries are more likely to occur in whiplash patients than are fractures. A 1994 study[43] found that 36% of 423 whiplash patients had asymmetrical left/right rotation at C0-C1 when evaluated using functional CT. The authors also found that the majority of those patients with asymmetrical rotation were hypermobile to the left as compared to the right, which they suggested could indicate that the right alar ligament is more commonly injured in individuals with whiplash injuries (Figure 5-6). A number of studies

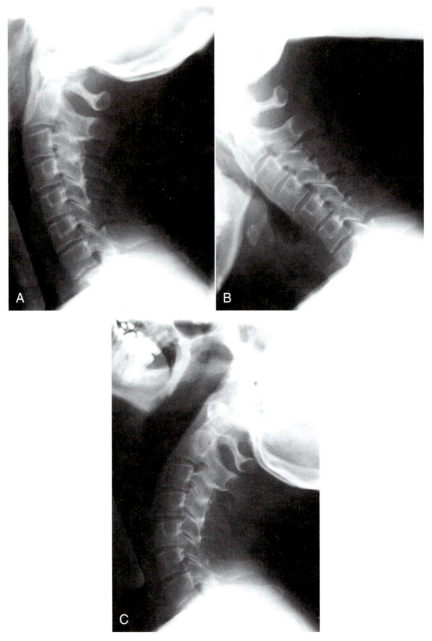

Figure 5-4 A 53-year-old female, 6 days post-MVA. **A,** The retrolisthesis at C2-C3 is present on the neutral lateral. **B,** These reduce on flexion with the C4-C5 level producing slight anterolisthesis. **C,** Minimal retrolisthesis is seen at C2-C3 through C5-C6 on extension. None of these reach the 4-mm threshold for radiographic evidence of instability. Osteophytes are present at the facets of C2-C3 through C4-C5 as well. Degenerative disease is the likely source of listhesis in this case.

evaluating 92 chronic WAD patients and 30 uninjured control patients found a higher number of lesions in either the alar ligaments or transverse ligament in the WAD patients as compared with the control group.[44-47] When evaluating the ligaments, the radiologist looks for abnormal high signal within one of the ligaments (which are normally black on MRI) or complete absence (rupture) of the ligament to indicate that a lesion is present (Figure 5-7). The visualized ligamentous lesions were given a grade of 0 to 3, indicating the severity of the lesion based on the signal characteristics of the ligaments.

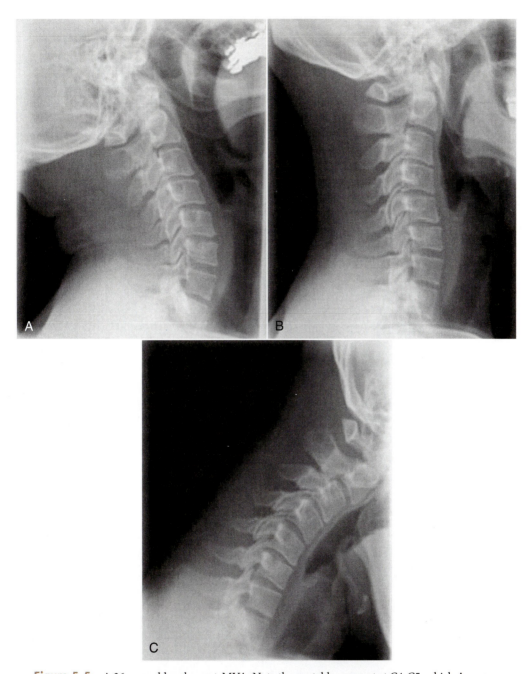

Figure 5-5   A 36-year-old male, post-MVA. Note the unstable segment at C4-C5, which **A,** moves posteriorly on extension, **B,** shows a reversal of the normal lordosis on the neutral lateral view, and **C,** shows slight anterior translation on the flexion view. The translation was measured to be 3.5 mm from extension to flexion.

For the alar ligaments, no grade 2 or 3 lesions were found in the control group, which would suggest that these lesions are caused by whiplash injury.[44] For the transverse ligament, only 36% of the injured group had a normal transverse ligament as compared to 73% normal transverse ligaments in the control group (Figure 5-8). Of the abnormal transverse ligament changes demonstrated in the WAD group, 23% had a moderately or markedly increased signal throughout the entirety of the ligament, which corresponds to a grade 2 or 3 lesion.[45] The greatest limitation of these studies is the fact that

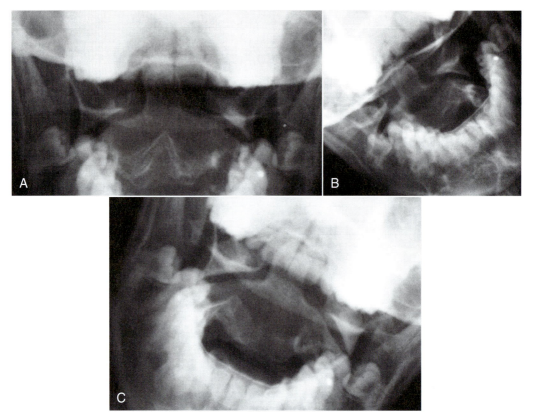

Figure 5-6 A 25-year-old female, post-MVA. **A,** Note the increased paraodontoid space on the left on the anteroposterior open-mouth view. **B, C,** This prompted lateral flexion views, which demonstrate lateral translation of C1 upon C2. Findings such as these should prompt MRI evaluation of the alar ligaments for rupture.

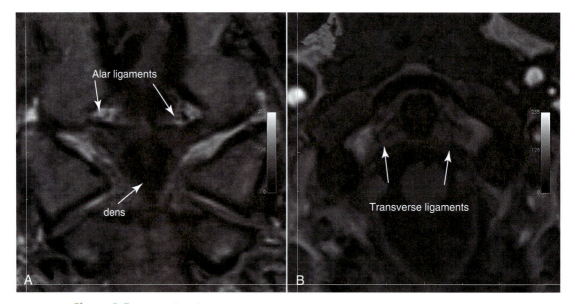

Figure 5-7 Examples of normal, intact alar and transverse ligaments on MRI evaluation.

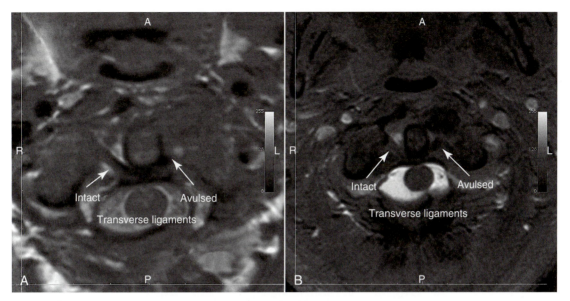

Figure 5-8   Rupture of the transverse ligament on the left in a WAD patient as seen on MRI with an **A,** T1-weighted sequence and **B,** T2-weighted sequence.

the alar and transverse ligaments can be very difficult to evaluate on MRI, and interobserver agreement is often fair at best. Proper detection and diagnosis of an alar ligament or transverse ligament tear depends largely on image quality as well as the expertise of the radiologist reading the images. A nonvisualized ligament could be due to complete tear or inadequate visualization (due to patient position, image acquisition, etc.), which often cannot be determined from the images obtained.

Of interest, another study examined the impairment rating of chronic WAD patients and compared this rating with their MRI findings of the alar and transverse ligaments as well as the tectorial and posterior atlanto-occipital membranes.[48,49] The study showed that patients with a grade 2 or 3 lesion report more difficulties in daily living as compared to those patients without demonstrated lesions. Those patients with demonstrated alar ligament lesions showed the most consistent association with the reported pain and disability scores. The disability scores also increased with an increase in the number of grade 2 and 3 lesions seen in multiple abnormal structures (more than one ligament or membrane injured), and multiple lesions were almost always in conjunction with an alar ligament lesion.[48]

Some authors do not agree with the necessity of evaluating the alar ligaments, however. A 2001 study by Wilmink and Patijn[50] found a high inter- and intra-observer disagreement when evaluating the alar ligaments. They also reported false positive reporting of alar ligament lesions due to anatomical differences side-to-side. Because of these findings, the authors suggest that MR evaluation of the alar ligaments is not a reliable method for diagnosing WAD.[50]

From a clinical standpoint, kinematic MR evaluation is the current trend for evaluation of the whiplash patient to determine abnormal motion or instability. When questioning MRI centers and radiologists in the field about a protocol used with whiplash patients, it was reported that flexion and extension MR evaluation is most widely utilized. The imaging centers do assess the alar ligaments, especially if there is a suspicion of a lesion; however, it seems that the main focus of evaluation is on evaluating instability, and this is best shown by the kinematic MR images. Whereas flexion and extension x-rays have long been the standard for plain film imaging of these patients, it has just begun being utilized with MR imaging in recent years. With kinematic MRI evaluation, the radiologist is able to assess each spinal level for instability to a degree that is not possible with plain film radiography. In addition to looking for movement or laxity at each spinal level, the radiologist evaluates the discs and ligamentous tissues for signal changes indicating a

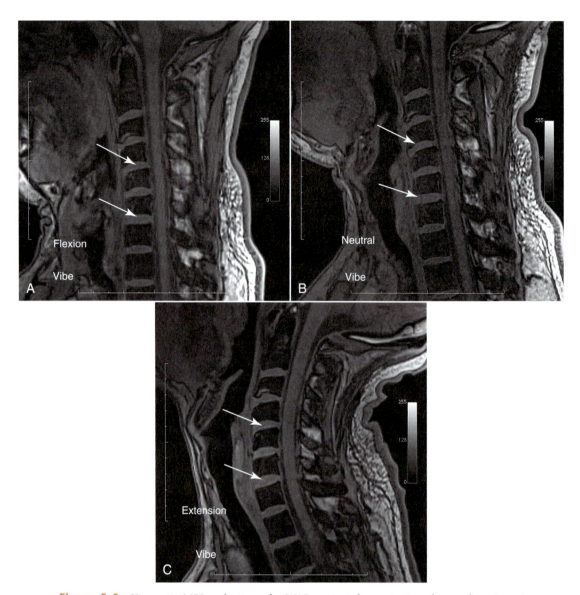

Figure 5-9   Kinematic MRI evaluation of a WAD patient demonstrating abnormal motion at C4-C5 and C6-C7. The abnormal motion is best visualized by noting the change in disc heights from **A,** flexion through **B,** neutral to **C,** extension while the unaffected disc heights remain unchanged. This type of change would be very difficult, if at all possible, to evaluate on plain film radiographs.

lesion (Figure 5-9). Although there was no literature found on this topic to date, it is helpful to remember that kinematic MR evaluation can be useful when assessing chronic WAD patients when plain film imaging has not provided enough information.

This systematic method of evaluation is beginning to change the treatment aspect of these patients as well. It has long been understood that a movement greater than 3.5 mm at any given segment, as seen on plain film radiographs when evaluating

flexion and extension studies, is considered to be an unstable segment (see earlier description). Anything less than that measurement has been considered to be either within normal limits or insignificant. However, through the use of kinematic MRI, it is now possible to evaluate and measure spinal levels with a smaller degree of movement as well as evaluate changes to the discs at these particular levels. It has been found through clinical experience that the discs actually change in size when going from flexion to extension in patients with abnormal motion. This change in disc size is a newer way of determining whether there is abnormal motion at a specific spinal level that can be monitored to see whether it progresses to degenerative changes with continued abnormal motion. This leads to the question of what to do with these patients clinically. Should these smaller measurements of abnormal motion be considered to be "unstable" or "normal" or somewhere in between? The answer to this question can come from continued clinical experience of monitoring these patients as well as future studies reported in the literature.

CONCLUSION

The role of imaging in the evaluation of WAD patients is determined by the extent of injury and the stage that the patient is in (acute vs. chronic). For the acute WAD patient, plain film imaging is the first step to rule in or out more significant injury, such as fracture, dislocation, or instability, and can prompt further imaging if necessary. If there is clinical suspicion of instability, flexion and extension views in the lateral position are warranted. Advanced imaging, such as CT or MRI, in the acute setting is indicated if significant injury has occurred and further evaluation is needed. For the chronic WAD patient, MRI may be warranted for evaluation of the alar and transverse ligaments and the cervical extensor musculature. Kinematic MRI can evaluate for abnormal motion that may not have been measurable by plain film. The information gained from the imaging obtained will help the clinician properly manage the WAD patient.

REFERENCES

1. Spitzer WO, et al: Scientific monograph of the Quebec Task Force on Whiplash-Associated Disorders: redefining "whiplash" and its management, *Spine* 20:2S-73S, 1995.
2. Eck JC, Hodges SD, Humphreys SC: Whiplash: a review of a commonly misunderstood injury, *Am J Med* 110:651-656, June 2001.
3. Bogduk N, Yoganandan N: Biomechanics of the cervical spine. Part 3: minor injuries, *Clin Biomech* 16:267-275, 2001.
4. Hunter OK, Freeman MD: Cervical sprain and strain: differential diagnosis and workup, Updated May 20, 2008 Emedicine.medscape.com.
5. Daffner RH, et al: ACR. appropriateness criteria: suspected spine trauma, 1999, Last reviewed 2007. www.acr.org.
6. Braddock E, et al: *Manual medicine guidelines for musculoskeletal injuries*, California, April, 1 2007. Academy for Chiropractic Education. www.guidelines.gov.
7. Stiell IG, et al: The Canadian C-spine rule versus the NEXUS low-risk criteria in patients with trauma, *N Engl J Med* 349:2510-2518, 2003.
8. Hoffman JR, et al: Selective cervical spine radiography in blunt trauma: methodology of the National Emergency X-radiography Utilization Study (NEXUS), *Ann Emerg Med* 32(4):461-469, 1998.
9. Dickinson G, et al: Retrospective application of the NEXUS low-risk criteria for cervical spine radiography in Canadian emergency departments, *Ann Emerg Med* 43(4):507-514, 2004.
10. Knopp R: Comparing NEXUS and Canadian C-spine decision rules for determining need for cervical spine radiography, *Ann Emerg Med* 43(4):518-520, 2004.
11. Mower WR, Hoffman J: Comparison of the Canadian C-spine rule and NEXUS decision instrument in evaluating blunt trauma patients for cervical spine injury, *Ann Emerg Med* 43(4):515-517, 2004.
12. Hoffman JR, et al: Validity of a set of clinical criteria to rule out injury to the cervical spine in patients with blunt trauma, *N Engl J Med* 343(2):94-99, 2000.
13. Touger M, et al: Validity of a decision rule to reduce cervical spine radiography in elderly patients with blunt trauma, *Ann Emerg Med* 40(3):287-293, 2002.
14. Woodring JH, Goldstein SJ: Fracture of the articular process of the cervical spine, *AJR* 139:341-344, 1982.
15. Hadida C, Lemire JJ: Missed upper cervical spine fractures: clinical and radiological considerations, *J Can Chiropr Assoc* 41(2):77-85, 1997.
16. Rowell RM, Stites J, Stone-Hall K: A case report of an unstable cervical spine fracture: parallels to the thoracolumbar Chance fracture, *JMPT* 29(7):586-589, 2006.
17. King SW, et al: Missed cervical spine fracture-dislocations: The importance of clinical and radiographic assessment, *JMPT* 25(4):263-269, 2002.
18. Daffner RH, Deeb ZL, Rothfus WE: The posterior vertebral body line: importance in the detection of burst fractures, *AJR* 148(1):93-96, 1987.
19. Herr CH, et al: Sensitivity of prevertebral soft tissue measurement of C3 for detection of cervical spine fractures and dislocations, *Am J Emerg Med* 16(4):346-349, July 1998.
20. DeBehnke DJ, Havel CJ: Utility of prevertebral soft tissue measurements in identifying patients with cervical spine fractures, *Ann Emerg Med* 24(6):1119-1124, Dec 1994.

21. Cothren CC, et al: Cervical spine fracture patterns mandating screening to rule out blunt cerebrovascular injury, *Surgery January* 141(1):76-82, 2007.
22. Wilberger JE, Maroon JC: Occult posttraumatic cervical ligamentous instability, *J Spin Dis* 3(2):156-161, 1990.
23. Cook C, et al: Identifiers suggestive of clinical cervical spine instability: a Delphi study of physical therapists, *Phys Ther* 85(9):895, 2005.
24. Shah VM, Marco RA: Delayed presentation of cervical ligamentous instability without radiologic evidence, *Spine* 32(5):E168-E174, 2007.
25. Hwang H, et al: Threshold cervical range-of-motion necessary to detect abnormal intervertebral motion in cervical spine radiographs, *Spine* 33(8):E261-E267, 2008.
26. Penning L: Normal movements of the cervical spine, *AJR February* 130:317-326, 1978.
27. Dvorak J, et al: Functional radiographic diagnosis of the cervical spine: flexion/extension, *Spine* 13(7):748-755, 1988.
28. Dvorak J, et al: Clinical validation of functional flexion/extension radiographs of the cervical spine, *Spine* 18(1):120-127, 1993.
29. Henderson DJ, Dormon TM: Functional roentgenometric evaluation of the cervical spine in the sagittal plane, *JMPT* 8(4):219-227, 1985.
30. Frobin W, et al: Sagittal plane segmental motion of the cervical spine. A new precision measurement protocol and normal motion data of healthy adults, *Clinical Biomechanics* 17:21-31, 2002.
31. Kristjansson E, et al: Increased sagittal plane segmental motion in the lower cervical spine in women with chronic whiplash-associated disorders, grades I-II, *Spine* 28(19):2215-2221, 2003.
32. Kristjansson E, Jonsson H: Is the sagittal configuration of the cervical spine changed in women with chronic whiplash syndrome? A comparative computer-assisted radiographic assessment, *JMPT* 25(9):550-555, 2002.
33. White AQA, et al: Biomechanical analysis of clinical stability in the cervical spine, *Clin Ortho and Rel Research* 109:85-96, June 1975.
34. Ronnen HR, et al: Acute whiplash injury: is there a role for MR imaging—a prospective study of 100 patients, *Radiology* 201:93-96, 1996.
35. Kongsted A, et al: Are early MRI findings correlated with long-lasting symptoms following whiplash injury? A prospective trial with 1-year follow-up, *Eur Spine J* 17:996-1005, 2008.
36. Parrish RW, et al: MRI evaluation of whiplash injuries. In DuBoilay G, editor: *Proceedings XIV*

Symposium Neuroradiologicum, London, England, 1990, Springer, pp 89.
37. Petterson K, et al: MRI and neurology in acute whiplash trauma: no correlation in prospective examination of 39 cases, *Acta Orthop Scand* 65:525-528, 1994.
38. Petterson K, et al: Disc pathology after whiplash injury: a prospective magnetic resonance imaging and clinical investigation, *Spine* 22(3):283-287, 1997.
39. Fagerlund M, et al: MRI in acute phase of whiplash injury, *Eur Radiol* 5:297-301, 1995.
40. Elliot J, et al: Fatty infiltration in the cervical extensor muscles in persistent whiplash-associated disorders: a magnetic resonance imaging analysis, *Spine* 31:E847-E855, 2006.
41. Elliot J, et al: MRI study of the cross-sectional area for the cervical extensor musculature in patients with persistent whiplash associated disorders (WAD), *Manual Therapy* 13:258-265, 2008.
42. Elliot J, et al: Fatty infiltrate in the cervical extensor muscles is not a feature of chronic, insidious-onset neck pain, *Clinical Radiology* 63:681-687, 2008.
43. Antinnes JA, et al: The value of functional computed tomography in the evaluation of soft-tissue injury in the upper cervical spine, *Eur Spine J* 3:98-101, 1994.
44. Krakenes J, et al: MRI assessment of the alar ligaments in the late stage of whiplash injury: a study of structural abnormalities and observer agreement, *Neuroradiology* 44:617-624, 2002.
45. Krakenes J, et al: MR analysis of the transverse ligament in the late stage of whiplash injury, *Act Radiol* 44:637-644, 2003.
46. Krakenes J, et al: MRI of the tectorial and posterior atlanto-occipital membranes in the late stage of whiplash injury, *Neuroradiology* 45:585-591, 2003.
47. Krakenes J, Kaale BR: Magnetic resonance imaging assessment of craniovertebral ligaments and membranes after whiplash trauma, *Spine* 31:2820-2826, 2006.
48. Kaale BR, et al: Whiplash-associated disorders impairment rating: neck disability index score according to severity of MRI findings of ligaments and membranes in the upper cervical spine, *J Neurotrauma* 22:466-475, 2005.
49. Kaale BR, et al: Head position and impact direction in whiplash injuries: associations with MRI-verified lesions of ligaments and membranes in the upper cervical spine, *J Neurotrauma* 22:1294-1302, 2005.
50. Wilmink JT, Patijn J: MR imaging of alar ligament in whiplash-associated disorders: an observer study, *Neuroradiology* 43:859-863, 2001.

Chapter 6

Management of Muscle Injury and Myofascial Pain Syndromes

Meridel I. Gatterman and Bonnie L. McDowell

I njury to the muscles of the cervical spine is extremely common from "whiplash" trauma, the most widespread being from motor vehicle collisions. When exposed to rapid stretch, individual muscle fibers may not have sufficient time to relax, resulting in rupture and damage to muscle and fascial structures.[1] Injured muscles, when left untreated, significantly prolong healing time and often result in unnecessary disability. The residual of muscle strain is characterized by tender areas known as "trigger points," readily palpable in the involved muscles.

HISTORICAL OVERVIEW OF MUSCLE PAIN LITERATURE

German Literature

Prior to the 20th century, references to muscle pain syndromes appeared most extensively in the German literature.[2] As early as 1843, the German literature referred to tendinous cords or wide bands in muscle as "muskelschwiele" (muscle callus).[2] In 1876, Helleday described a myalgic condition characterized by nodules near the origin of muscles that were tender on palpation. The phenomenon of pain spreading from nodules in muscles was also reported by German students of the Dutch masseur Mezger.[3]

In 1912, Muller discussed fiber hardenings and insertion nodules on palpation of injured muscles. His unique contribution to the early German literature was the identification of insertion nodules, which he described as pressure sensitive. He reported that with pressure, some hardenings radiated pain to far-reaching areas, while others were even spontaneously painful. He noted that these hardenings were predictably found in specific locations in specific muscles.[3] Muller pointed out that they were liable to be overlooked because doctors tend not to search for them in a systematic and skillful manner.[4] Schmidt, in 1914, implicated muscle spindles as responsible for the painfulness of the muscle hardenings, because of the anatomical location and known sensory function of spindles.[2]

American Literature

The terms "trigger point" and "myofascial pain" permeate the American literature that describes muscle pain syndromes. As early as 1936, Edeiken and Wolferth[5] used the term "trigger zone" to describe pain reported by coronary thrombosis patients referred to the shoulder and down the left arm in response to pressure over the upper part of the left scapula. Steindler,[6] in 1940, used the phrase "trigger point" to describe areas from which pain was referred. He described the treatment of chronic pain by injection of trigger points with procaine. In 1942, Travell, with coauthors Ringler and Herman,[7] first reported on her many studies on trigger points. Travell's interest in myofascial pain stemmed from a painful muscle strain that she suffered in the course of her work. She reported in her autobiography that she could touch spots in the muscle that reproduced and intensified the pain that radiated from the trigger area.[4] Since that time, Travell has written extensively on this topic, publishing, with Simons in 1983, *Myofascial Pain and Dysfunction: The Trigger Point Manual.*[8] In addition to procaine injections, they described the less invasive treatment of trigger points, recommending stretching of the affected muscles, following topical spraying with vapocoolant. The vapocoolant acts as a distraction while stretching the affected muscle is the desired action.[8]

Good, who previously published under the names Gutstein and Gutstein-Good, reported in 1950 and 1951 that the patterns of pain referral from tender points in individual muscles are the same in everyone, mapping these in well-executed illustrations.[4]

Writing in the *Journal of the National Chiropractic Association* in 1957, Nimmo[9] discussed the concept that excessive contraction produced by muscle strain, or other trauma, engages numerous receptors, producing a vicious cycle of noxious impulses. He developed a therapy in which pressure is applied to trigger points to interrupt the pain-spasm-pain cycle. Referred to by Travell and Simons[8] as "ischemic compression," this type of therapy has been widely used by chiropractors in the treatment of muscular trigger points.

THEORETICAL MODELS OF MUSCLE AND MYOFASCIAL PAIN

An early model of pain put forward by Descartes postulated that there was a direct line between the peripheral tissues and the brain. He based this on philosophical reflections rather than experimental evidence.[10] Von Frey, after correctly identifying pain receptors ("nociceptors"), concluded that the intensity with which pain arising in these structures is felt is in direct proportion to the strength of stimulus applied to them. Goldscheider theorized that the build-up and prolongation of the pain experience, often after a period of time, may be some form of pain-summation mechanism in the spinal cord.[10] Livingston,[11] in 1943, suggested the possibility of the initiation of activity in closed self-exciting

neuronal loops he called "reverberating circuits." He put aside the long-held view that pain signals pass uninterrupted to the brain and considered the possibility that they may be either augmented or suppressed as they pass through the peripheral and central nervous system. This is supported by the observation that the amount of pain suffered by individuals varies widely and that even seemingly innocuous stimuli may be pain producing.[10]

Local Response and Muscular Pain

The physical response to painful stimuli is determined by the responsiveness to the nociceptive and modulating system of the individual. Locally, muscle nociceptors take the form of free nerve endings markedly sensitive to chemical stimuli. The degree of pain perception for a given-strength stimulus depends first on the sensitivity of the receptor. Receptors may be sensitized by two different mechanisms, prior stimulation and a variety of chemical agents. These include histamine, prostaglandins, bradykinin, and serotonin.[12] The results of their action locally may be not only sensitization of the pain receptors but also local inflammation and hyperirritability of myofascial trigger points. Bradykinin is one of the most potent inflammatory exudates found in damaged tissues. It not only activates nociceptors but also sensitizes them. Serotonin is released from platelet and mast cells as part of the inflammatory response to muscle tissue damage. Both bradykinin and serotonin have a strong vasodilatory effect that leads to the development of edema. It is because of the chemical sensitization of nociceptors that there is a lowering of the pain threshold, making them responsive not only to high intensity noxious stimuli but also to low intensity, mildly noxious or innocuous stimuli.[13] In addition bradykinin has the effect of releasing prostaglandins from damaged tissue cells. These in turn have a powerful nociceptor sensitizing effect.[10] The sensitization of nociceptors in the damaged muscle makes the myofascial trigger points exquisitely tender, provoking the patient to flinch involuntarily when pressure is applied.

Central Sensitization

Central sensitization can be defined as an exaggerated response of the central nervous system (CNS) to a peripheral stimulus that is normally painful (hyperalgesia) or nonnociceptive, such as touch (allodynia), denoting hyperexcitability and hypersensitivity of the CNS neurons. Characteristic of central sensitization is the persistence of pain.[14] It is thought that noxious mechanical and chemical stimulation of nociceptors in the cervical muscles, sensitized by input in their respective fields, shows dramatic expansion of their neuronal activity in the spinal cord. Similar processes were described in the osteopathic literature by Korr,[15] and later Patterson and Steinmetz,[16] referred to the neurophysiological effect as the "facilitated state." The reason for the development of secondary hyperalgesia is that the sensory afferent barrage set up by the activated and sensitized trigger point nociceptors causes neurons in the dorsal horn to develop a marked increase in excitability now known as central sensitization.[14]

The current view of the cellular mechanisms underlying neuroplastic changes indicates that sensitization is caused, at least in part, by changes in the intrinsic characteristics of the spinal neurons involved in addition to changes in the damaged peripheral tissues.[17] The process appears to be dependent on an initial activation of nociceptive afferents and the subsequent release of excitatory amino acids and neuropeptides.[10,18] Animal studies have demonstrated that the excitatory amino acids, glutamate and aspartate, and neuropeptides, substance P and calcitonin gene-related peptide, for example, trigger a cascade of cellular changes leading to enduring increases in neuronal excitability.[19]

This increased excitability with the consequent neuroplasticity is thought to lead to central sensitization.[17] From other animal studies,[20] it is believed that the sensitization of dorsal horn neurons brought about as a result of the sensory afferent barrage, developed in response to the activation and sensitization of nociceptors at the trigger point sites, has the following effects: (a) an increase in the receptive fields of dorsal horn neurons leading to the spread and referral of trigger point pain, (b) the development of secondary hyperalgesia in the zone of the trigger point referred pain, and (c) the perpetuation of dorsal horn neuronal activity, with, as a consequence, the persistence of the pain.[10]

Referred Pain from Myofascial Trigger Points

Referred pain originating from trigger points is felt at a distance, often entirely remote from its source of origin. The distribution of referred trigger point pain rarely coincides with the entire distribution of peripheral nerve or dermatomal segment. The pain initiated by muscle nociceptors is referred to an area served by other somatic receptors that converge on the spinothalamic tract neurons. This mechanism of pain production places the active myofascial trigger point in the position of acting as a peripheral pain generator perceived in a distant location.

Lewis, in 1942, described pain that develops as a result of injury to muscle and perceived by the brain as arising some distance away from the affected site.[10] This concept was first put forward in 1909 by Mckenzie and reintroduced by Ruch in 1940.[10] The subsequent hypothesis put forward by Mense[21] is the assumption that afferent fibers from a muscle's nociceptors not only make synaptic connections with dorsal horn neurons responsible for conducting nociceptive information from that muscle upward, but also connect with neighboring neurons that normally transmit sensory information from other muscles. It is understood that one-to-one synaptic transmission is the exception rather than the rule in the CNS. A single neuron is acted upon by many other neurons and in turn acts upon multiple neurons. Based on this, it is reasonable to believe that pain originating in myofascial trigger points not only converges and sensitizes the afferent barrage in the dorsal horn neurons primarily responsible for transmitting nociceptive information upward, but also activates and sensitizes dorsal horn neurons that are responsible for transmitting information from distal muscles. The brain, through this mechanism, receives confusing messages and mislocates the pain, perceiving it as originating from a distal muscle and not just the pain-generating trigger point.

Inhibitory Controls

It has been demonstrated that the body produces endogenous pain-suppressing substances that produce analgesic effects in the CNS. These various substances are referred to as "opioid peptides" and include endorphins, dynorphins, and enkephalins.[22] These morphine-like substances, which work as inhibitory mechanisms, use both GABA and opioidergic transmitter pharmacologies to suppress nociceptive neuron excitability.[17] It is thought that mechanical forces produced by various therapies are of sufficient magnitude to coactivate both low threshold mechanoreceptors and high threshold nociceptive afferents that simultaneously activate antinociceptor systems, suppressing hyperexcitability of myofascial structures. These central antinociceptive mechanisms may operate in conjunction with peripheral antinociceptive mechanisms, particularly when there is inflammation in damaged peripheral tissues.

Pain Patterns from Myofascial Pain Syndromes

Myofascial pain syndromes are characterized by hypersensitive trigger points described as hard, indurated nodules in the muscle, which refer pain in patterns consistent from person to person. Single or multiple trigger points with a twitch response and accompanying taut band are characteristic of muscle exhibiting myofascial pain syndromes.[8] Palpation across the muscle fiber reveals the taut band that includes the trigger point, whereas deep palpation along the length of the same muscle fibers gives the impression of a nodule at the trigger point. The local twitch response is seen or felt as a contraction of the fibers in the taut band and lasts as long as 1 second. A sustained burst of electrical activity that resembles motor unit action potentials has been monitored on electromyography (EMG).[8]

Once established in injured muscles, trigger points may persist for decades, restricting range of motion and recurrently referring pain in characteristic patterns when left untreated. Travell and Simons[8] classified trigger points as either active or latent. When referred pain elicited by pressure applied to the trigger point is recognized by the patient as corresponding to his or her clinical complaint, then the trigger point is said to be active. A latent trigger point may persist for years after apparent recovery from injury. The latent trigger points are clinically silent but can become active, with minor overstretching, overuse, or chilling, predisposing to acute attacks. Active trigger points, when left untreated, can become latent and contribute to a poor prognosis or late whiplash syndrome. (See Chapter 11.)

Common Myofascial Pain Patterns from Whiplash Injuries

The muscles most frequently strained during whiplash trauma are the anterior strap muscles: the sternocleidomastoid (SCM) muscles and the scalene muscles. These muscles form the first line of defense, protecting from hyperextension by lengthening as they contract until the forces of impact become stronger than the muscle contraction can control. This eccentric contraction makes the neck muscles as vulnerable to strain as are the muscles of the lower back that become strained when a weight is lowered while bending forward with the knees straight. In this case the forces of gravity on the weight overcome the controlled muscle contraction, leading to injury.

Trigger points in the SCM, in addition to those found in the upper trapezius, temporalis, posterior cervical, and suboccipital muscles, can be the cause of headaches following whiplash injuries. The scalene muscles, on the other hand, commonly refer pain down the upper extremity from entrapment of the lower trunk of the brachial plexus as a result of tautness of the scalene anterior and medius. (See Chapter 8.) This entrapment can cause ulnar pain, tingling, numbness, and dysesthesia. No nerve or vascular entrapment has been recognized as due to trigger points in the levator scapulae, but complaints of neck stiffness following whiplash injury to this muscle is common as both muscles acting together checkrein neck flexion.[8] Pain drawings are useful tools that can suggest the location of trigger points and areas of referred pain. Figures 6-1 through 6-24 indicate the location of typical trigger points (*) and areas of referred pain (x).

Sternocleidomastoid (SCM) Muscle

Anatomically, the sternocleidomastoid is a complex muscle with two divisions, the sternal, which is more medial and superficial, and the clavicular, which lies lateral and deeper (Figure 6-1). The muscle is attached above by a short tendon into the lateral surface of the mastoid process and to the lateral half of the superior nuchal line of the occipital bone. Below, the medial or sternal head is attached to the manubrium sterni running obliquely upward, laterally, and backward. The lateral or clavicular head attaches below to the medial third of the superior border of the anterior surface of the clavicle. It passes almost vertically upward behind the sternal head and blends, with its deep surface forming a thick rounded belly.[23]

The sternocleidomastoid is innervated by the accessory nerve, which arises within the spinal column from the ventral roots of the motor fibers of the upper five cervical segments. The motor nerve fibers ascend through the foramen magnum and then descend through the jugular foramen, where they unite with sensory fibers from the anterior primary division of the second and sometimes third cervical nerves.[24]

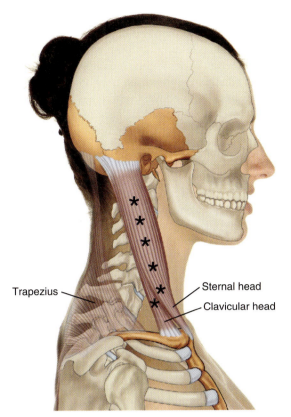

Figure 6-1 Lateral view of the sternocleidomastoid muscle illustrating the typical locations of trigger points (*).

Acting unilaterally, the sternocleidomastoid muscle tilts the head toward the ipsilateral side while rotating the face to the contralateral side. Acting with the upper trapezius, it laterally bends the neck, drawing the ear toward the ipsilateral shoulder. It acts along with the scalene and trapezius muscles to compensate for head tilt due to postural distortion. Acting together, the two muscles draw the chin forward, assisting the longi colli in neck flexion, checking hyperextension of the neck, and resisting forceful backward movement of the head. Acting with the trapezius, the two muscles stabilize the head during talking and chewing. If the head is fixed, they assist in elevating the thorax in forced inspiration. The two muscles are also active when the head is raised while the body is supine.[23]

Trigger points in the SCM generate complaints of "soreness" of the neck and, most commonly, headaches. Figure 6-2 illustrates the typical site of trigger points and pain referral in the SCM. To palpate the SCM with the patient seated or supine, the neck and head are rotated contralaterally. As the head and neck are lifted, the SCM will visibly contract. The SCM can then be palpated along its length. Trigger points can be palpated when the muscle is slackened by laterally flexing the patient's head toward the shoulder on the symptomatic side and rotating the face slightly to the contralateral side. Trigger points can then be located by grasping the muscle between the thumb and fingers.

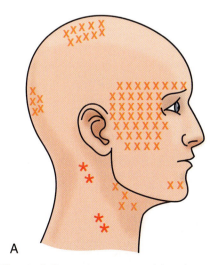

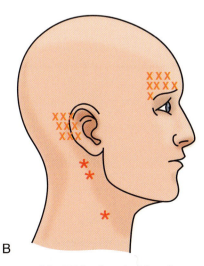

Figure 6-2 **A,** Trigger points (*) in the sternal division of the SCM refer pain (x) to the vertex of the occiput, across the cheek, over the eyes to the throat and the sternum. **B,** Trigger points (*) in the clavicular division refer pain (x) to the eye and face as well as the ipsilateral suboccipital region.

Ischemic compression can be applied to the trigger points exerted by a pincer-like grasp rather than by direct pressure on the trigger point. The clavicular division of the SCM muscle can be stretched by extending the head and neck while rotating the face to the opposite side. To stretch the sternal division, the head is first rotated toward the side of complaint, and at full rotation, the chin is tipped downward toward the shoulder, elevating the occiput and mastoid to provide maximum stretch.[8]

Scalene Muscles

Pain from trigger points in the scalene muscles can refer anteriorly, laterally, or posteriorly into the shoulders, chest, arm, and hand. This muscle group, along with the sternocleidomastoideus muscles, is frequently strained in whiplash-type injuries that produce painful trigger points.

The anterior scalene muscle attaches above to the anterior transverse processes of C3 through C6 and below to the first rib (Figure 6-3). The middle scalene muscle attaches above to the posterior transverse processes of C2 through C7 (occasionally to only C4 and C5). This muscle runs diagonally and attaches below to the cephalad surface of the first rib. (See Figure 6-3.) The posterior scalene muscle attaches above to the posterior transverse processes of the lowest two or three cervical vertebrae and below to the lateral surface of the second and sometimes third rib. It lies deep to the levator scapulae muscle and posterior to the medial scalene muscle. (See Figure 6-3.) Innervation of the scalene muscles is by motor branches of the anterior primary rami of the spinal nerves C2 through C3, corresponding to the segmental level of muscular attachment.

The action of the scalene muscles varies according to whether they are fixed from above or below. When fixed from above, the scalenes act as auxiliary muscles of inspiration. They help to support and elevate the upper rib cage when lifting, carrying, or pulling heavy objects. When fixed from below, the scalene muscles, acting unilaterally, laterally flex the cervical spine, moving the head obliquely forward and sideways. Acting bilaterally, the anterior scalene muscles assist neck flexion. The contralateral scalene muscles act as agonists, stabilizing the neck during lateral flexion.

Patients with a history of trauma to the neck should be examined for scalene muscle injury. Muscle strain of the scalene muscles frequently results from hyperextension from whiplash injuries. If the head is turned during impact or is hit from the side, the injury will be unilateral. The characteristic pain pattern referred from trigger points in the scalene muscles extends over the deltoid area, down the front and back of the arm (over the biceps and triceps), and along the radial side of the forearm, thumb, and index finger (Figure 6-4). When it occurs on the left side, it may be mistaken for referred pain from the heart. Posteriorly, the pain may be referred over the upper half of the vertebral border of the scapula and interscapular area. (See Figure 6-4.)

Entrapment of the brachial plexus between the anterior and middle scalene muscles refers pain down the ulnar side of the hand, with numbness due to sensory impairment. (See Figure 6-4.) With

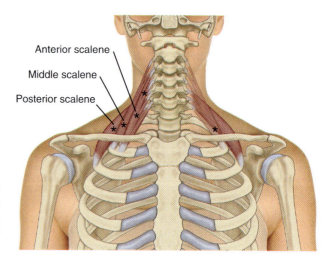

Figure 6-3 Anterior view of the scalenes. All three scalenes are seen on the right of the patient; the posterior scalene and ghosted-in middle scalene are seen on the left. The (*) indicate typical locations of trigger points.

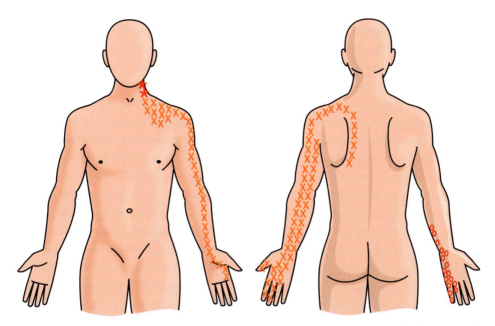

Figure 6-4 Trigger points (*) in the scalene muscles refer pain (x) anteriorly to the chest, laterally to the upper extremity, and posteriorly to the medial scapular border and adjacent interscapular region. Brachial plexus entrapment from swollen scalene muscles produces numbness and tingling (o) in the ulnar distribution, affecting the fingers, hand, and forearm.

swollen and taut scalene muscles, referred pain and entrapment pain may be present along with active trigger points. Motion palpation of the first rib will differentiate costovertebral joint restriction, which should be differentiated.

Examination will reveal restricted lateral bending of the neck to the contralateral side. Placing the ipsilateral forearm across the forehead while raising and pulling the forearm forward lifts the clavicle off the underlying scalene muscles and brachial plexus, may relieve the pain,[8] and may be used to differentiate cervical radiculopathy.

Trigger points in the anterior scalene are palpated beneath the posterior border of the clavicular division of the sternocleidomastoid muscle. Trigger points in the middle scalene can be palpated against the transverse processes of the cervical vertebrae, while those in the posterior scalene muscle are palpated medial to the levator scapulae, which must be pushed aside. Pressure on the trigger points in the scalene muscles produces ischemic compression and brings rapid relief of the patient's symptoms.

Stretching to prevent recurrence can be performed by the patient at home. To stretch the anterior scalene muscle, the head and neck are tilted toward the opposite side, and the head is pressed in a posterolateral direction. To stretch the middle scalene muscle, the head and neck are tilted toward the opposite side and pressed toward the contralateral shoulder. To stretch the posterior scalene muscle, the head and neck are not turned but are pressed in an anterolateral direction along the lines of the muscle fibers.[8] Exercises to stretch the scalene muscles can be performed supine if the patient lacks the strength to perform them seated. Resistance exercise to improve strength should not be prescribed before the muscle has been stretched to its optimal length and range of motion restored.

Superficial Muscles of the Neck and Back

Two superficial muscles of the neck and back commonly strained in whiplash accidents are the trapezius and levator scapulae muscles. These muscles are vulnerable to forces produced by whiplash from the side or when the head is turned to one side on impact. The trapezius is the most superficial, with the levator scapulae comprising part of the second layer of back and neck muscles.[23]

Trapezius Muscle

The trapezius is a tripartite muscle with upper, middle, and lower fibers that often function

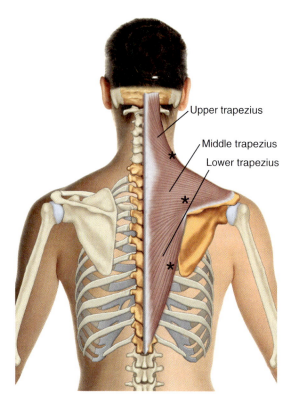

Figure 6-5   Posterior view of the right trapezius. The (*) indicate locations of typical trigger points.

independently (Figure 6-5). It is a flat, triangular muscle extending over the back of the neck and upper thorax. It is probably the muscle most often beleaguered by trigger points,[8] possibly because of its function as a stabilizer of the upper extremities. Once injured, trigger points often become chronic because of the frequent static loading of this muscle.

Anatomically, the right and left trapezius muscles form a large trapezium from which they are named. They are attached to the medial one third of the superior nuchal line of the occipital bone, the external occipital protuberance, the ligamentum nuchae, the seventh cervical and all the thoracic spinous processes, and the corresponding supraspinous ligaments. The superior fibers pass downward, attaching to the outer third of the clavicle. The middle fibers attach laterally to the acromion and superior border of the spine of the scapulae. The lower fibers proceed upward, attaching to the tubercle at the medial end of the spine of the scapula, just lateral to the lower attachment of the levator scapulae muscle. (See Figure 6-5.)

The motor innervation of the trapezius muscle is supplied by the spinal accessory nerve (cranial nerve XI) arising from the ventral roots of the first

five cervical segments, which ascend through the foramen magnum and exit the skull through the jugular foramen. This nerve joins a plexus beneath the trapezius with sensory (proprioceptive) fibers from spinal nerves (C3 and C4).

The upper fibers act with the levator scapulae to elevate the scapulae and with it the point of the shoulder. Acting with the serratus anterior, the trapezius rotates the scapula in a forward direction, so that the arm can be raised above the head. Acting bilaterally, the upper fibers may extend the head and neck when the shoulder is fixed. The middle fibers abduct and retract the scapula (move it toward the midline). They also assist in rotating the glenoid fossa upward, allowing the arm to abduct, especially near the end of its full range. The lower fibers of the trapezius retract the scapula and rotate the glenoid fossa upward by depressing the vertebral border of the scapula. These fibers also assist in flexion and abduction of the arm.

Patients with trigger points in the upper fibers of the trapezius muscle complain of pain unilaterally upward along the posterolateral aspect of the neck to the mastoid process (Figure 6-6). These trigger points are a common source of neck ache and temporal headache on the ipsilateral side. Occasionally the pain may be referred to the angle of the jaw with a resultant misdiagnosis of cervical radiculopathy or atypical facial neuralgia.[8] Trigger points in the upper fibers of the trapezius are found near the medial end of the spine of the scapula, just lateral to the attachment of the levator scapulae. (See Figure 6-6.)

Examination may reveal slight restriction of motion on contralateral lateral flexion and flexion of the neck as well as abduction of the arm due to the restricted upward rotation of the scapula. These patients may also complain of pain on contralateral rotation at the extreme range of motion.

To locate and deactivate trigger points in the upper fibers of the trapezius, the patient is either supine or seated, with the ipsilateral ear drawn slightly toward the shoulder. A pincer grasp is then applied to the muscle mass that harbors the trigger point, lifting it off the underlying supraspinatus muscle. The muscle can then be rolled firmly between the thumb and fingers. These trigger points in the upper fibers of the trapezius often refer pain to the neck, occiput, and temple.

Trigger points in the middle fibers of the trapezius muscle produce a burning pain that is referred medially from the trigger points located near the upper border of the scapula. This pain may radiate

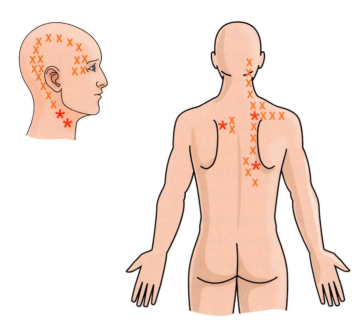

Figure 6-6 Trigger points (*) in the upper trapezius fibers (lateral view) characteristically refer pain (x) along the posterolateral aspect of the neck, behind the ear, and to the temple. Trigger points (*) in the middle trapezius refer pain (x) medially to the spinous processes and laterally to the top of the shoulder. Trigger points (*) in the lower fibers refer pain (x) mainly to the neck, suprascapular, and intrascapular region.

upward as far as C7. Trigger points found near the acromion refer aching pain to the top of the shoulder or acromial process.

Trigger points in the lateral lower trapezius fibers can refer pain downward along the vertebral border of the scapula. Those located more medially refer pain upward to the cervical region of the paraspinal muscles, the adjacent mastoid area, and the acromion (Figure 6-7). The lower fibers are strained by prolonged bending and reaching forward while sitting.

To examine for trigger points in the middle and lower fibers of the trapezius, the patient is seated with the arms folded in front of the body to protract the scapula and the trunk slightly flexed to place the muscle on stretch. The patient's head can then be tractioned to the contralateral side to add further stretch, while deep pressure is applied directly to the trigger points.[8] The patient may apply ischemic compression at home by lying on a tennis ball that is positioned to press on tender spots.[8] Stretching of the trapezius muscles can be achieved by having the patient bend forward in a seated position.

Levator Scapulae

The levator scapulae are a common site of trigger points that produce complaints of a stiff neck and restricted range of cervical motion. They are

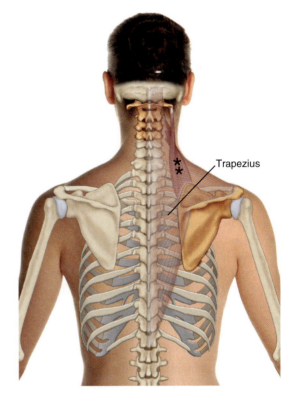

Figure 6-7 Posterior view of the right levator scapula. The trapezius muscle has been ghosted in. The (*) indicate locations of typical trigger points.

frequently strained in whiplash injuries when the head is turned to one side.[8] Neck motion is moderately restricted, as the patient tends to look sideways by turning the eyes or body rather than the neck. The head may be tilted slightly to the involved side.

The levator scapulae are attached above by tendinous slips to the transverse processes of the atlas and axis and the posterior tubercles of the transverse process of the third and fourth cervical vertebrae. They descend diagonally to attach below to the medial border of the scapula. They twist so that the C1 digitation is superficial to the others with the fibers vertical. The C4 digitation lies deepest and passes more diagonally to attach to the superior angle of the scapulae.[8] Innervation is supplied directly by the third and fourth cervical spinal nerves and by the fifth cervical through the dorsal scapula nerve.

The levator scapulae act in association with other muscles to stabilize the shoulder during movements of the upper extremity. When the cervical part of the spine is fixed, the levator scapulae act with the trapezius to elevate the scapulae or to sustain a weight carried on the shoulder. If the shoulder is fixed, the muscle inclines the neck to the same side. Both muscles acting together resist neck flexion. Acting with the rhomboid muscles and the latissimus dorsi, the levator scapulae rotate the glenoid fossa of the scapulae downward, while pulling the inferior angles of the scapulae together. The levator scapulae, in conjunction with the upper trapezius and uppermost fibers of the serratus anterior, elevate the scapulae, as when shrugging the shoulders.

Trigger points develop in the levator scapulae just cephalad to the attachment of the muscle to the superior angle of the scapula and at the angle of the neck where the muscle emerges from the upper fibers of the trapezius. To locate the trigger points, the patient is seated with the neck turned toward the opposite side to stretch and tighten the muscle and to lift it toward the palpating fingers. To locate the lower trigger point, a stroking action back and forth across the muscle may be necessary. These trigger points are exquisitely tender to pressure and refer pain upward to the upper cervical region[8] (Figure 6-8).

Repeated manipulation of the ipsilateral upper cervical vertebrae should be avoided. Although manipulation provides temporary relief of symptoms (up to 2 hours), as with any muscular joint restriction, treatment is more effective when

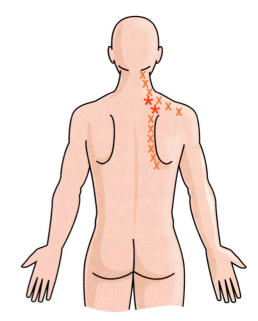

Figure 6-8   Trigger points (*) in the levator scapulae refer pain up the neck, into the shoulder, and along the vertebral border of the scapulae.

directed to the muscle rather than to the joints. Active stretching of the levator scapulae can be achieved with the patient in a seated position by stretching the head forward and to the opposite side. In addition to pressure therapy, home stretching under a hot shower with the contralateral arm pulling the head down brings more effective relief.

Intermediate Layers of Muscles that Act on the Posterior Cervical Spine

Both the splenius capitis and the splenius cervicis are susceptible to the trauma of a rear-end collision, especially if the head and neck are somewhat rotated at the time of impact. These muscles are not always protected by the more superficial neck muscles and are often associated with trigger points in the trapezius and levator scapulae, and SCM. Patients with trigger points in the splenius capitis and cervicis often complain of an "ache inside the skull."[8]

Splenius Capitus

The splenius capitis attaches to the lower part of the ligamentum nuchae and spinous processes of C7 through C3 or C4 and inserts into the mastoid

process, temporal bone, and occiput. The muscle passes upward and laterally under cover of the sternocleidomastoid muscle (Figure 6-9). Bilaterally, the two splenii capitii extend the head. Acting unilaterally, they laterally flex and rotate the face toward the same side.[8]

Trigger points in the splenius capitus, which overlies the occipital triangle, refers pain to the vertex of the head (Figure 6-10). Splenius capitus trigger points can be located by flat palpation within the upper portion of the muscular triangle bounded by the trapezius behind, the SCM in front, and the

levator scapulae below and at the insertion of the muscle on the mastoid process.

To stretch the splenius capitus, the patient is seated in a chair with arm rests to relax the shoulder girdle musculature. The head is rotated 20 to 30 degrees toward the opposite side while the head is gently pressed forward and sideways to the opposite side, slightly more laterally than forward. Patients may obtain a more effective stretch by using their own hands to grasp the back of the head, while turning the face to the other side and pulling the head down in the opposite direction. By actively applying stretch to this muscle, the patient thus learns how to stretch this muscle at home.

Splenius Cervicis

The splenius cervicis originates from the spinous processes of T3-T6 inserting on the transverse processes of C1 through C3 or C4. Acting bilaterally, they extend the neck. When they contract unilaterally, they laterally flex and rotate the face toward the same side. Each is therefore synergistic with the contralateral sternocleidomastoid (Figure 6-11).

Trigger points in the upper splenius cervicis refer pain to the ipsilateral orbit with the pain seeming to shoot through the inside of the head to

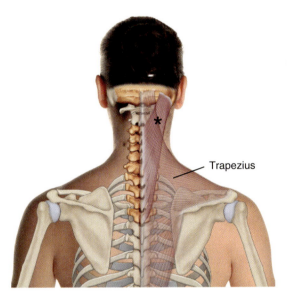

Figure 6-9   Posterior view of the right splenius capitus. The trapezius muscle has been ghosted in. The (*) indicate locations of typical trigger points.

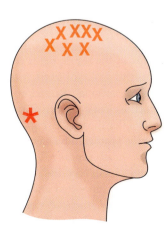

Figure 6-10   Trigger points in the splenius capitus (*) refer pain (x) to the vertex of the head.

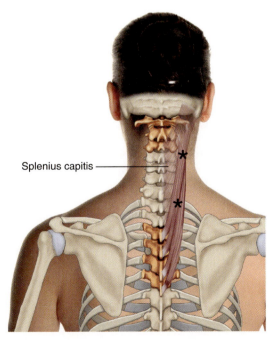

Figure 6-11   Posterior view of the right splenius cervicis. The (*) indicate locations of typical trigger points.

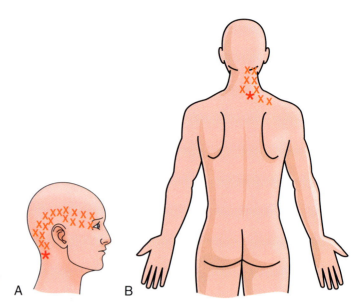

Figure 6-12 **A,** Trigger points (*) in the upper splenius cervicis refer pain (x) to the orbit. **B,** Trigger points (*) in the lower splenius cervicis refer pain (x) to the angle of the neck.

A   B

the back of the eye[8] (Figure 6-12A). The lower splenius cervicis trigger points refer pain to the angle of the neck (Figure 6-12B).

To palpate the splenius cervicis trigger points, the patient's head and neck are flexed toward the side to be examined in order to slacken the upper trapezius and levator scapulae. The free border of the upper trapezius is then displaced and the levator scapula pressed anterolaterally. Trigger points in the lower splenius cervicis can be located by rotating the head and neck to the opposite side, stretching the muscle to the desired degree of tautness to allow for palpation. To palpate the upper trigger points, the finger is slid cephalad along the muscle fibers between the upper trapezius and levator scapula.

To stretch the splenius cervicis, the patient is seated as above with the head dropped forward and the face turned 30 to 40 degrees toward the opposite side. The head is then pressed more forward than laterally flexed. The patient can actively apply stretch by latching the fingers over the back of the head, pulling it forward and downward while the head is turned slightly to the side opposite the stretched splenius cervicis. The patient can perform this exercise at home while seated in a hot shower.

Deep Layers of Muscles That Act on the Posterior Cervical Spine

The deep muscles that act on the posterior cervical spine produce complaints of neck stiffness. If

entrapment of the greater occipital nerve is present, there may be complaints of numbness, tingling, and burning pain in the scalp over the ipsilateral occipital region (occipital neuralgia). The deep posterior cervical muscles checkrein neck and head flexion and to a lesser extent contralateral rotation. Caution is advised when needling or injecting these muscles because of the hazard to the vertebral arteries.[8]

Semispinalis Cervicis

The semispinalis cervicis is a thick mass of muscle that originates from the transverse processes of the upper five or six thoracic vertebrae and may also arise from the articular processes of the lower four cervical vertebrae. It inserts onto the spinous process of the axis and the spinous processes of C3 to C5. The semispinalis cervicis extends the neck and, acting alone, rotates the head to the opposite side.[6]

Trigger points in the semispinalis cervicis refer pain upward to the posterior head with painfully restricted cervical motion. Palpation of trigger points in the semispinalis cervicis is facilitated by having the patient flex the neck to enhance the tautness. Relaxation is promoted by having the patient seated with the head supported. To bilaterally stretch the semispinalis cervicis, the patient is seated with the arms supported and the head and neck hanging forward. The head is gently pressed forward and downward. To unilaterally stretch the muscle, the head is gently flexed and rotated to the opposite side.

Semispinalis Capitis

The semispinalis capitis is a thick powerful muscle that arises from the transverse processes of C7 to T6 and the articular processes of C4 to C6 and inserts onto the occiput. Acting together, the muscles extend the thoracic and cervical portions of the spine. Acting alone, the muscle rotates the vertebral bodies to the opposite side.[6] Trigger points in the semispinalis capitis refer pain in a band across the head just above the orbit. Trigger points in the upper splenius cervicis refer pain to the ipsilateral orbit with the pain seeming to shoot through the inside of the head to the back of the eye.[8] The lower splenius cervicis trigger points refer pain to the angle of the neck.

To stretch the splenius capitus, as with the splenius cervicis, the patient is seated in a chair with arm rests. The head is also rotated 20 to 30 degrees toward the opposite side while the head is gently pressed forward and sideways to the opposite side. Patients can effectively stretch the muscle by using their own hands to grasp the back of the head, while turning the face to the other side and pulling the head gently down in the opposite direction.

Suboccipital Muscles (Rectus Capitis Posterior Minor and Major, Obliquus Inferior and Superior)

The rectus capitis posterior minor arises from the posterior tubercle of the atlas and attaches into the medial part of the area between the inferior nuchal line and the foramen magnum. It extends the head at the atlantooccipital joint. The rectus capitis posterior major starts with a pointed tendon from the spine of the axis and fans out, attaching to the lateral part of the inferior nuchal line of the suboccipital bone lateral to the rectus capitis posterior minor. (See Figure 6-13.) It extends the head and turns the face toward the ipsilateral side. The obliquus capitis superior attaches below to the transverse processes of the atlas, running almost vertically to insert above, between the superior and inferior nuchal lines of the occiput. It is narrow below and wide and expanded above. (See Figure 6-13.) The obliquus capitis superior extends the head and laterally flexes it to the ipsilateral side. The obliquus capitis inferior attaches medially and below to the spinous process and adjacent part of the lamina of the axis, running obliquely to fasten laterally and above to the transverse process of the

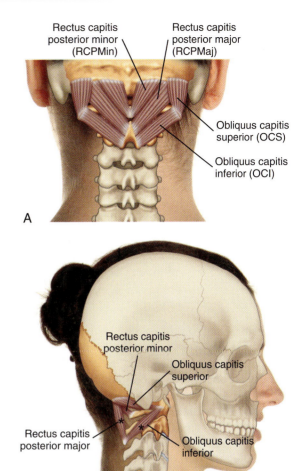

A, Posterior view of the suboccipital muscles. Labels: Rectus capitis posterior minor (RCPMin); Rectus capitis posterior major (RCPMaj); Obliquus capitis superior (OCS); Obliquus capitis inferior (OCI).

B, Lateral view. Labels: Rectus capitis posterior minor; Obliquus capitis superior; Rectus capitis posterior major; Obliquus capitis inferior.

Figure 6-13 **A,** Posterior view of the suboccipital muscles (rectus capitis posterior minor and major, obliquus inferior and superior). **B,** Lateral view of the suboccipital muscles (rectus capitis posterior minor and major, obliquus inferior and superior). The (*) indicate locations of typical trigger points.

atlas. (See Figure 6-13.) This muscle turns the face toward the ipsilateral side.

Trigger points in the suboccipital muscles are a common source of "headaches" that are difficult to distinguish from the symptoms produced by trigger points in the overlying posterior cervical muscles. (See Figure 6-13.) The differential diagnosis must be made since the suboccipital muscles are a common source of posttraumatic headache.[25] Palpation of trigger points in the suboccipital muscles is difficult but may elicit the characteristic pain referral pattern. (See Figure 6-14.) Examination by flat palpation elicits a deep tenderness without evidence of a palpable band or local twitch response. Ischemic compression is particularly

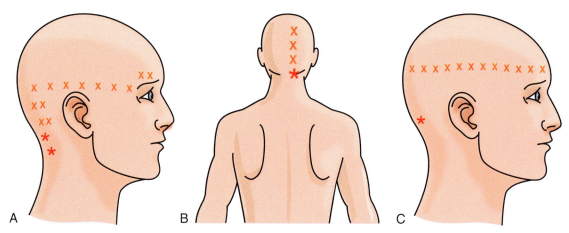

Figure 6-14   Trigger points (*) in the suboccipital muscles refer pain (x) from the occiput to the orbit.

effective to inactivate trigger points in the suboccipital muscles close to their attachments to the occiput.[8] To stretch the suboccipital muscles, the head must be tilted on top of the neck in specific directions to stretch either those muscles that flex and extend the head, the ones that tilt it to one side, or the ones that rotate it. The patient can actively stretch the suboccipital muscles by pulling the head down with the hands clasped behind the head and the upper back and neck maximally flexed.

Trigger Points in the Muscles of the Temporomandibular Joint (TMJ)

The signs and symptoms of traumatic temporomandibular joint (TMJ) dysfunction typically appear within 48 hours.[26] Consideration must be given to the seriousness and intensity of patients' other symptoms, however, as they may not be aware of TMJ dysfunction within that time period. The differential diagnosis between pain from joint dysfunction and that of myofascial origin may require arthrography before treating trigger points in the muscles. It is important to determine through an adequate history (see Chapter 3) whether TMJ dysfunction was present prior to the whiplash trauma. It is just as important to examine the patient for strain of the TMJ muscles because this often goes undetected, causing head and jaw pain to persist when this condition is not addressed. Trigger points in the masseter, temporalis, digastric, and internal and external pterygoid muscles should not be overlooked. Pain in the muscles of the TMJ in many

instances is related to muscle dysfunction rather than derangement of the jaw itself.[8]

Masseter Muscle

The masseter muscle is a complex muscle with superficial and deep layers. Both layers attach above to the zygomatic process of the maxilla and zygomatic arch below; the superficial layer attaches to the external surface of the mandible at the angle and to inferior half of the ramus. The deep layer attaches to the superior half of the ramus (Figure 6-15). The primary action of the muscle is to elevate the mandible and close the jaw. The deep fibers of the muscle also retrude the mandible.

Referred pain from trigger points in the various parts of the masseter muscle may be projected to the eyebrow, jaw, and the ear (Figure 6-16). Unilateral tinnitus may be associated with trigger points in the upper posterior portion of the deep layer of the muscle. For examination of trigger points in the masseter, the jaw must be open far enough to tauten the muscle within the limit of pain. Palpation of trigger points in the masseter muscle can be performed by pressing the muscle against the mandible with the mouth open. Trigger points in the deep layer are located by palpation against the posterior portion of the ramus and along the zygomatic buttress.

To actively stretch the masseter muscle, the patient inserts two fingers of one hand behind the lower incisor teeth and with the thumb hooked behind the mandible under the chin, pulls the mandible forward and downward to fully open the

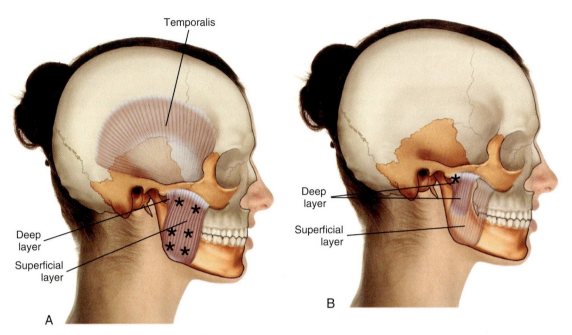

Figure 6-15   Lateral views of the right masseter. **A,** The temporalis has been ghosted in. **B,** The superficial head of the masseter has been ghosted in. The (*) indicate locations of typical trigger points.

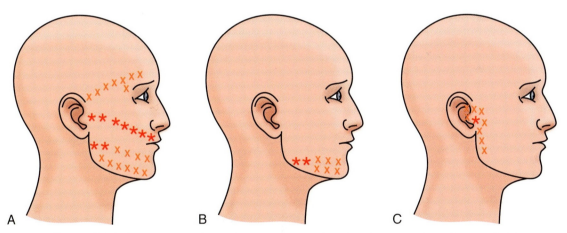

Figure 6-16   Trigger points (*) in the masseter muscle refer pain (x): **A,** from the superficial portion to the eyebrow, maxilla, mandible anteriorly, and to the eyebrow; **B,** from the mid-portion of the superficial layer to the mandible; and **C,** from the deep layer to around the temporomandibular joint.

jaw. The other hand stabilizes the head by pressing on the forehead. This stretch can be performed in the supine position to eliminate postural reflexes or in the seated position. Yawning is also an effective home exercise to stretch the masseter muscle.

Temporalis Muscle

The temporalis muscle attaches above to the bone and fascia in the temporal fossa, superior to the zygomatic arch, and below to the coronoid process of the mandible and along the mandibular ramus

(Figure 6-17). The temporalis muscles primarily close the jaw while the middle fibers bilaterally retrude the mandible. Acting unilaterally, the temporalis muscle deviates the mandible to the same side.

Trigger points in the temporalis muscle are a common cause of headache with a pain referral throughout the temple, along the eyebrow, behind the eye, and into the upper teeth. When the trigger points are in the anterior portion of the muscle, they refer pain along the supraorbital ridge and downward to the incisor teeth (Figure 6-18A). Trigger points in the intermediate portion of the muscle refer pain upward to the mid temple area and downward to the maxillary teeth on the same side (Figure 6-18B). Trigger points in the posterior section refer pain backward and upward (Figure 6-18C). Deep fibers in the mid region of the temporalis may refer pain to the maxilla and TMJ.

Trigger points in the temporalis are palpated with the mouth partly open to place the muscle fibers on stretch. Trigger points in the anterior and intermediate fibers are palpated just above the upper border of the zygomatic arch. Trigger points in the posterior fibers are palpated above the ear. Trigger points at the insertion on the inner surface of the coronoid process inside the mouth are palpated by pressing outward against the coronoid process.

To actively stretch the temporalis muscle in the supine position, the patient inserts two fingers behind the lower incisor teeth and with the thumb under the chin gently pulls the mandible forward and then downward, gradually increasing the stretch. The head is stabilized by the opposite hand. This stretch can also be performed by the patient in a seated position.

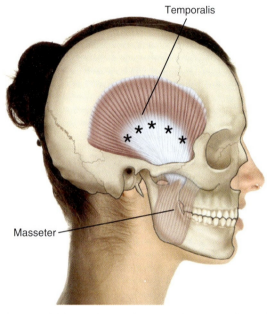

Figure 6-17   Right lateral view of the temporalis and masseter muscles. The masseter muscle has been ghosted in with the typical location of trigger points (*) in the temporalis muscle indicated.

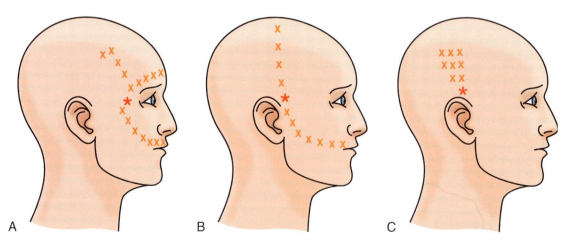

Figure 6-18   **A,** Trigger points (*) in the anterior fibers of the temporalis muscle refer pain (x) forward along the supraorbital ridge and downward to the upper incisor teeth. **B,** Trigger points (*) in the middle fibers refer pain (x) upward to the mid-temple area and downward to the intermediate maxillary teeth on the same side. **C,** Trigger points (*) in the posterior fibers refer pain (x) backward and upward.

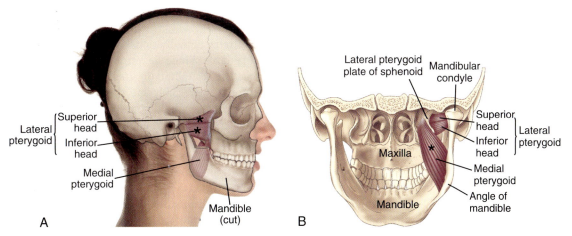

Figure 6-19   Views of the right lateral and medial pterygoids. **A,** Lateral view with the mandible partially cut away. **B,** Posterior view of the lateral and medial pterygoids with the cranial bones cut away and illustrating typical locations of trigger points (*).

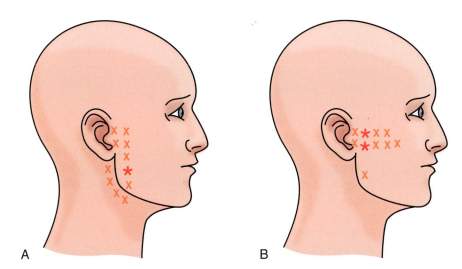

Figure 6-20   **A,** Trigger points (*) in the medical pterygoid muscle refer pain (x) to the mouth and pharynx and below the TMJ. **B,** Trigger points (*) in the lateral pterygoid muscle are felt strongly in the TMJ and maxilla.

Medial Pterygoid

The medial pterygoid muscle attaches to the angle of the mandible and to the lateral pterygoid plate to form a sling with the masseter muscle that suspends the mandible (Figure 6-19). The primary action is to elevate the mandible and laterally deviate it to the opposite side. It can assist in protrusion of the mandible. Referred pain from the medial pterygoid is poorly circumscribed in regions of the mouth and hard palate and below and behind the TMJ (Figure 6-20A).

Examination for trigger points in the medial pterygoid is performed both inside and outside the mouth with the patient in a supine position. To palpate from outside the mouth, the head is tilted slightly to access the muscle. Palpation with one finger locates trigger points on the inner surface of the mandible by pressing upward at its angle. Palpation of the mid-belly is performed inside the mouth with the pad of the palpating index finger. A finger cot protects the finger that faces out and slides over the molar teeth until it encounters the bony edge of the ramus of the mandible behind the last molar tooth. The muscle is palpated as a vertical mass, and pressure on trigger points in it elicits exquisite tenderness. To ensure the safety of the examining finger, the examiner's other hand can push from the outside to push the patient's opposite cheek inward between the back teeth. The patient will then bite his or her own cheek before biting the finger.

To actively stretch the medial pterygoid, the patient lies supine and places two fingers behind the lower incisor teeth and the thumb under the chin, and by pulling the mandible forward and down, the patient opens the jaw fully. The opposite hand is placed on the forehead to stabilize the head and neck. The medial pterygoid responds well to ischemic compression and stretching.[8]

Lateral Pterygoid

The lateral pterygoid is important in understanding TMJ dysfunction because active trigger points in the muscle disturb the position of the mandible and its incisal path when opening and closing the mouth. The inferior division of the muscle is strongly implicated in TMJ dysfunction syndromes. The superior division of the lateral pterygoid attaches in front to the sphenoid bone and behind to the articular disc and capsule of the TMJ. The inferior division attaches in front to the lateral pterygoid plate and behind to the neck of the mandible. (See Figure 6-19.) The action of the superior division pulls the articular disc forward and checks its backward movement, assisting in elevation of the mandible. The inferior division protrudes and depresses the mandible with lateral deviation to the opposite side.[8]

Trigger points in the lateral pterygoid refer pain around the ipsilateral TMJ and into the maxilla. (See Figure 6-20B.) Trigger points in the inferior lateral pterygoid can be palpated intraorally by pressing the finger backward as far as possible along the roof of the cheek pouch. After sliding the finger along the outer side of the cul de sac to reach as high as possible along the inner surface of the coronoid process, pressure is applied inward toward the lateral pterygoid plate. Pressure on the trigger points is exquisitely tender and care must be taken to work to patient tolerance. Tenderness to pressure directed upward and slightly forward indicates trigger points in the mid portion of the superior division. Tenderness to downward pressure and forward toward the mouth is indicative of

trigger points in the mid portion of the inferior division.

To stretch both divisions of the lateral pterygoid, the mandible should be retruded as far as possible against the restraining ligaments without opening the mouth appreciably and then rocking it gently from side to side, holding the jaw open only a few millimeters. This is best done with the patient in the supine position. The patient grasps the point of the chin with one hand, gently pushing the mandible backward and upward. A gently sideways rocking motion is added to ensure maximum retrusion. The patient should practice full active range of motion by maximally protruding and retruding the mandible. Opening the jaw as far as possible without translation and in maximum voluntary retrusion slightly stretches the upper division of the lateral pterygoid. This involves opening the mouth while retruding the mandible and preventing condylar translation by placing the tip of the tongue against the roof of the mouth, as far back as possible. The mouth is then opened and closed alternately about 1 inch.

Digastric Muscle

When not addressed, trigger points in the digastric muscle may be mistaken for referred pain from the SCM. The anterior and posterior bellies of the digastric attach below, by a common tendon, to the hyoid bone. Behind and above, the posterior belly attaches to the mastoid notch deep to the attachments of the splenius capitus and SCM muscles. In front and above, the anterior belly attaches to the inferior border of the mandible, close to the symphysis (Figure 6-21). Both bellies of this muscle assist depression and retrusion of the mandible.

Trigger points in the posterior digastric muscle refer pain into the upper part of the SCM (Figure 6-22). They also refer pain under the chin and sometimes into the occiput. Less frequently, trigger points in the anterior belly of the digastric refer pain to the lower incisors.

Trigger points in the digastric muscle are palpated in the supine position. The posterior belly is palpated between the angle of the jaw and the mastoid process by applying pressure against the underlying neck structures. Trigger points in the anterior belly are palpated with the neck extended further and the head tilted back. The jaw is closed to stretch the muscle as pressure is applied to palpate trigger points against the underlying soft tissue.

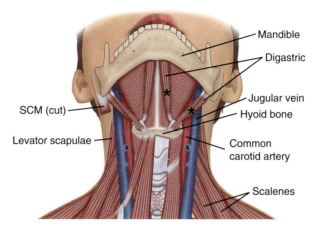

Figure 6-21   Anterior view of the neck illustrating the two bellies of the digastric muscle and the fibrous loop that attaches to the hyoid bone.

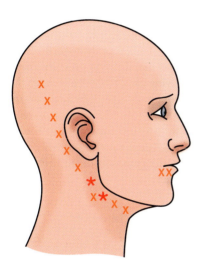

Figure 6-22   Trigger points (*) in the posterior belly of the digastric muscle refer pain (x) to the upper part of the SCM. Trigger points in the anterior belly of the digastric muscle project pain into the lower incisor teeth refer pain to the lower incisors.

To passively stretch the posterior belly of the digastric, the patient leads the head back against the practitioner in a relaxed position with the teeth nearly approximated. For stretching of the right posterior digastric, the patient's head is turned to the right to move the mastoid process away from the hyoid bone. The head and neck are extended to tense the anterior belly and tension is increased on the posterior belly by pressing on the hyoid bone down and to the left. To stretch the anterior belly, the head is tipped back with the mandible protruded in a nearly closed position. Both bellies of the digastric muscle are responsive to ischemic compression.[8] The patient should actively do self stretches in the supine position by protruding the jaw.

Shoulder Muscles

Shoulder injuries frequently occur in motor vehicle accidents. Less common than injury to neck muscles, rotator cuff muscles should also be checked for trigger points. Often overlooked if the patient complains of shoulder pain and points to the more commonly injured trapezius muscle, actual shoulder injury can occur from direct trauma, producing a contusion if the shoulder strikes a door, or more commonly from torquing produced by interaction with the seatbelt. The driver may have tensed the shoulder muscles by grasping the steering wheel to brace against the impact, or reaching across to protect a passenger. Trigger points in the rotator cuff muscles (subscapularis, supraspinatus, infraspinatus, and teres minor) may be mistaken for cervical radiculopathy because of the pattern of referred pain from trigger points in these muscles. When cervical radiculopathy is ruled out, patients may be branded as malingerers or suffer much unnecessary treatment if trigger points in shoulder girdle muscles are overlooked.

Infraspinatus Muscle

The infraspinatus attaches medially to the infraspinatus fossa of the scapula and laterally to the greater tubercle of the humerus (Figure 6-23A). The infraspinatus is innervated by the suprascapular nerve through the upper trunk from spinal nerves C5 and C6. The infraspinatus externally rotates the arms at

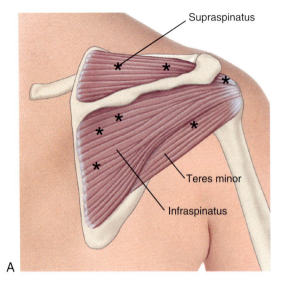

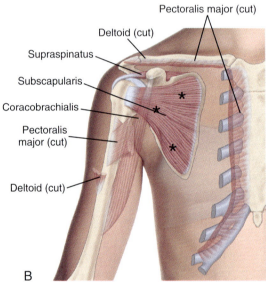

Figure 6-23   Muscles of the rotator cuff. **A,** Posterior view showing the supraspinatus, infraspinatus, and teres minor. **B,** Anterior view showing the subscapularis, illustrating the typical location of trigger points (*).

the shoulder and assists in the stabilization of the head of the humerus in the glenoid fossa during upward movement of the arms.

Trigger points in the infraspinatus muscle produce complaints that the patient cannot reach upward and back to pull down an automobile seat belt. Sleep disturbances occur because lying on the involved shoulder produces referred pain due to compression and stimulation of the trigger points. Lying on the uninvolved side stretches the infraspinatus, also disturbing sleep. The patient is unable to

internally rotate and adduct the arm at the shoulder. Complaints of shoulder fatigue are common. Trigger points in the infraspinatus muscle produce pain deep in the shoulder joint (Figure 6-24A).

Examination for trigger points is performed with the patient seated and the muscle stretched by bringing the hand and arm across the front of the chest. Trigger points in the infraspinatus muscle are commonly found just caudal to the spine of the scapula and the midpoints about mid muscle along the vertebral border of the scapula and at the tendinous insertion of the humerus. Abduction and external rotation are restricted due to pain.

Stretching the infraspinatus can be accomplished actively by grasping the elbow on the involved side and tractioning the shoulder, with the elbow close to the chest or by having the patient reach backward, attempting to reach for the opposite shoulder blade. Stretching under a hot shower directed on the involved muscle is beneficial. Travell and Simons[8] recommend home pressure therapy with the patient lying on a tennis ball under the trigger point, utilizing body weight to maintain increasing pressure for 1 to 2 minutes. They also recommend that a pillow be placed under the involved arm with the patient sleeping on the uninvolved shoulder. This relieves the pain-producing stretch that interferes with sleep.

Teres Minor Muscle

The teres minor muscle is sometimes fused with the infraspinatus. It attaches medially to the dorsal surface of the scapula just below the infraspinatus and inserts laterally into the greater tubercle of the humerus. (See Figure 6-23A.) It is innervated by the axillary nerve through the posterior cord from C5 and C6 spinal nerves. Like the infraspinatus, it externally rotates the arm at the shoulder and helps to stabilize the head of the humerus in the glenoid fossa during arm movement.

The patient is positioned for examination of the teres minor as for examination of the infraspinatus. Trigger points are found in the belly of the muscle, with tenderness at the insertion into the humerus. (See Figure 6-24A.) Trigger points in the teres minor rarely occur alone and are activated by strain of the infraspinatus muscle. These trigger points produce complaints of localized pain deep under the deltoid muscle in the belly of the teres minor. Stretching and corrective action for the teres minor are the same as those described for the infraspinatus.

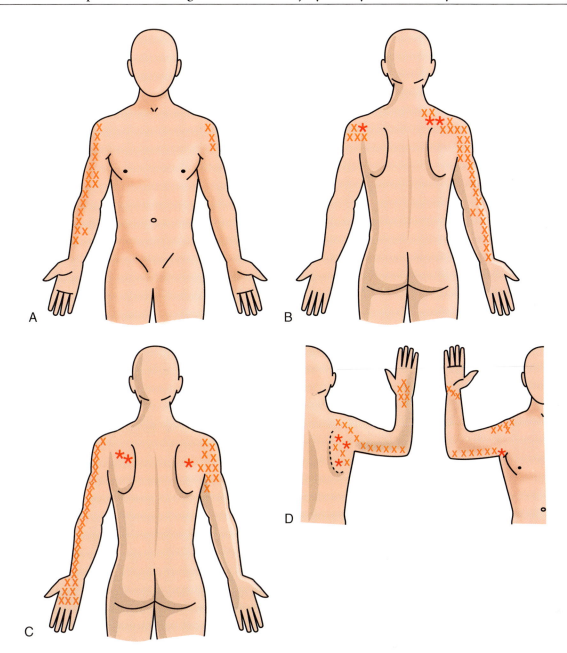

Figure 6-24   **A,** Trigger points (*) in the left infraspinatus muscle refer pain (x) to the anterior deltoid region of the left shoulder, extending down the front and lateral aspect of the arm and forearm, occasionally including the radial half of the hand. Trigger points (*) in the right teres minor muscle refer pain (x) to the right posterior deltoid region (right side). **B,** Trigger points (*) in the subscapularis refer pain (x) to the posterior area, medially over the scapula, and down the posterior aspect of the arm, skipping to a band around the wrist. **C,** Trigger points (*) in the left supraspinatus tendon refer pain (x) to the mid-deltoid region (anterior view). **D,** Those trigger points (*) located in the belly of the muscle refer pain (x) around the shoulder and down the arm and forearm (right side).

Subscapularis Muscle

The subscapularis forms the major part of the posterior wall of the axilla. It is a long, triangular muscle that arises from the inner surface of the scapula, filling the subscapular fossa from the vertebral border to the axillary border of the scapula. It converges laterally into a tendon that attaches to the lesser tubercle of the humerus and the front of the capsule of the shoulder joint. (See Figure 6-23B.) It is innervated by the upper and lower subscapular nerves: C5, C6, and C7. The actions of the subscapularis are primarily internal rotation and adduction of the arm at the shoulder. It also assists in the stabilization of the humerus in the glenoid fossa and thus assists in abduction of the arm.

Subscapularis trigger points cause severe shoulder pain both at rest and in motion. The pain is concentrated in the posterior deltoid area and may extend medially over the scapula and down the posterior aspect of the arm. (See Figure 6-24B.) It commonly produces a strap-like distribution of referred pain around the wrist.[8]

Examination reveals restriction of motion on abduction and internal rotation of the arm at the shoulder. Locating trigger points in the subscapularis muscle is difficult and should be performed with the patient supine and the involved arm abducted away from the chest wall. In this position, trigger points can be palpated along the axillary border of the scapula. Travell and Simons[8] warn that in patients with severe subscapularis involvement, deep tenderness in this muscle is usually so exquisite that they can tolerate only very light digital pressure on the trigger points. Patients with trigger points in the supraspinatus muscle complain of pain during abduction of the arm as well as a dull ache at rest. They may also complain of shoulder stiffness and sleep disturbances with nocturnal pain. Activities requiring the use of the arm overhead may be restricted. Some patients complain of a scraping crepitus or catch in the shoulder joint. This is thought to be due to interference with the normal glide of the head of the humerus in the glenoid fossa.

Stretching the subscapularis can be performed with the arm raised over the head, grasping the elbow with the opposite hand and drawing the elbow toward the opposite side.

Supraspinatus Muscle

Anatomically, the supraspinatus attaches medially to the supraspinatus fossa of the scapula and laterally to the greater tubercle of the humerus. (See Figure 6-23A.) It is innervated by the suprascapular nerves (C4, C5, and C6). The supraspinatus muscle abducts the arm and pulls the head of the humerus into the glenoid fossa. This prevents downward displacement of the humerus when the arm is dependent.

Examination reveals restriction of abduction of the arm. Palpation will locate trigger points at the attachment of the tendon and through the trapezius muscle in the belly of the supraspinatus muscle. Pressure on the trigger points refers pain down the arm and often to the forearm or over the lateral epicondyle of the elbow (see Figure 6-24C). To stretch the supraspinatus, the forearm of the seated patient is placed behind the back at waist level or across the front of the chest with the patient grasping the elbow and actively stretching the muscle.

Diagnosis of Myofascial Pain Syndromes Related to Whiplash Injuries

Following a history of trauma involving a whiplash mechanism, the patient's primary complaint is often neck stiffness and decreased range of motion. Discomfort generally increases for the first 72 hours until the initial swelling subsides. This gradual worsening may account for the paucity of symptoms reported by the patient when initially seen, which subsequently appear in the succeeding days. The initial swelling delays the diagnosis of trigger points in specific muscles. Although the diagnosis of muscle strain is not inaccurate, it does not give a definitive diagnosis as to which structures are damaged. Therefore substituting "muscle strain" for "whiplash" as a diagnostic term is no more enlightening as to the patient's true condition than the latter.[27] A thorough history will help point to the most likely tissues injured. (See Chapter 3.) Different muscles will be injured if patients were looking in the rearview mirror at the time of impact than if they were looking straight ahead. Observation of the patient's movement and posture at rest helps to determine which tissues are injured. Guarding of injured neck muscles causes patients to turn their body rather than their head when looking around. They may assume an antalgic tilt of the head to minimize discomfort, and movement is likely to be slow and protective. Contraction of strained muscles produces pain and differentiates muscle strain from ligamentous sprain.

Once the initial swelling has subsided, diagnosis of trauma-induced trigger points can be effectively palpated in the injured muscles. Often those unskilled in palpation find if difficult to identify the generator of nociceptive input causing a patient's referred pain. Whereas some dismiss the diagnosis of trigger points as subjective,[28] those skilled in palpatory techniques have little difficulty determining the location of the triggering sites. Both Sciotti[29] and Gerwin[30] have demonstrated good to excellent clinical precision among experienced clinicians in diagnosing the presence of myofascial trigger points. A training period was found to be essential, emphasizing the need for sufficient preparation for clinicians to adequately address myofascial pain syndromes. Manual palpatory skills require considerable practice and, when coupled with patient feedback, provide for reliable diagnosis in the absence of more sophisticated diagnostic imaging or other criteria[28] that are based on the hegemony of vision.

PAIN DIAGRAMS

A pain diagram is a useful tool, providing that the clinician remembers that the referred pain from myofascial trigger points does not characteristically follow known dermatomal or sclerotomal patterns. The typical pain drawing[31] is filled out by the patient using different symbols to indicate the type of pain that they are experiencing. (See Chapter 4.) The typical pain referred from trigger points is described as a steady, dull, and deep ache.[8] Verbal descriptions are often imprecise and can be misleading if the patient is unable to accurately verbalize his or her complaint. Patients may say, "My head hurts," or "My neck is stiff," neither of which is definitive of their complaint. Localizing the pain by having the patient point with one finger to the problem area is helpful, adding to the information gleaned from the pain drawing. With knowledge of characteristic pain patterns associated with specific muscles, the practitioner has a basis to begin searching for specific trigger points. When several muscles are involved, the pattern of pain is more difficult to interpret, and the patient-centered practitioner is always cognizant of individual variations between patients.

TECHNIQUES FOR DIAGNOSING TRIGGER POINTS

Location of trigger points first requires knowledge of the location and direction of the various muscle fibers. Travell[8] describes several ways of detecting trigger points, including a local twitch response, palpation of a taut band and the trigger point itself, and observation of a jump sign. She reported, in 1955,[32] a localized twitch of part of the muscle when the trigger point was rolled under the fingers. The twitch could be vigorous enough to cause a perceptible jerk of the body part. She also observed this twitch response when a needle was inserted into the trigger area.[8] Simons reported, in 1976, EMG characteristics of the local twitch response.[33] Associated with trigger points, the local twitch response is a transient contraction to those muscle fibers in the tense band that harbors the trigger point. The response is elicited by a sudden change of pressure on the trigger point that can be produced by rolling the trigger point under the finger,[34] a transverse snapping palpation of the taut band, or needle contact with the trigger point. Most muscles with active trigger points exhibit a vigorous local twitch response.

PALPATION OF THE TAUT BAND AND LOCALIZED TRIGGER POINT

To locate the taut band, the muscle is stretched until the fibers of the band are under tension and the uninvolved fibers remain slack. The stretch should evoke localized discomfort on the verge of causing pain. The palpable band feels like a taut cord of tense muscle fibers among the normally slack fibers. The band palpates like a rope or cord 1 to 4 mm in diameter.[8]

To palpate the trigger point within the taut band, the finger slides along the band until the point of maximum tenderness is located. Direct pressure on the trigger point with the pad of the index finger or thumb produces pain referred to the area of the patient's complaint, confirming the diagnosis of myofascial pain.[34] An active trigger point palpates as an area of increased turgor similar to a grape. When there is nothing underlying the trigger point such as those found in the SCM, a pincer palpation is performed by grasping the belly of the muscle between the thumb and fingers.

THE JUMP SIGN

The jump sign is the tendency for the patient to flinch or recoil disproportionally to the amount of pressure being applied. This exquisite sensitivity is characteristic of light pressure applied to the nidus trigger point. The location of this jump sign tenderness is highly reproducible for a given trigger point.[8]

MANAGEMENT OF MYOFASCIAL PAIN SYNDROMES

There is a plethora of modalities used in the treatment of myofascial pain, ranging from some that are noninvasive to those that inject various substances into the trigger point locus. The effectiveness of the vast majority of these is dependent on the ability of the clinicians to accurately palpate the trigger points. The required high level of palpation skills must be accompanied by a high degree of kinesthetic perception.[28] A systematic review of the literature[35] listed the following interventions: transcutaneous electrical nerve stimulation (TENS), electrical muscle stimulation (EMS), ischemic compression, myofascial release therapy, stretch with vapocoolant spray, interferential current, stretch, ultrasound, direct dry needling, trigger point injection (with various solutions and medications), neuro-reflexotherapy, deep pressure soft tissue massage, hydrocollator superficial heat, exercise, yoga, acupuncture, ice massage, magnetic stimulation, laser therapy, injection of botulinum toxin, topical anesthetic preparation, passive rhythmic release, active rhythmic release, counterstrain, high-velocity low-amplitude thrust, biofeedback, and clinical psychophysiology. Not all of the treatment modalities are equally effective, each requiring different skills, levels of training, and licensing.[35]

Although evidence based on randomized controlled trials of a single treatment procedure is considered the strongest form of evidence, patients may benefit from a combination of modalities. For example, hydrocollator superficial heat and ultrasound help to relax patients, facilitating palpation of trigger points. Applied singly or together they might not resolve the patient's myofascial pain, but in combination with other therapies, they can contribute to effective treatment. Given that myofascial pain is a multidimensional problem, greater attention should be given to the suggestion that it requires a structured multimodal approach to treatment.[35] Failure to administer adequate treatment is a potential pitfall following motor vehicle accidents.[36] Patients frequently present for independent medical examinations and impairment rating without the benefit of adequate treatment.[36] If the examining physician is not skilled at locating myofascial trigger points, the patient may be dismissed as exhibiting no objective residuals of whiplash injury. For

patients to have reached maximum medical improvement, they must have received the benefit of adequate treatment for the residuals of muscle strain incurred as the result of whiplash injuries.

TREATMENT

It is common for treatment modalities to be combined. The modalities that follow have a demonstrated effectiveness alone, but it is common for more than one modality to be utilized.

Ischemic Compression

Ischemic compression is one of the least invasive trigger point therapies and has been employed by chiropractors since 1957.[9] Chiropractic therapy has been reported to be among the most effective measures in the treatment of muscle pain syndromes.[37] In addition to the application of ischemic compression, the patient is encouraged to actively stretch the involved muscles. This approach to patient-centered care of muscle pain syndromes encourages patients to contribute to their own rehabilitation rather than be party to passive therapy alone that encourages patients to be dependent on others for their recovery.

Ischemic compression is a mechanical treatment of myofascial trigger points that consists of application of sustained pressure for a long enough time to inactivate the trigger points. Travell and Simons[8] termed this therapy "ischemic compression" because, on release of pressure, the skin is at first blanched and then shows reactive hyperemia. These changes correspond to circulatory changes in the underlying muscle, which is subjected to the same pressure. Pressure can be applied with a thumb, finger, knuckle, or elbow depending on the size, depth, and thickness of the muscle being compressed. Specific pressure is applied directly to the center of the trigger point to the patient's tolerance. Care must be taken not to exceed the patient's tolerance, and if the patient tenses or pulls away, then a lighter pressure should be applied. If the pressure is too painful, the patient will respond with muscle tightening in the area.[38] It is crucial to apply the pressure to the nidus of the trigger point. This requires considerable palpatory skill and it is important not to slip off of the center of the trigger point because this causes needless pain. Pressure is sustained for 10 to 20 seconds and gradually increased as the trigger point releases. A "melting" away of the trigger point monitors the effectiveness of the treatment. A thumb or finger from the other hand may be used for reinforcement. Pressure is most effective when applied straight into the trigger point. The patient will generally be happy to confirm the exact site of pressure application, often with the statement that "it hurts good" or "that is the spot" or other indication that it is uncomfortable but on target. Mechanical devices can be used, but these do not give the necessary feedback as the trigger point releases.[34] Ischemic pressure therapy may have to be repeated every 2 to 3 days for several weeks, depending on the chronicity of the problem and the patient's response to treatment. Acute cases frequently respond with 3 to 4 treatments. Treatment time varies and may be extended in a patient with a long-standing history of pain and pain referral.[38]

Fryer and Hodgson[39] have demonstrated through monitoring of pressure that sustained manual pressure produces a reduction in perceived pain and a significant increase in tolerance to treatment pressure. This appeared to be the result of a change in tissue sensitivity, rather than an unintentional reduction in pressure by the examiner. As pressure is sustained, the practitioner can feel a decrease in turgor as the trigger point "melts" away, and when the size and texture of the trigger point changes, pressure can gradually be increased to the patient's tolerance. This is monitored by observing the patient carefully to see if they grimace or pull away. Monitoring the patient in this way requires a sensitivity that balances effective pressure with the patient's discomfort.

The effectiveness of ischemic compression as a treatment of myofascial trigger points in the trapezius muscle has been demonstrated through a change in pressure pain threshold using a pressure algometer (expressed in kg/cm^2) and a decrease in visual analogue scores.[40] A comparative study[41] of spray and stretch, hydrocollator superficial heat, ultrasound deep heat, and deep pressure soft tissue massage demonstrated significantly higher scores on the Index of Threshold Change (the ratio of post-treatment pain threshold scores to pre-treatment pain threshold) for the deep pressure soft tissue massage than the other three modalities and the controls. All four therapeutic modalities showed significant treatment effects, with spray and stretch more effective than thermotherapy. Because of the environmental effects of using a vapocoolant spray, stretch alone is now recommended. Travel and Simons[8] emphasized that stretch is the action while the spray is a distraction. Although the spray makes the patient more comfortable, they stress that stretch is the effective component of spray and stretch therapy. Whenever possible, active stretching by the patient is preferable to a passive stretch by a therapist. When force is applied by the therapist, it does not allow patients to stretch to their pain tolerance.

Laser Therapy

The term "laser" is an acronym for "light amplification by stimulated emission radiation." The biological effects are a direct function of the light emissions. The biostimulatory action is thought to be analgesic, attributed to its anti-inflammatory and neuronal effects. These neuronal effects include depressed neuronal and lymphocytic respiration, stabilization of membrane potential, and release of neurotransmitters.[42] Three types of lasers are described in the studies of laser therapy used to treat myofascial trigger points: gallium-arsenide -aluminum (Ga-AS-Al),[43-45] helium-neon (He-Ne),[46,47] and infrared diode.[48] These studies have demonstrated a statistically significant difference between the treatment and placebo groups in the treatment of pain from myofascial trigger points. Long term, a significant effect was demonstrated at a 3-month follow-up in two studies,[43,48] with equivocal results at 6 months.[45,47] Rickards concluded that the quality of these trials is high,[28] with demonstrated effectiveness of laser therapy for the treatment of trigger points in muscles of the cervical spine. Although laser therapy may have some side effects, it is not as invasive as needling.

Needling

A comparison of dry and wet needling suggests that the effect is due to the needle itself, or due to placebo, rather than to the injection of saline or drugs.[35] Myofascial trigger point injections have been performed with a variety of injectables, such as procaine, lidocaine, and other local anesthetics; isotonic saline solutions; nonsteroidal anti-inflammatories; corticosteroids; bee venom; botulinum toxin; and serotonin antagonists.[49] Dry needling of trigger points is also referred to as "intramuscular stimulation." It is an invasive procedure in which an acupuncture needle is inserted into the skin and muscle directed at the trigger point. It is within the scope of practice of chiropractors and physical therapists in some states as well as being performed by medical practitioners.

The popularity of dry needling as a treatment of myofascial pain is relatively recent, although Lewit described the results of treating 241 patients with myofascial pain with this technique during the years 1975 to 1979.[50] His treatment consisted of inserting a needle into what he described as sites of maximum tenderness, trigger zones, and pain spots. The analgesia produced by needling he referred to as the "needle effect." He concluded that the pain-relieving effect previously ascribed to local anesthetics might be due to the needling itself. Like ischemic compression, dry needling is dependent upon the ability of the therapist to accurately palpate the trigger points. A high degree of kinesthetic perception is required to use the needle effectively and to appreciate the changes in the firmness of those tissues pierced by the needle.

Dry needling is recommended because it is less invasive and safer than injecting substances into the trigger point although it may cause more discomfort for the patient. Proper sterilization procedures are essential, and side effects may include slight bleeding. Dry needling is a relatively new technique and is often used in combination with other physical therapy interventions.

Exercises

Stretching exercises are used to improve range of motion and to prevent recurrence of trigger points in injured muscles. It is important that muscles be stretched to pre-injury length before resistance exercises are prescribed.[51] Exercises to stretch injured muscles that exhibit myofascial trigger points promote the deactivating nociceptive process.[51] Progressive stretching is facilitated by passive stretching to demonstrate the desired stabilization and line of stretch. Patients are then encouraged to actively stretch the muscle to tolerance, progressively increasing the stretch until full range of motion is obtained. Patients must be monitored to ensure that correct stretching procedures are being performed. Having the patient demonstrate the prescribed stretching regime each visit will ensure that optimal technique is being performed. (See Box 6-1.)

Strengthening Exercises

Active isometric exercises are an important part of the rehabilitation program to strengthen the neck muscles of patients with whiplash injuries.[52] These

---

BOX 6-1 | **General Goals of Rehabilitation**

Emphasis on increased function and decreased pain
Patient-centered education that involves patients' active participation in their rehabilitation program based on specific goals
Restoration of pre-injury range of motion, flexibility, and strength
Postural training that develops optimal balance and alignment during activities of daily living
Encouragement of early return to work and recreational activities

should be started as soon as pre-injury range of motion is achieved. The clinician can demonstrate these passively to ensure the correct line of resistance is followed and then monitor active exercises to ensure that the patient is performing them correctly and to reinforce the importance of returning strength to the neck.[53] Soft tissues injured in whiplash accidents no longer provide adequate support for the movements and weight of the head (10-15 pounds). In the early phase of treatment, the amount of movement during each exercise should be limited to avoid further pain and discomfort.[52] A cervical collar should not be worn continuously or beyond the first 2 weeks post injury when pain is acute.[51] The purpose of the collar is not immobilization but for support of injured muscles. When riding in a vehicle, wearing a collar is prudent for a short time beyond the 2 weeks until the cervical muscles are strengthened to prevent re-injury. It is essential that patients do not become dependent on a cervical collar because it reinforces the notion that they have permanent disability when the majority of patients can be returned to pre-injury status with appropriate care.

Dynamic exercising using progressive resistance to stimulate the muscles and the nerves is a useful form of active exercise.[54] During isotonic exercising, the joints move (stimulating the mechanoreceptors) and the opposing muscles relax through reciprocal inhibition. This form of exercise has the advantage of developing neurological coordination through neuromuscular adaptation. Cervical exercises performed in the position of neck function (upright) develop skills that transfer to normal daily activities. Regular monitoring of exercise programs is essential to ensure that exercises are performed optimally and to encourage the patients to perform them regularly.

Posture

The patient's posture should be assessed following whiplash injuries. It is important that optimal spinal curves be promoted. Initially, a flattening of the cervical lordotic curve is common due to the protective muscle spasm. It is also common to see an obvious forward head posture from anterior translation of the head.[52] This posture is secondary to the damaging "S-curve" motion that injures the lower and upper spinal regions in the different vectors of force produced by the whiplike motion. Without correction, this posture aggravates myofascial trigger points in the neck, upper back, and shoulders.[52] A forward head carriage has been demonstrated to restrict rotation[55] with a permanent restriction on activities of daily living, including the inability to adequately turn the head when driving. The residuals found in patients suffering from neck trauma are a significant limitation in their various ranges of cervical motion.[56,57] (See Chapter 8.) Restriction of cervical flexion-extension and rotation is directly associated with neck pain and headache.[58] Rehabilitation of the cervical spine should include rotation exercises whereby the eyes look in the direction of rotation to help reestablish the neurological coordination between neck muscle activity and the ocular reflexes (the eye-head-neck interaction).[59] (See Box 6-2.)

BOX 6-2	**General Postural Advice**

Avoid prolonged period of static posture.
Optimize balance and alignment (correct forward head).
Ensure optimal spinal curves.
Seated posture should emphasize 90-degree angles at the hips, knees, and ankles.
Avoid asymmetric postures (use head set instead of cradling the phone).
Ensure an ergonomically correct work station (chairs with arm rests and lumbar support, computer monitor at eye level, and a foot rest when sitting for prolonged periods).
Avoid carrying heavy bags of purses slung over one shoulder.
Use firm couches, chairs, and mattresses that offer support.

FIBROMYALGIA

Fibromyalgia has long been controversial, with little general agreement among health professionals about this syndrome.[60-72] Too often the widespread and multiple complaints, recently labeled fibromyalgia, have been considered to be "all in the patient's head" and have not been seriously considered when treating patients complaining of chronic muscle pain. With the establishment of criteria for diagnosis of fibromyalgia in 1990[73] and the recent development of theories of central sensitization,[51] we now have a better understanding of the mechanism of fibromyalgia. Now classified as a sensitization syndrome,[51] fibromyalgia has been linked to whiplash injuries in some patients. Buskila[74] found that fibromyalgia may develop as a late complication of a whiplash injury. He compared patients with neck injuries from whiplash accidents (90% involving rear-impact vehicle collisions) with a control group made up of patients with leg fractures. He found that 21.6% of the patients with neck injuries met the criteria of the American College of Rheumatology for the diagnosis of fibromyalgia syndrome[73] whereas only 1.7% of patients with leg fractures showed signs of fibromyalgia syndrome 3.2 months after the trauma. From this study, Buskila concluded that patients are 13 times more likely to develop fibromyalgia syndrome following trauma to the neck than following lower extremity injury.

Symptoms of Fibromyalgia

The most common subjective complaints of patients suffering from fibromyalgia syndrome include an aching-type pain, stiffness, and overbearing fatigue. Location of the major complaint shifts from one muscle group to another, which can confound the diagnostician and eventually end in misdiagnosis and inappropriate treatment. In addition to a shifting in the site of pain, there is marked fluctuation in day-to-day severity. This causes some to discount the severity of patients' complaints, pointing out that they were "fine yesterday, so why are they complaining today." A history of complete but transient remission of symptoms is an important clue to the diagnosis of fibromyalgia. Patients may also report a stabbing or "knife-like" pain, burning, and numbness. The complaints of numbness frequently fail to follow dermatomal patterns and are often inconsistent with sensory testing. It is typical for a person to experience the complete range of painful sensations, with dull, diffuse achiness at one time and sharp, stabbing, more localized pains at another. The pain is particularly severe in the morning and late evening and is accompanied by marked diffuse stiffness. The pain is exacerbated by activity and exercise but is not reliably relieved by rest. Severe ancillary manifestations are often present, such as headaches (tension or migraine), joint pain, and peripheral vascular instability resembling Raynaud's phenomenon, with hypersensitivity to cold or heat. The patient will also report a sensation of stiffness, which does not correlate with the severity of fibromyalgia but is usually in the same location as the painful areas. The stiffness is usually present in the morning, lasting longer than 15 minutes. Extreme fatigue is one of the most characteristic symptoms of fibromyalgia, with most patients with the syndrome complaining of a reduced sense of energy (i.e., lassitude), or global feeling of generalized weakness.

About 75% of patients with fibromyalgia syndrome complain of sleep disturbances. Poor sleep may be indicated by difficulty falling asleep, frequent awakening, light sleep, and morning fatigue. The nonrestorative sleep pattern found in fibromyalgia patients aggravates their pain and contributes to their overall fatigue. Significant

psychological distress (varying degrees of anxiety, depression, mental stress, and poor coping skills) has been observed in 30% to 40% of fibromyalgia patients.

Clinical Characteristics of Fibromyalgia

Fibromyalgia is a chronic, noninflammatory, diffuse muscle pain disorder. Patients typically complain of generalized aching and stiffness involving multiple muscle groups with well-defined tender points in consistent locations. Unlike myofascial trigger points, these tender points are not always located in the muscle and do not refer pain in consistent patterns as do trigger points.[75,76]

This distinction is used to differentiate myofascial pain syndrome, characterized by referred pain from trigger points in a localized muscle group, from the more generalized fibromyalgia syndrome, which involves multiple muscle groups and nonreferring tender points. (See Table 6-1.) Differentiation becomes clouded when patients exhibit characteristics of both myofascial pain and fibromyalgia.[34,76] Myofascial pain may lead to fibromyalgia, with unresolved localized muscle

TABLE **6-1**

Comparison of Myofascial Pain and Fibromyalgia Syndromes

Characteristic	Myofascial Pain Syndrome	Fibromyalgia Syndrome
Tenderness	Trigger points: belly and insertion	Multiple tender points
Pain	Referred pain	Generalized aching
Duration	Muscle specific—if untreated becomes chronic	Chronic—more than 3 months
Sex	Equal number of males and females	90% female
Prevalence	Common, 50% male and female	Uncommon, 2% 3.4% female, 0.5% male
Disturbed sleep pattern	Common secondary to discomfort due to position	Sleep disorder by definition greater than 80%
Treatment	Local muscle massage ice/heat, ultrasound, stretching exercises, ischemic compression, spray and stretch, nutritional support	Systemic light aerobic exercise, rest, decreased stress, psychological support, nutritional support, chiropractic

Modified from Simons DC: Fibrositis/fibromyalgia: a form of myofascial trigger points, *Am J Med* 81:93-98, 1986.

pain ultimately involving multiple muscle groups in addition to CNS involvement.[65]

Diagnostic Criteria for the Fibromyalgia Syndrome

The American College of Rheumatology criteria for diagnosis of fibromyalgia syndrome[73] provided consistent criteria promoting standardized methodology for epidemiological investigations. The criteria for classification of fibromyalgia were derived from a sample of 558 rheumatic disease patients who had other rheumatic conditions included in the differential diagnosis of fibromyalgia. The new classification proved to have acceptable sensitivity and specificity, thus raising

fibromyalgia to a recognizable syndrome. Thus the condition is no longer diagnosed by way of exclusion.

The diagnosis of fibromyalgia was based on the following criteria:

1. Widespread pain (left and right side of the body, above and below the waist, and axial [cervical spine anterior chest, thoracic spine or low back]) for at least 3 months
2. Presence of tenderness at 11 or more of the 18 specific tender point sites (Figure 6-25)

A tender point has been defined as an area of prominent localized tenderness that elicits a verbal response, physical withdrawal, or facial expression on palpation. (See Table 6-2.) Nine paired points exist:

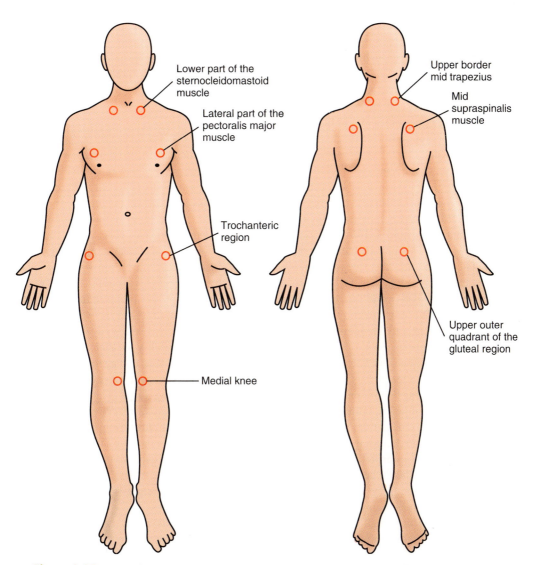

Figure 6-25 Sites of the seven most common pairs of trigger points noted in fibromyalgia patients.

TABLE **6-2**

Comparison of Trigger Points and Tender Points

	Trigger Points	Tender Points
Characteristic of	Myofascial pain	Fibromyalgia
Common sites	Belly and insertion of traumatized muscles or muscle groups	Prescribed locations in multiple areas
Referral pattern	Source of consistent referred pain	Localized tenderness without referral pattern

Modified from Simons DG: Fibrositis/fibromyalgia: a form of myofascial trigger points, *Am J Med* 81:93-98, 1986.

1. Occiput at the suboccipital muscle insertion
2. Lower cervical spine, at the anterior aspects of the intertransverse spaces at C5-C7
3. Trapezius, at the midpoint of the upper fold
4. Supraspinatus at origin (medial border of the scapula)
5. Second costochondral junction
6. Lateral epicondyle (2 cm distal)
7. Gluteal, at the upper outer quadrant
8. Greater trochanter, posterior to the trochanteric prominence
9. Medial fat pad of the knee (see Figure 6-25)

A careful history of the duration and location of symptoms is necessary to determine the diagnosis of fibromyalgia.[75] Subjective aching and stiffness of more than 3 months duration is a necessary component.[76] This makes the diagnosis following whiplash injury fall more into the category of late whiplash syndrome. (See Chapter 11.) A careful history is necessary to determine the onset of the patient's symptoms. The most definitive physical finding is localized, exaggerated tenderness (tender point) on pressure at specific periarticular, muscle, spinal, and muscle insertion sites. The digital palpation of tender points is a learned skill. Variability can exist when determining the presence of a tender point, such as force of palpation, number of fingers used for palpation, rate of palpation, gender of the patient, specific site palpated, muscle mass and adiposity of the patient, and interpretation of patient responses.[77] The pressure should be applied perpendicularly, gradually increasing by 1 kg force/s over a period of 4 seconds.[78] This is equivalent to enough pressure "to blanch the fingernail" (4 kg of pressure). The thumb pad of the dominant hand should be used to palpate each site. Wolfe has indicated that tenderness may occur in a radius of 1 cm from the specified site, and that a rolling sliding palpation produces tenderness when straight palpation pressure does not.[77] To be considered positive, the patient's response must be that it is "painful" and not just "tender." Similar pressure applied to control points (e.g., forehead, middle phalanx of the fingers) should not be painful.

Management of Fibromyalgia

The key to management of fibromyalgia is a firm diagnosis, followed by assurance that the condition is noncrippling and may eventually remit.[79] Fibromyalgia has yet to respond long term to a single therapeutic modality, and thus the management must be comprehensive. Nevertheless the condition requires a multidisciplinary approach to treatment. This must include education, behavior modification, physical modalities to reduce pain, manipulation to restore proper biomechanics, exercise, and a comprehensive approach to "wellness."[80]

Patients must be educated about fibromyalgia and take responsibility for their own care.[81] A necessary component in management is a change in attitude.[81] Patients must be encouraged to remain active and to strive for a greater level of physical fitness. Most patients with fibromyalgia allow their muscles to become chronically unfit through disuse. Others may cause a flare-up of symptoms by pursuing a too-vigorous exercise program. Patients must learn to pace activity levels, such that they can maintain enough weight-bearing activity to avoid accelerated bone loss.

Fibromyalgia is not a crippling disorder, but patients frequently restrict activity out of fear of aggravating their condition. Because the window is very small between sufficient activity and too much exercise that causes a worsening of the symptoms, patients with fibromyalgia often avoid activity that is essential for their well-being. Gentle, progressive exercise can usually ease the symptoms of fibromyalgia and provide weight control; however, there is a fine line dividing the amount of exercise that is helpful and the amount that aggravates this condition. McCain[82] found that increased cardiovascular fitness significantly improved objective measurements of pain in 34 fibromyalgia patients who met Smythe's original criteria. McCain documented that fibromyalgia patients who attain high levels of physical exercise commonly report not only an improvement in self-esteem but also a sense of control over the painful experience. The exercise program cannot be expected to have the desired effects before 12 weeks and as long as 20 weeks. McCain notes that it is not effective to have fibromyalgia patients training at 75% to 80% aerobic thresholds. Resting heart rates of 55 to 65 beats/min may be targeted for most patients between 20 and 50 years of age.[82] It is thought that exercise leads to significant alterations in opioid and nonopioid as well as neural and hormonal intrinsic pain-regulating systems that decrease pain sensitivity. McCain[82] cautioned, however, that strenuous exercise at sustained levels not only induces physiological changes but also may be responsible for the development of a stress response that appears to perpetuate the fibromyalgia syndrome. Consequently the exercise program should be monitored carefully to determine the appropriate exercise intensity (percentage of maximal heart rate), duration, and frequency. The patient should be aware that the exercise prescription will be gradual and progressive toward a lifelong program.

Alternative and Complementary Medicine Treatment of Fibromyalgia

Chiropractors are the most frequently consulted alternative and complementary medicine practitioners by patients with fibromyalgia syndrome.[84] Blunt[85] reported an increase in cervical and lumbar ranges of motion, straight leg raise, and decreased pain levels in patients treated with chiropractic management compared with controls. Treatment included soft tissue massage, stretching, spinal manipulation, and education administered 3 to 5 times a week for 4 weeks. Hains and Hains[86] evaluated the efficacy of chiropractic treatment that included ischemic compression and spinal manipulation in patients with fibromyalgia. Sixty percent of the patients were classified as responders with a minimum of 50% improvement in total pain score and less fatigue.

Cognitive Therapy

Cognitive behavioral therapy includes relaxation training, reinforcement of healthy behavior patterns, reducing pain behavior, coping skills training, and the restructuring of maladaptive beliefs about a person's ability to control pain. Cognitive therapy can be effective in relieving the patient's depression as well as dealing directly with any underlying anger. Changing the fibromyalgia patients' perspectives of themselves and their attitudes toward others can have a dramatic effect on them. These patients frequently think of themselves as helpless and hopeless. Their future becomes unrealistically bleak, and they are often not only negative but also illogical. Cognitive therapy works to change thought patterns and can help these patients to see more positive explanations for stressful situations. A well-trained cognitive therapist can help change the patient's "doomed-to-fail" attitude or help the patient deal with a difficult situation in specific, realistic terms. Patients must strive to reduce stressful factors that seem to exacerbate their symptoms, be these emotional or physical stressors.

Pharmacological Management of Fibromyalgia

Studies of pharmacological agents in the treatment of fibromyalgia have focused mainly on serotonergic drugs. Several studies have demonstrated limited effectiveness in double-blind controlled trials. Amitriptyline at a dose of 10 to 50 mg at bedtime may be beneficial in treating sleep disorders associated with fibromyalgia. Amitriptyline combined with fluoxetine has been reported to be more effective than either agent alone, but when combined, dosage of both drugs should be kept low. Cyclobenzaprine and trazodone have also been used.[87]

Prognosis

Nies[88] believes the prognosis for patients with fibromyalgia is good when the onset of symptoms is clearly defined and the history of the symptoms is short (less than 1 year). Factors for poor prognosis include a long history of symptoms, patient inability to take responsibility for his or her health, and patient involvement in adversarial actions.[88] Clearly the stress of drawn-out legal proceedings should be avoided.[89] The most effective management of fibromyalgia is reassurance, mild to moderate activity, and working with the patient to minimize stressful activities that lead to exacerbation.

REFERENCES

1. Foreman SM, Croft AC: *Whiplash injuries: the cervical acceleration/deceleration syndrome*, 3rd ed, Baltimore, 2002, Lippincott Williams & Wilkins.
2. Simons DG: Muscle pain syndromes, part I, *Am J Phys Med* 54:289-311, 1975.
3. Reynolds MD: The development of the concept of fibrositis, *J Hist Med Allied Sci* 38:5-35, 1983.
4. Baldry P: The evolution of current concepts. In Baldry P, editor: *Myofascial pain and fibromyalgia syndromes*, London, 2001, Churchill Livingstone, pp 3-15.
5. Edeiken J, Wolferth CC: Persistent pain in the shoulder region following myocardial infarction, *Am J Med Sci* 191:201-210, 1936.
6. Steindler A: The interpretation of sciatic radiation and the syndrome of low-back pain, *J Bone Joint Surg* 22:28-34, 1940.
7. Travell J, Ringler S, Herman M: Pain and disability of the shoulder and arm, *JAMA* 120:411-422, 1942.
8. Travell JG, Simons DG: *Myofascial pain and dysfunction: the trigger point manual*, Baltimore, 1983, Williams & Wilkins.
9. Nimmo RL: Receptors, effectors and tonus … a new approach, *J NCA* 27:21-23, 60-64, 1957.
10. Baldry P: Relevant neurophysiologic mechanisms. In Baldry P, editor: *Myofascial pain and fibromyalgia syndromes*, London, 2001, Churchill Livingstone, pp 3-15.
11. Livingston WK: *Pain mechanisms*, New York, 1943, Macmillan.
12. Dwarakanatz GK, Warfield CA: The pathophysiology of acute pain, *Hosp Pract* 64B-64R, 1986.
13. Mense S: Nociception form skeletal muscle in relation to clinical muscle pain, *Pain* 54:241-289, 1993.
14. Yunus MB, Inanici F: Fibromyalgia syndrome: clinical features, diagnosis, and biopathophysiologic mechanisms. In Rachlin ES, Rachlin SI, editors: *Myofascial pain and fibromyalgia: trigger point management*, 2nd ed, St Louis, 2002, Mosby, p 31.
15. Korr IM: The neural basis of the osteopathic lesion, *J Am Osteopath Assoc* 47:191-198, 1947.
16. Patterson MM, Steinmetz JE: Long-lasting alterations of spinal reflexes: a potential basis for somatic dysfunction, *Manual Med* 2:38-42, 1986.
17. Gillette RG: Spinal cord mechanisms of referred pain and related neuroplasticity. In Gatterman MI, editor: *Principles of chiropractic: subluxation*, St Louis, 2005, Mosby, pp 349-370.
18. Simons DG: Review of microanalytical in vivo study of biochemical milieu of myofascial trigger points, *J Bodyw Mov Ther* 10:10-11, 2006.
19. Gerwin RD, Dommerholt J, Shah JP: An expansion of Simons' integrated hypothesis of trigger point formation, *Curr Pain Headache Rep* 8:468-475, 2004.
20. Mense S: Pathophysiologic basis of muscle pain syndromes. An update, *Phys Med Rehabil Clin N* 8:23-53, 1997.
21. Mense S: Referral of muscle pain. New aspects, *Am Pain Soc J* 3:1-9, 1994.
22. Thompson JW: Opioid peptides, *BMJ* 288:259-260, 1984.
23. Salmons S: Muscle. In Williams PL, editor: *Gray's anatomy*, 38th ed, British. Philadelphia, 1995, Churchill Livingstone, pp 737-900.
24. Cramer GD, Darby SA: *Basic and clinical anatomy of the spine, spinal cord and ANS*, St Louis, 1995, Mosby, p 202.
25. Rubin D: Myofascial trigger point syndromes: an approach to management, *Arch Phys Med Rehabil* 62:107-110, 1981.
26. Curl D: Whiplash and temporomandibular joint injury: principles of detection and management. In Foreman SM, Croft AC, editors: *Whiplash injuries: the cervical acceleration/deceleration syndrome*, 3rd ed, Baltimore, 2002, Lippincott Williams & Wilkins, pp 452-498.
27. Baldry P: The evolution of current concepts. In Baldry P, editor: *Myofascial pain and fibromyalgia syndromes*, London, 2001, Churchill Livingstone, pp 3-15.
28. Rickards LD: The effectiveness of non-invasive treatments for active myofascial trigger point pain: A systematic review of the literature, *Int J Osteopath Med* 9(4):120-136, 2006.
29. Sciotti VM, et al: Clinical precision of myofascial trigger point location in the trapezius muscle, *Pain* 93:259-266, 2001.
30. Gerwin RD, et al: Inter-rater reliability in myofascial trigger point examination, *Pain* 69:65-73, 1997.
31. Finseth R: Examination. In Gatterman MI, editor: *Chiropractic management of spine related disorders*, 2nd ed, Baltimore, 2004, Lippincott Williams & Wilkins, p 88.
32. Travell J: Referred pain from skeletal muscle: the pectoralis major syndrome of breast pain and soreness and the sternomastoid syndrome of

headache and dizziness, *NY State J Med* 55:331-339, 1955.

33. Simons DG: Electrogenic nature of palpable bands and "jump sign" associated with myofascial trigger points. In Bonica JJ, Albe-Fessard D, editors: *Advances in pain research and therapy*, New York, 1976, Raven Press, pp 913-918.

34. Gatterman MI, Blunt KL, Goe D: Muscle and myofascial pain syndromes. In Gatterman MI, editor: *Chiropractic management of spine related disorders*, Baltimore, 2004, Lippincott Williams & Wilkins, pp 319-369.

35. Dommerholt J, Mayoral del Moral O, Gröbli C: Trigger point dry needling, *J Man Manip Ther* 14:E70-E87, 2006.

36. Alvarez DJ, Rockwell PG: Trigger points: diagnosis and management, *Am Fam Physician* 65:1-11, 2002.

37. Wolfe F: The clinical syndrome of fibrositis, *Am J Med* 81:7-14, 1986.

38. Sandman KB: Myofascial pain syndromes: their mechanism, diagnosis and treatment, *J Manipulative Physiol Ther* 4:135-140, 1981.

39. Fryer G, Hodgson L: The effect of manual pressure release on myofascial trigger points in the trapezius muscle, *J Bodyw Mov Ther* 9:248-255, 2005.

40. Fernández-de-las Peñas C, et al: The immediate effect of ischemic compression technique and transverse friction massage on tenderness of active and latent myofascial trigger points: a pilot study, *J Bodyw Mov Ther* 10:3-9, 2006.

41. Hong CZ, et al: Immediate effects of various physical medicine modalities on pain threshold of an active myofascial trigger point, *J Musculoskel Pain* 1:37-53, 1993.

42. Harris DM: Biomolecular mechanisms of laser biostimulation, *J Clin Laser Med Surg* 277-280, 1991.

43. Gur A, et al: Efficacy of 904 nm gallium arsenide low level laser therapy in the management of chronic myofascial pain in the neck: a double blind and randomize-controlled trial, *Lasers Surg Med* 35:229-235, 2004.

44. Hakguder A, et al: Efficacy of low level laser therapy in myofascial pain syndrome: an algometric and thermographic evaluation, *Lasers Surg Med* 33:339-343, 2003.

45. Altan L, et al: Investigation of the effect of GaAs laser therapy on cervical myofascial pain syndrome, *Rheumatol Int* 25:23-27, 2003.

46. Snyder-Mackler L, et al: Effects of helium-neon laser irradiation on skin resistance and pain in patients with trigger points in the neck or back, *Phys Ther* 69:336-341, 1989.

47. Ilbuldu E, et al: Comparison of laser, dry needling and placebo laser treatments in myofascial pain syndrome, *Photomed Laser Surg* 22:306-311, 2004.

48. Cecherelli F, et al: Diode laser in cervical myofascial pain: a double-blind study versus placebo, *Clin J Pain* 5:301-304, 1989.

49. Dommerholt J, Mayoral del Moral O, Gröbli C: Trigger point dry needling, *J Man Manip Ther* 14:E70-E87, 2006.

50. Lewit K: The needle effect in the relief of myofascial pain, *Pain* 6:83-90, 1979.

51. Baldry P: The neck. In Baldry P, editor: *Myofascial pain and fibromyalgia syndromes*, London, 2001, Churchill Livingstone, pp 121-150.

52. Gatterman MI, Hyland JK: Whiplash. In Gatterman MI, editor: *Principles of chiropractic: subluxation*, St Louis, 2005, Mosby, pp 429-447.

53. Rosenfeld M, et al: Active intervention in patients with whiplash-associated disorders improves long-term prognosis, *Spine* 38:2491-2498, 2003.

54. Berg HE, Bergren G, Tesch PA: Dynamic neck strength training effect on pain and function, *Arch Phys Med Rehabil* 75:661-665, 1994.

55. Walmsley RP, Kimber P, Culham E: The effect of initial head position on active cervical axial rotation in two age populations, *Spine* 21:2435-2442, 1996.

56. Osterbauer PJ, et al: Three-dimensional head kinematics and cervical range of motion in the diagnosis of patients with neck trauma, *J Manipulative Physiol Ther* 19:231-237, 1996.

57. Dall'Alba PT, et al: Cervical range of motion discriminates between asymptomatic persons and those with whiplash, *Spine* 26:1246-1251, 2001.

58. Kasch H, et al: Headache, neck pain, and neck mobility after acute whiplash injury, *Spine* 26:1246-1251, 2001.

59. Fitz-Ritson D: Phasic exercises for cervical rehabilitation after whiplash trauma, *J Manipulative Physiol Ther* 18:21-24, 1995.

60. Bennett KM: Fibrositis: does it exist and can it be treated? *J Musculoskel Med* June:52-72, 1984.

61. Goldenberg DL: Fibromyalgia syndrome: an emerging but controversial condition, *JAMA* 257:2782-2787, 1987.

62. Bennett KM: The fibrositis/fibromyalgia syndrome: current issues and perspectives, *Am J Med* 81:1-114, 1986.

63. Wolfe F: Workshop on criteria for diagnosing fibrositis/fibromyalgia, *Am J Med* 81:114-115, 1986.

64. Simons DG: Myofascial pain syndromes: where are we? Where are we going? *Arch Phys Med Rehabil* 69:207-221, 1988.

65. Bennett KM: Fibromyalgia, *JAMA* 257:2802-2803, 1987.

66. Masi AT, Yunus MB: Concepts of illness in population as applied to fibromyalgia syndromes, *Am J Med* 81:19-23, 1986.

67. Campbell SM, et al: Clinical characteristics of fibrositis, *Arthritis Rheum* 26:817-824, 1983.

68. Smythe HA: Non-articular rheumatism and psychogenic musculoskeletal syndromes. In McCarty DJ, editor: *Arthritis and allied conditions*, 9th ed, Philadelphia, 1979, Lea & Febiger, pp 881-891.

69. MacNab I: Acceleration injuries of the cervical spine, *J Bone Joint Surg* 46-A:1797-1799, 1964.

70. Kraft GH, Johnson EW, LaBon MM: The fibrositis syndrome, *Arch Phys Med Rehabil* 49:155-161, 1968.

71. Smythe HA: Fibrositis and other diffuse musculoskeletal syndromes. In Kelley WH, et al, editors: *Textbook of rheumatology*, Philadelphia, 1980, Saunders, pp 485-493.

72. Wolfe F: Development of criteria for the diagnosis for fibrositis, *Am J Med* 81:99-104, 1986.

73. Wolfe F, et al: The American College of Rheumatology 1990 criteria for classification of fibromyalgia: report of the Multicenter Criteria Committee, *Arthritis Rheum* 33:160-172, 1990.

74. Buskila D, et al: Increased rates of fibromyalgia following cervical spine injury. A controlled study of 161 cases of traumatic injury, *Arthritis Rheum* 40:446-452, 1997.

75. Wolfe F: Workshop on criteria for diagnosing fibrositis/fibromyalgia, *Am J Med* 81:114-115, 1986.

76. Simons DG: Myofascial pain syndromes: where are we? Where are we going? *Arch Phys Med Rehabil* 69:207-221, 1988.

77. Wolfe F: Diagnosis of fibromyalgia, *J Musculoskel Med* 7(7):53-69, 1990.

78. Okifuji A, et al: A standardized manual tender point survey. I. Development and determination of a threshold point for the identification of positive tender points in fibromyalgia syndrome, *J Rheumatol* 24:377-383, 1997.

79. Yunus M, et al: Primary fibromyalgia (fibrositis): clinical study of 50 patients with matched normal controls, *Semin Arthritis Rheum* 11:151-170, 1981.

80. Bennett KM: Fibrositis: does it exist and can it be treated? *J Musculoskel Med* 1:57-72, 1984.

81. Sandman KB, Backstrom CJ. Psychophysiological factors in myofascial pain, *J Manipulative Physiol Ther* 7:237-241, 1984.

82. McCain GA: Role of physical fitness training in the fibrositis/fibromyalgia syndrome, *Am J Med* 81:73-79, 1986.

83. Yunus MB: Fibromyalgia syndrome and myofascial pain syndrome: Clinical features, laboratory tests, diagnosis, and pathophysiologic mechanisms. In Rachlin ES, editor: *Myofascial pain and fibromyalgia: trigger point management*, New York, 1994, Mosby.

84. Pioro-Boisset M, Esdaile JM, Fitzcharles MA: Alternative medicine use in fibromyalgia syndrome, *Arthritis Care Res* 1996:9:13-17.

85. Blunt KL, Rajwani MH, Guerriero RC: The effectiveness of chiropractic management of fibromyalgia patients: A pilot study, *J Manipulative Physiol Ther* 20(6):389-399, 1997.

86. Hains G, Hains F: A combined ischemic compression and spinal manipulation in the treatment of fibromyalgia: a preliminary estimate of dose and efficacy, *J Manipulative Physiol Ther* 23:225-230, 2000.

87. Inanici F, Yunas MB: Management of fibromyalgia syndrome. In Baldry P, editor: *Myofascial pain and fibromyalgia syndromes*, London, 2001, Churchill Livingstone, pp 379-398.

88. Nies KM: Treatment of the fibromyalgia syndrome, *J Musculoskel Med* 9(5):20-26, 1992.

89. Kraft GH, Johnson EW, LaBon MM: The fibrositis syndrome, *Arch Phys Med Rehabil* 49:155-161, 1968.

Chapter 7

Headache in Whiplash: A Comprehensive Overview

Christina Peterson

The impact of headache associated with whiplash is significant but has thus far proven difficult to quantify.

Accessing data about whiplash-associated headache disorders is difficult at best. The National Accident Sampling System (NASS) lists only the top six injuries that have occurred in a crash resulting in a tow-away. This may not include a soft tissue injury such as a whiplash, let alone a resultant headache. And, of course, many such injuries do not result from a crash that results in a tow-away.

Acquiring data from emergency department records is also problematic. Post-whiplash headache may not appear in the first 24 or 48 hours, and even if it does, it may not be the chief complaint and may not be recorded clearly or prominently. Furthermore, not everyone involved in a car crash will present to the emergency department. Prevalence data of whiplash-associated headache are thus estimates and have been reported as varying from 32% to 80%.[1] Whereas costs of whiplash have been estimated at $4.5 billion annually in the United States, the costs of whiplash-associated headache are unknown.

TAKING A HEADACHE HISTORY

Studies of doctors and patients have found that the best way to elicit history is to ask open-ended questions and allow the patient to tell their story. The American Migraine Communication Study, in particular, found this was especially important in taking a headache history.[2] Ask patients to describe when their headaches began and how their headaches feel. Allow them to speak, uninterrupted, until they are finished. You will find that with most patients, this takes only about 2 minutes or less. Then you may begin to ask more specific questions to fill in the gaps of what you need to know.

Major historical features to cover in a headache history are frequency of headache, severity of pain, quality of pain, duration of headache, and degree of disability. Location of pain is also important; it is most important if it *never* changes. Associated headache features should also be determined, meaning presence of nausea, avoidance of light and/or sound, dizziness, difficulty with concentration due to head pain, or visual disturbances.

Frequency of headache may at first be daily. However, as recovery progresses, the headache disorder usually becomes intermittent, and it is important to see the frequency and duration of headache attacks. Headache diaries can be useful in this regard (Figure 7-1).

These may be as simple as a grid to record yes/no for headache, and estimated time of pain, or may be very complex, with room to record detail such as associated symptoms or treatments tried. The

Headache Diary

Date/time headache started	How long did the pain last?	Where did you feel the pain?	Headache severity 0=none 1=mild 2=moderate 3=severe	What did you do to relieve the pain?	How long did it take?	Day of menstrual cycle (if appropriate)	Stress level	Weather change? Yes/No	Possible trigger (Foods, etc.)
		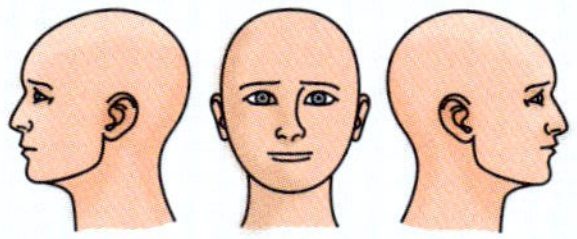							
		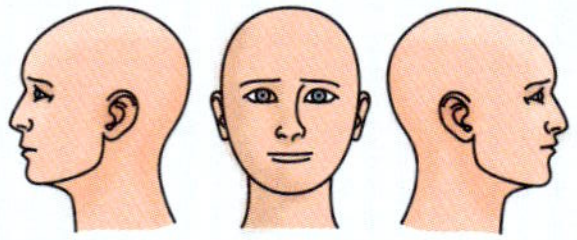							
		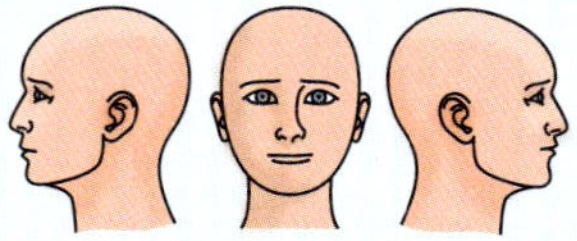							
		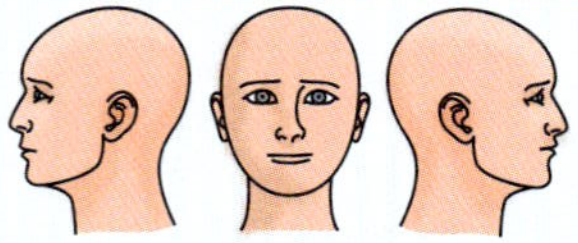							
		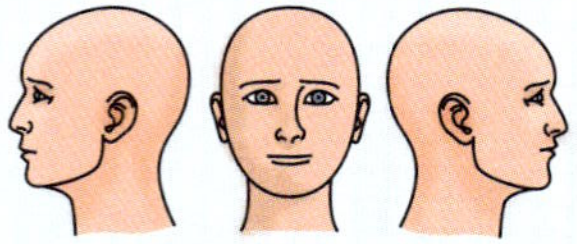							
		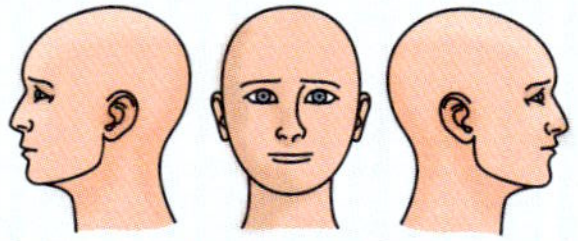							
		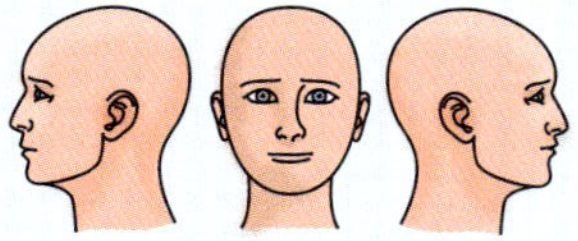							

Figure 7-1   Headache Diary.

Headache Impact Test (MIDAS Questionnaire)

INSTRUCTIONS: Please answer the following questions about ALL the headaches you have had over the last 3 months. Write your answer in the box next to each question. Write zero if you did not do the activity in the last 3 months. (Please refer to the calendar below, if necessary.)

1. On how many days in the last 3 months did you miss work or school because of your headaches? _____ days

2. How many days in the last 3 months was your productivity at work or school reduced by half or more because of your headaches? (Do not include days you counted in question 1 where you missed work or school) _____ days

3. On how many days in the last 3 months did you not do household work because of your headaches? _____ days

4. How many days in the last 3 months was your productivity in household work reduced by half or more because of your headaches? (Do not include days you counted in question 3 where you did not do household work) _____ days

5. On how many days in the last 3 months did you miss family, social, or leisure activities because of your headaches? _____ days

A. On how many days in the last 3 months did you have any headache? (If a headache lasted more than one day, count each day) _____ days

B. On a scale of 0-10, on average, how painful were these headaches? _____ days

---

Figure 7-2   Headache Impact Test (MIDAS Questionnaire).

patient should use the diary format that best suits their needs. No diary will work if it is not used.

Many patients do not understand the term "quality of pain"; just ask them "What does the pain feel like?" Sometimes, it may be necessary to prompt with adjectives, such as squeezing, dull, sharp, or throbbing, but it is best to avoid this if possible, and allow patients to express it in their own terms. Severity of pain is often expressed in descriptive terms rather than a numeric scale. One person's "3" may be another person's "6." A standard practice in headache medicine is to grade headache pain as none, mild, moderate, or severe. Others prefer a 0-10 pain scale such as the Visual Analogue Scale (VAS). Both scales are useful in the ongoing evaluation of headache to monitor progress of individual patients. Pain scales are subjective and not reliably reproducible between patients. If more objective measures are desired, it should be realized that current technology does not support objective measurement of the experience of pain. The best that can be done is the standardization of subjective reports, and for that, the Headache Impact Test (HIT-6) can be used.[3] Although the HIT-6 is a measure based on subjective reporting by the

patient, it is a standardized method that yields a numeric value and thus means the same thing to everyone. The Migraine Disability Assessment Scale (MIDAS), devised for measuring disability related to migraine headache, can also be adapted for other headache types and provides a quantifiable scale as well[4] (Figure 7-2).

Degree of disability should be discussed with the patient. Are there things they are no longer able to do because of head pain? Are they avoiding social activities? Is it affecting home life? Are they able to work? Headache disorders have been socially stigmatized, and many patients will go to work with pain and simply be less productive, or even call in with the "flu" before they will admit disability due to headache pain.

Associated symptoms may or may not be present in whiplash-associated headaches. Nausea can be a concomitant of headache and does not in itself necessarily denote concussion. Whether or not nausea indicates concussion depends on timing, and on the presence of cognitive symptoms. Avoidance of light or sound, or aggravation of headache pain by bright light or noise, is a fairly common associated symptom. Dizziness is often reported in whiplash-associated headache. This may manifest as true vertigo, described as a spinning sensation, especially with head tilting or turning, or may manifest as dysequilibrium, in which there is a sense of feeling unsteady or off-balance.

Visual disturbances also occur in association with headache disorders. Some visual disturbances are intrinsic to the headache itself, which usually occurs in migraine headaches. Existing migraine headaches may be exacerbated by a whiplash injury and can certainly be exacerbated by head injury.[5] However, visual blurring, double vision, or changes in visual processing can occur as a consequence of mild head trauma or whiplash in those who have never experienced migraine.[6,7]

Although not specific to headache, it is important to be certain that there have been no episodes of loss of consciousness, which could indicate a posttraumatic seizure disorder.

And, finally, at the conclusion of the patient encounter, it is useful to ask if the patient has additional issues or questions. Research done at UCLA in primary care indicates that it is more effective to ask, "Is there something else you want to address in the visit today?" than to ask, "Is there anything else you want to address in the visit today?" Surprisingly, this single word change brought out answers in an additional 40% of patients.[8]

TYPES OF HEADACHE THAT MIGHT BE ENCOUNTERED

Posttraumatic Headaches

The posttraumatic headache is defined as a headache following head trauma. There are a variety of grading systems for head injury. In terms of classifying posttraumatic headache, the International Classification of Headache Disorders, second edition (ICHD-2) of the International Headache Society (IHS) has divided posttraumatic headaches into acute and chronic and into mild and moderate-severe (Table 7-1). In this scheme, moderate or severe head injury requires loss of consciousness for more than 30 minutes, a Glasgow Coma score of less than 13, or posttraumatic amnesia for more than 48 hours. Mild head injury in the ICHD-2 requires all these: no loss of consciousness or loss of consciousness less than 30 minutes, a Glasgow coma score ≥13, and symptoms or signs diagnostic of concussion.[9]

Posttraumatic headaches occur in a high proportion of head-injured individuals. Motor vehicle collisions are the most common cause of head injuries, constituting 42%. Earlier estimates indicated that between 30% and 50% of those who sustained mild head injury would experience headache lasting 2 months or more; more recent data suggest acute posttraumatic headache affects up to 80%.[10,11] Mild head injury is associated with an increased risk of chronic posttraumatic headache.[12] Paradoxically, the severity of head injury is inversely proportional to the severity of posttraumatic headache.[13] Posttraumatic headache results in more disability than the primary headaches do (migraine, tension-type headache, cluster headache, and others).[14]

There is no usual headache type that characterizes posttraumatic headache. The pain may be constant or intermittent, pulsating or non-throbbing, sharp or dull. In some patients, there may be more than one type of headache pain reported. Photophobia, phonophobia, nausea, and vomiting are fairly common in posttraumatic headache. The presence of double vision, anosmia, or other neurological abnormalities indicates a higher likelihood of chronic posttraumatic headache. Anosmia, memory loss, dizziness, irritability, depression, anxiety, and personality change occur in 20% to 25% of those with chronic posttraumatic headache.[11]

The exact pathogenic mechanisms of posttraumatic headache remain unclear. Historically, "chronic" posttraumatic headache had to last more than 2 months. More recently, the IHS ICHD-2 somewhat arbitrarily declared 3 months as the cut-off for chronic posttraumatic headaches.[9] Approximately 20% of posttraumatic headaches will last more than 1 year, and a substantial number of these may become permanently chronic headache.[15]

Whiplash-Associated Headache

Headache occurs frequently as a consequence of whiplash and may affect up to 80% of individuals in the first 4 weeks. Continued symptoms are more likely if there are abnormal neurological findings, degenerative joint disease seen on x-rays, or a prior headache history.[11] Headache is often more severe if the occupant of the vehicle is unprepared for the collision. Headache and neurological symptoms are more likely to occur in rear-end collisions.[16]

There is no specific headache type that characterizes the whiplash-associated headache. The headache symptoms may mimic either tension-type headache or migraine headache and, in one

TABLE 7-1

International Headache Society (IHS) Classification of Headache

IHS Number	Diagnosis	ICD-10	Diagnostic Criteria	Comment
5.2	Chronic posttraumatic headache	G44.3		Chronic posttraumatic headache is often part of the posttraumatic syndrome, which includes a variety of symptoms, such as equilibrium disturbance, poor concentration, decreased work ability, irritability, depressive mood, sleep disturbances, etc. The relationship between legal settlements and the temporal profile of chronic posttraumatic headache is not clearly established, but it is important to assess patients carefully who may be malingering and/or seeking enhanced compensation.

5.2.1	Chronic posttraumatic headache attributed to moderate or severe head injury [S06]	G44.30	A. Headache, no typical characteristics known, fulfilling criteria C and D
			B. Head trauma with at least one of the following:
			  1. Loss of consciousness for >30 min
			  2. Glasgow Coma Scale (GCS) <13
			  3. Posttraumatic amnesia for >48 hours
			  4. Imaging demonstration of a traumatic brain lesion (cerebral hematoma, intracerebral and/or subarachnoid hemorrhage, brain contusion, and/or skull fracture)
			C. Headache develops within 7 days after head trauma or after regaining consciousness following head trauma
			D. Headache persists for >3 months after head trauma	

5.2.2	Chronic posttraumatic headache attributed to mild head injury [S09.9]	G44.31	A. Headache, no typical characteristics known, fulfilling criteria C and D
			B. Head trauma with all the following:
			  1. Either no loss of consciousness, or loss of consciousness of <30 min
			  2. Glasgow Coma Scale (GCS) ≥13
			  3. Symptoms and/or signs diagnostic of concussion
			C. Headache develops within 7 days after head trauma
			D. Headache persists for >3 months after head trauma
				Mild head injury may give rise to a symptom complex of cognitive, behavioral, and consciousness abnormalities and a GCS of ≥13. It can occur with or without abnormalities in the neurological examination, neuroimaging (CT scan, MRI), EEG, evoked potentials, CSF examination, vestibular function tests, and neuropsychological testing. There is no evidence that an abnormality in any of these changes the prognosis or contributes to treatment. These studies should not be considered routine for patients with ongoing posttraumatic headache. They may be considered on a case-by-case basis or for research purposes.

Continued

TABLE 7-1

International Headache Society (IHS) Classification of Headache—Cont'd

IHS Number	Diagnosis	ICD-10	Diagnostic Criteria	Comment
5.3	Acute headache attributed to whiplash injury [S13.4]	G44.841	A. Headache, no typical characteristics known, fulfilling criteria C and D B. History of whiplash (sudden and significant acceleration/deceleration movement of the neck) associated at the time with neck pain C. Headache develops within 7 days after whiplash injury D. One or other of the following: 　1. Headache resolves within 3 months after whiplash injury 　2. Headache persists but 3 months have not yet passed since whiplash injury	The term "whiplash" commonly refers to a sudden acceleration and/or deceleration of the neck (in the majority of cases due to a road accident). The clinical manifestations include symptoms and signs that relate to the neck, as well as somatic extracervical, neurosensory, behavioral, cognitive, and affective disorders whose appearance and modes of expression and evolution can vary widely over time. Headache is very common in this post-whiplash syndrome. The Quebec Task Force on Whiplash-Associated Disorders has proposed a classification in five categories that may be useful in prospective studies. There are important differences in the incidence of post-whiplash syndrome in different countries, perhaps related to expectations for compensation.
5.4	Chronic headache attributed to whiplash injury [S13.4]	G44.841	A. Headache, no typical characteristics known, fulfilling criteria C and D B. History of whiplash (sudden and significant acceleration/deceleration movement of the neck) associated at the time with neck pain C. Headache develops within 7 days after whiplash injury D. Headache persists for >3 months after whiplash injury	Chronic post-whiplash injury headache is often part of the posttraumatic syndrome. There is no good evidence that ongoing litigation, with settlement pending, is associated with prolongation of headache. It is important to assess patients carefully who may be malingering and/or seeking enhanced compensation.

From *IHS Classification ICHD-II: Chronic posttraumatic headache.* International Headache Society. http://www.ihs-classification.org/en/02_klassifikation/03_teil2/05.02.00_necktrauma.html. Accessed June 14, 2010.
CSF, cerebral spinal fluid; CT, computed tomography; EEG, electroencephalography; ICD-10, International Classification of Diseases (10th ed.); MRI, magnetic resonance imaging.

study, were reported in equal proportions. In another study, however, headaches reported were either generalized, dull, aching pain, a mixture of aching and tightness, or more typical tension-type headaches. Only 3% described headache pain typical of migraine. Unlike posttraumatic headache, continuous headache was short-lived, and lasted only 3 weeks in 85% of cases.[17]

A 2001 study found a fairly even distribution of headache types following whiplash, with 37% reporting tension-type headache, 27% migraine headache symptoms, 18% cervicogenic headache by IHS criteria, and 18% not fulfilling specific headache criteria. Most importantly, however, 93% of patients reported neck pain in conjunction with headache pain.[18]

Cervicogenic Headache: A Matter of Terminology

To many, the term "cervicogenic headache" simply means a headache arising from cervical structures. The term has a far richer, and more contentious, history. It is beyond the scope of this book to trace that history, but the reader should be aware that the term, when encountered in the literature, may carry differing connotations, depending on author and author's background, date of publication, and country of origin.

There have been diagnostic criteria established by the IHS, as well as by the Cervicogenic Headache International Study Group (CHISG).[9,19] The difficulty at present is that it has been determined that upper cervical and posterior head pain is common in primary headache disorders such as migraine, tension-type headache, and even trigeminal autonomic cephalgias. The mere existence of neck pain is not sufficient for a diagnosis of cervicogenic headache. Moreover, existing criteria do not adequately address biomechanical concerns.

The CHISG diagnostic criteria have, since 1998, been somewhat muddied by various reports of migraine symptom patterns. The criterion requiring unilateral neck pain has been eroded by several reports of migraine presenting with neck pain. There has also been a recent study describing reduced cervical range of motion in women with migraine, casting some lack of clarity on that criterion for cervicogenic headache.[20] The IHS criteria have, in the revised version, been simplified to the point of a danger of lack of specificity. In the CHISG criteria, the underlying principle is that the diagnosis is not proved without invasive diagnostic

anesthetic nerve blockade of C2, the "third occipital nerve," or other suspected cervical structures, including facets.

Opposing opinions in the headache field have arisen, pointing out emerging evidence of trigeminal pathways within the cervical spinal cord, as well as other areas of diagnostic uncertainty due to symptom overlap between various headache syndromes. Again, it is not the scope of this book to debate these issues in detail. This trigeminocervical complex and its role in headache and neck pain will be discussed in further detail later in this chapter.

Pre-existing Headache Syndromes Exacerbated by Whiplash

A pre-existing headache syndrome is prone to worsening when subjected to a whiplash injury. The argument has been made, in fact, that whiplash headache is solely due to a transitory worsening of a pre-existing primary headache.[21] This conclusion was based on the logic that both the collision group and the matched controls had the same long-term prognosis (at 1 year), and that therefore the headaches were primary headaches, with worsening most likely induced by the stress of the accident situation. Given that this study was conducted in Lithuania by the same investigators who did the original Lithuanian study, it would be reasonable to conclude that there might be some bias present.[22]

A retrospective records review of 2,771 headache patients, looking for correlation with trauma, found a trauma history in 1.3% of migraine patients, 1.5% of tension-type headaches, and 15% of cervicogenic/neck-associated headaches. The majority of the traumatic incidents were believed to include a whiplash action. Some of the headaches occurred remote to the trauma history. This data set suggests that worsening of migraine, if present, is not likely to be long-lasting on the basis of whiplash injury.[23] Anecdotally, many headache experts will state that pre-existing headache disorders will be exacerbated by whiplash injuries. Unfortunately, this population is often excluded from study populations, and thus, many questions remain.

Temporomandibular Dysfunction

Temporomandibular dysfunction, also called temporomandibular joint disorder (TMJD) can occur as the sequelae of whiplash injury, even without direct trauma to the jaw. If the individual does not see the collision coming, for example, and has the mouth open, perhaps in conversation, the forces involved in a whiplash can cause sudden forcible closure of the jaw. In lateral collisions, there is increased risk of direct trauma to the jaw.

Either bruxism, which is clenching or grinding, or frank temporomandibular dysfunction can exacerbate or trigger any co-occurring headache type. There are two types of temporomandibular disorders recognized by the American Academy of Orofacial Pain: myogenous temporomandibular disorder (TMD) and arthrogenous TMD. Myogenous TMD is due to bruxism, clenching, or both, and lacks evidence of joint pathology. Arthrogenous TMD is secondary to some level of articular disorder and may include disc derangement or degeneration. Symptoms may overlap, and some individuals may have both conditions.

TMD occurs more frequently in women, with a 4 to 1 ratio reported.[24] In the setting of trauma, there has often been a tendency to attribute TMD primarily to personality factors rather than to sequelae of trauma, similar to the tendency to dismiss chronic TMD in nontrauma patients as a function of personality factors or psychiatric disorders.

Clearly, not everyone with TMD is depressed. There is a study that shows no difference in pain levels between depressed TMD patients who received intervention for depression and nondepressed individuals with TMD.[25] Most significantly, it has recently been discovered that individuals with TMD are more likely to have an abnormality in the serotonin transporter gene, which indicates that there may be an inherited predisposition to abnormal pain processing in at least some TMD patients.[26]

Arthrogenous TMD often results in the popping, clicking, and loss of parafunction often associated with TMD, such as inability to fully open the jaw. This can result in a variety of symptoms, not always listed as the cardinal diagnostic features. These include ear pain, tinnitus, a sense of fullness in the ear, hyperacusis (hypersensitivity to ordinary sound levels), and dizziness.

Both patients with myogenous TMD and arthrogenous TMD should be monitored for signs and symptoms of a worsening condition, heralded by increasing or new sounds generated by the use of the jaw, decreased jaw range of motion, decreased function, and increasing pain. Onset of new ear symptoms may also be a clue.

The National Institute of Dental and Craniofacial Research in a 1996 consensus statement recommended that treatment measures for TMD should be reversible when at all possible, citing the lack of universally accepted, scientifically based diagnostic guidelines and the need for further study. The use of stabilization splints (night guards, bite splints), although used widely, remains controversial.

Self-care measures for myogenous TMD causing myofascial pain include the use of moist heat, avoidance of chewing gum, and in marked cases, a soft diet. Self-awareness of clenching, which can be difficult to reinforce, is important in order to reduce this behavior. Physical therapy or relaxation training measures may be of assistance. For a discussion of manual techniques used in the treatment of TMD, see Chapter 6.

Low Pressure Headaches

Low pressure headaches associated with cerebrospinal fluid (CSF) leaks can occur in the setting of head and neck trauma. Acute CSF leaks are infrequent, but they present in a relatively straightforward fashion for those diagnosticians who retain a high index of suspicion. Low pressure headaches are typically diffuse, dull headaches that become worse within 15 minutes of sitting or standing and that generally are accompanied by at least one of the following: neck stiffness, tinnitus, hypacusia, nausea, or photophobia.

The condition that may well be more common in the setting of whiplash is the low pressure headache due to a subacute CSF leak. This will present with essentially the same symptoms as the acute CSF leak headache but is less likely to be affected by position. There is considerable symptom overlap between low pressure headaches, also known as intracranial hypotension, and whiplash-associated headache. An interesting study, noting this overlap, looked at 66 patients with chronic whiplash-associated disorder and performed radioisotope cisternography in all in search of a CSF leak. A surprising 56% (37) were positive. Symptoms in the positive group were—in addition to headache—dizziness, memory loss, visual impairment, and nausea. Symptoms were markedly improved after epidural blood patch, and half were able to return to work.[27]

The work-up of low pressure headache should begin with cranial MRI with contrast. Pachymeningeal enhancement can be seen in intracranial hypotension but is not always present. If clinical suspicion persists, the next diagnostic study to be pursued is either myelography or cisternography. Lumbar puncture will need to be performed for either of these studies, and it is essential that an opening pressure be measured. A pressure of less than 60 mm H_2O in the sitting position is diagnostic of intracranial hypotension.[9] Low pressure headaches tend to be resistant to medication and are treated with an epidural blood patch.

Headache with Autonomic Symptoms

Although infrequent, sometimes headache syndromes with autonomic features can be seen in the setting of either posttraumatic or whiplash-associated headaches. Both cluster headache and hemicrania continua have been reported.[28,29]

Hemicrania continua is an infrequently seen headache, manifesting with a baseline underlying headache of mild to moderate severity with superimposed exacerbations of severe pain. Exacerbations often center in the temporal and orbitofrontal regions. There may be stabbing pains. The headache is "side-locked," meaning that it does not switch sides. Typically, there are associated autonomic features, which include nasal congestion, eyelid edema, tears, conjunctival injection, and ptosis. Often, ocular discomfort will be present, reported as a gritty sensation or foreign body sensation. There may be associated features of nausea, photophobia, and phonophobia.

Classically, hemicrania continua has been held to be so dramatically responsive to indomethacin that an absolute response to indomethacin was felt to be diagnostic. More recently, however, there have been reports of indomethacin-unresponsive hemicrania continua. Patients may respond to other nonsteroidal anti-inflammatory agents.

Cluster headache can also occur as a consequence of trauma, and has been reported in the setting of whiplash as well as head injury.[29] Cluster headache is a severe headache, sometimes colloquially known as "the suicide headache" because of the excruciating nature of the pain that occurs during attacks. Cluster headache is so named because of the periodicity of headache attacks, which often occur in clusters. Headaches tend to be relatively short, usually lasting 30 to 60 minutes, although they may last up to 3 hours. It is common for cluster headache sufferers to experience two or three attacks per day; up to eight attacks per day have been noted. Often, one of the attacks will occur at night and may correlate with the first rapid eye movement (REM) period of sleep.

The pain in the cluster headache attack is unilateral and focuses in the orbital region or the temporal region. The pain, which may be described as constant, stabbing, burning, or throbbing, is always severe or very severe. Most cluster headache sufferers feel restless or agitated during attacks. There may or may not be associated nausea, photophobia, or phonophobia. The characteristic autonomic features of cluster headache are tears and conjunctival injection on the same side as the headache, which occur in 80% of cases, and nasal congestion or clear drainage, also ipsilateral, which occurs in 75% of cases. Other autonomic symptoms that may be seen are forehead sweating, eyelid edema, ptosis, and pupillary constriction. The prevalence of head trauma in cluster headache has been reported ranging from 5% to 37%. The onset of cluster headaches may be somewhat remote to the occurrence of whiplash or head trauma.

EXAMINING THE HEADACHE PATIENT

The examination of the headache patient should include vital signs and an assessment of mood and orientation. Fever is not normal and should lead to further investigation. Blood pressure elevation can be an indicator of pain but may also herald other problems. Trends in blood pressure over time are a better indicator of clinical status than is a single reading in the office.

If the patient is disoriented, further assessment of mental status is warranted with either the Mini-Mental State Examination or the St. Louis University Mental Status Examination.[30-33] If abnormalities are detected, the patient should be closely monitored and consideration given to further diagnostic testing. If cognitive difficulties persist over time and are not attributable to an acute process, referral to a neuropsychologist may be in order.

If the patient seems anxious or depressed, there are office-based screening tools that can be useful in making a provisional diagnosis and assessing severity and need for referral.[34] Concurrent management of anxiety or depression is essential in achieving good control of headaches. Physical evaluation of the headache patient should include a cardiovascular evaluation, head and neck examination, and a neurological examination.

Deciding What the Diagnoses Are

Most headaches are diagnosed on the basis of clinical diagnostic criteria. A broad subdivision is made between primary and secondary headaches. Primary headaches are those that are not a symptom of, or caused by, another condition. (Migraine, tension-type headache, and cluster headache are the most common primary headaches.) Secondary headaches are caused by another underlying condition. The headaches discussed in this chapter are, for the most part, secondary headaches. Diagnostic testing is performed to rule out ominous forms of secondary headaches when suspected.

There are a few secondary headaches of an ominous nature that must be ruled out acutely after head or neck trauma. These include intracerebral, epidural, and subdural hemorrhage from acute head trauma, and dissection of the carotid or vertebral arteries.

The emergency department evaluation of acute head trauma should assess for epidural, subdural, and intracranial hemorrhages. In the acute setting, a cranial CT scan gives adequate information in most cases, and cranial MRI is not also necessary. It is important, however, for the clinician to retain a high index of suspicion in the subacute period. A negative CT scan does not always guarantee a lack of findings. It is essential to listen to the patient at all times. In the case of an epidural hematoma, for example, there may have been trivial findings on CT and a clear mental status exam. Within hours or a day or two, there may be clinical deterioration that may warrant repeat imaging. Lumbar puncture should be performed if there is clinical suspicion of subarachnoid hemorrhage.

Subdural hematomas may appear isodense to brain parenchyma on CT and can be missed on initial scans. Subdural hematomas can also ooze slowly and grow in size over time, particularly in the patient who is taking aspirin, ibuprofen, ginkgo biloba, or other platelet-inhibiting supplements. A slowly deteriorating mental status in the face of ongoing headache complaints may warrant additional imaging studies.

Dissections of the carotid and vertebral arteries in the cervical spine are underrecognized and underdiagnosed. These have been reported to occur spontaneously as well as in relationship to trauma, some of which has been fairly trivial, such as looking up, looking over one's shoulder, or bumping into another person.[35-37] Thus, it behooves us to maintain a high index of suspicion when the trauma has been less than trivial. Cervical artery dissections have been reported in connection with seatbelt injuries in individuals of short stature; they have also been reported in conjunction with airbag injuries.[38,39]

An excellent review study of this condition sorts through the variety of possible risk factors that have been put forward as predisposing factors for cervical artery dissection syndromes, including minor trauma, cervical manipulation, connective tissue disorders, oral contraceptive use, migraine, vascular risk factors, or gene polymorphisms. Many of the case-control studies analyzed were either underpopulated or contained some sort of selection bias. The strongest associations found were for risk factors associated with genetic factors and for trivial trauma; one study of homocysteine, which found a weak association with cervical artery dissection, had the lowest risk of biased results.[40]

The headache associated with cervical arterial dissection will often present in a subacute fashion. This can present as a nonspecific headache with neck pain. However, it can also be misleading, with a presentation mimicking a cluster headache.[41]

Most individuals who have a whiplash-associated headache do not, of course, have an ominous process. (See Chapter 8.) The majority of the headaches encountered will be one or more of the headache types discussed in this chapter. Although many people, particularly those who are otherwise young and healthy, will see resolution of whiplash-associated or posttraumatic headaches in a few months, this is not always the case and cannot be assumed to be the norm.[42,43] For a more detailed discussion of prognostic factors in whiplash, see Chapter 11.

Risk factors for the late whiplash syndrome, which often includes whiplash-associated headache, include psychological factors, lack of a headrest in the vehicle, and poor cervical range of motion, which of course does not speak directly to causation.[43,44]

In the subacute setting, it is important for the clinician to remain vigilant for symptoms suggestive of either carotid or vertebrobasilar dissection, either of which can occur as the result of whiplash injury and which can present in a delayed fashion. Although transient ischemic attacks may herald vascular dissection, these may be as subtle as episodes of bilateral blurred vision. A high index of suspicion is essential. CT angiography and/or MR angiography are useful in the work-up of this condition.

Evaluation of suspected low pressure headache should begin with contrasted MRI. This, again, can be a condition that requires a strong clinical index of suspicion, although the outcome may not be as dire. If there is no clear-cut diagnosis yielded by MRI, yet clinical suspicion still suggests low pressure headache, consideration could be given to a blind lumbar autologous epidural blood patch. If symptoms are not controlled, further diagnostic radiology may be necessary. CT myelography may reveal the source of a CSF leak. If this is still not the case, it may (rarely) be necessary to proceed to radionuclide cisternography. It is in these instances that a consulting radiologist can be your guide. A more detailed discussion of imaging the whiplash patient is available. (See Chapter 5.)

WHAT ARE POSSIBLE MECHANISMS OF WHIPLASH-ASSOCIATED HEADACHE?

This question has been widely debated, and no clear answers are agreed upon. Pretraumatic headache has been identified as a risk factor for whiplash-associated headache, but only in those who also exhibit clinically relevant cervical spine injury.[45] The evidence to support psychiatric disorders as a sole cause of whiplash-associated headache is lacking. A biopsychosocial model of whiplash has been proposed, but it has been stressed as being distinct from a "psychosomatic" mechanism. Ferrari and Schrader,[46] strong proponents of the biopsychosocial model, do not perceive late whiplash syndrome to be a chronic injury, but rather a matter of symptom magnification based principally on cultural expectations and personality factors.

It has been flatly stated in the past that the lack of abnormalities on MRI, brainstem evoked potentials, or conventional radiographs constitutes conclusive evidence against "any theory that invokes anatomical disruption as the explanation for the continuation of symptoms."[44] This opinion is still held by some, but certainly not by many others. Functional MRI studies are more commonplace; high field MRI studies are detecting much finer detail, and with emergent techniques like diffusion tensor imaging tractography, it may not be long before such statements are disproved definitively. Certainly, there are both anatomical and physiological bases to explain a putative mechanism for the whiplash-associated headache.

In 1981, Bogduk et al described the anatomy and physiology of the vertebral nerve in relation to a syndrome then known as "cervical migraine," also previously referred to as posterior cervical sympathetic syndrome, Barré-Liéou syndrome, or Bärtschi-Rochaix syndrome.[47-49] This syndrome, which consisted of vertigo, nausea, tinnitus, visual disturbances such as scotomata, arm paresthesias, and cognitive difficulty, was first thought to be due to

cervical arthritis but later attributed to almost any cervical vertebral disorder. Bärtschi-Rochaix argued instead for compression of the vertebral artery as causation. Because of the poorly described understanding of the anatomical relationships of this region in the literature at the time, Bogduk's group set out to better define them, studying the monkey as well as human cadavers.

Their findings were that there was no individual nerve that could be referred to as the "vertebral nerve." The portion of the vertebral artery that is within the foramina is accompanied by a repeating system of neural arcades; the third part of the vertebral artery was found to be separately innervated by nerve filaments from the C1 ventral ramus. The results of the 1981 study provided neither anatomical nor physiological support that irritation of the "vertebral nerve" was a cause of cervical migraine, and opined that "on anatomical grounds the proposition that irritation of grey rami by mid and lower cervical lesions could influence the tone of distal branches of the vertebrobasilar system cannot be entertained. Physiologically, the vertebral artery is minimally responsive to stimulation of either the 'vertebral nerve' or the sympathetic trunk."[47] Thus, the terms Bärtschi-Rochaix syndrome and Barré-Liéou syndrome have fallen into disuse by some disciplines. This does not, however, leave us closer to a mechanism for whiplash-associated headache.

In 1992, Bogduk proposed the existence of the trigeminocervical nucleus, which served as the neuroanatomical basis for cervicogenic headache by receiving convergence input from afferents of the trigeminal nerve and the receptive fields of the first three cervical nerves.[50] This concept can be expanded to understand headache in general: in fact, Bogduk later states, "All headaches are mediated by the trigeminocervical nucleus, and are initiated by noxious stimulation of the endings of the nerves that synapse on this nucleus, by irritation of the nerves themselves, or by disinhibition of the nucleus."[51]

This concept has been further refined by Goadsby et al, who defined the trigeminocervical complex as the caudal trigeminal nucleus (in the brainstem) and dorsal horns of the C1-C2 cervical spinal cord.[52] Migraine physiology is not our primary focus here, but it does play a role in the understanding of the whiplash-associated headache in that there are shared pain mechanisms that share common anatomical structures and physiological pathways. Thus, whether in migraine or in whiplash-associated headache, nociceptive spinal cord neurons can become sensitized and hyperexcitable, resulting in an increased responsiveness to afferent stimuli, an enlargement of receptive fields or the emergence of new receptive fields, and recruitment of otherwise silent nociceptive afferents.[53] This results in spontaneous pain, hyperalgesia, and cutaneous allodynia. Bartsch states, "The mechanisms of convergence and central sensitization…are important to understanding the clinical phenomena of spread and referral of pain by which pain originating from an affected tissue is perceived as originating from a distant receptive field that does not necessarily involve a peripheral pathology in the cervical innervation territory."[53]

Convergent input from various pain sources that are ultimately received in the trigeminal and upper cervical neurons that comprise the trigeminocervical complex are thus thought to explain, in part, referred pain. Also important in this is the concept of central sensitization, in which a central hyperexcitability is evoked. In spinal cord neurons, this is due to the release of neuropeptides such as calcitonin gene-related peptide (CGRP), or due to glutamate release, which acts at the NMDA receptor. Afferent stimulation may also cause a decrease in local segmental spinal inhibition.[54] Central sensitization has also been shown to occur in the dura.[55] This relationship is complex, as sensitization of neurons in the dura has been shown to cause a subsequent increased excitability to stimulation of neck muscle and the greater occipital nerve.[56] This is important in the consideration of chronic neck pain after whiplash. If neck pain can be generated from dural inputs, there may therefore be no definitive pathology in the neck at all to account for the ongoing pain. Central sensitivity, whether spinal or brainstem, may result in clinical patterns of spontaneous pain, hyperalgesia, and allodynia.[57]

Central sensitization in the brainstem has been accepted as a mechanism for migraine pain and has been described extensively in experimental models of migraine with confirmation in neurophysiological studies in humans.[57-62] These studies have found that trigeminal activation produces symptoms in the trigeminal and cervical territories, and cervical activation produces symptoms in the cervical and trigeminal territories.[62]

Lessons from returning Iraq and Afghanistan US combat troops are also instructive. Although the chronic headaches in this population are more often related to blast exposure, about a third did experience neck trauma alone or additionally. The resultant headache type was usually a migraine-type headache.[63-66] This underscores the emerging opinion many authorities in the field have, which is that migraine-like head pain is the default, regardless of the etiology or proximate pathophysiological mechanism, and that the trigeminocervical pathways serve as a final common pathway for the transmission of head pain.

Before we leave this discussion thinking that all chronic whiplash-associated headaches are due to either psychosocial factors or mechanisms of referred pain and central sensitization, we cannot exclude the possibility that some do indeed have an underlying structural issue that may have been missed. (See Chapter 8.) Many clinicians worry about missing disc pathology. This is rarely a significant consideration in the headache patient. Most disc disruptions will occur in the lower cervical spine, well below the region of the trigeminocervical complex. However, there have been reports of disc disruption as a cause of cervicogenic headache.[67]

The remaining mechanism worthy of mention is chronic CSF leak. A recent study of 66 patients with whiplash-associated disorder complaining of headache, dizziness, and nausea lasting more than 3 months were studied with radioisotope cisternography. Of these, 37 (56%) were found to have a CSF leak, and 36 were treated with epidural blood patch therapy. All symptoms were improved (nausea, dizziness, visual impairment, headache, and memory impairment); it was notable, however, that headache improved from 100% of cases to 17% of cases, and benefit was maintained at 6 months post treatment.[68] Clearly, additional studies are warranted, but this is a cautionary study that should perhaps raise our clinical suspicion for this disorder.

MANAGING HEADACHE IN THE WHIPLASH PATIENT

The management of headache in the whiplash patient is no less contentious than the matter of whiplash-associated headache itself. Too often, turf battles have erupted. The proceduralists will wish to whip out their needles—some to perform diagnostic blocks at C2 and C3; others wish to perform prolotherapy for suspected ligamentous laxity. Those who perform hands-on therapy are sometimes inclined to view the whiplash patient in those terms only, and those who prescribe also have to guard against the tendency to think just in terms of medications and must avoid medication overuse headache. A patient-centered approach is called for.

There is no agreement on the natural history of whiplash-associated headache. A good many individuals with whiplash will experience some degree of headache initially, and for many, that will resolve in a few weeks. As will be seen in Chapter 9, which addresses epidemiology, there are significant cultural differences that undoubtedly affect the natural history of whiplash-associated headache. It is unclear who will go on to become a chronic headache sufferer. Nevertheless, once prudent diagnostic measures have been taken, patients may be reassured that their headaches do not herald anything serious.

Management of Acute Headache

Early reassurance is important in the reduction of symptoms. In a Danish study, Kongsted et al found that an initial acute stress response was associated with an increased risk of considerable persistent pain, although it did not predict chronicity.[69] Many individuals with whiplash-associated headache or posttraumatic headache will experience daily or near-daily headache pain in the first week or two, and then experience a decrease in headache frequency and severity thereafter. In this early phase, analgesics and reassurance are important. Adjunctive anti-nausea agents may also be useful. Utility of muscle relaxers has not been clearly established.

After the first month, if headaches are not decreasing, it may be helpful to have the patient keep a headache diary to document frequency and severity of pain. (See Figure 7-1.) This can help to determine the later necessity for preventive therapy and can assess the possible development of medication overuse headache.

Management of Chronic Headache

The mainstays of treatment for chronic whiplash-associated headache and posttraumatic headache are education and multidisciplinary efforts, including exercise, biofeedback, and counseling.[70,71] Lenaerts, Couch, and Couch state the following: "A holistic approach is not only useful but it is necessary for a therapeutic success."[70] Stewart et al found that a combined program of exercise and advice was "slightly more effective than advice alone for people with persisting pain and disability following whiplash." This was found to more true for those with higher baseline levels of pain and disability.[72] A retrospective analysis of biofeedback in the treatment

of posttraumatic headache found that over half reported at least modest improvement in headache 3 months (or more) later, and most noted some improvement in ability to cope.[73] Cognitive behavioral therapy can also serve as a useful adjunctive tool in the management of chronic headache.[74]

The headaches themselves, as noted previously in this chapter, may be difficult to classify and may take on mixed characteristics, most commonly of tension-type and migraine headaches. To date, there have been no randomized controlled trials of preventive medications for posttraumatic headache or whiplash-associated headache. Thus, there is little in the way of evidence-based recommendation. Anecdotal reports document the efficacy of amitriptyline, propanolol,[75,76] and valproate,[77] and mixed evidence on the efficacy of botulinum toxin chemodenervation.[78-80]

Most authorities in the field advocate the use of the preventive medications generally used for the type of headache the whiplash-associated or posttraumatic headache most closely resembles in symptomatology.

There is, however, more clear evidence to advise against analgesic overuse in this population. Individuals with posttraumatic headache are at risk of developing medication overuse headache. Indeed, detractors who are skeptical about the existence of prolonged posttraumatic headache or whiplash-associated headache have expressed the opinion that these chronic cases are attributable *solely* to analgesic overuse. Baandrup and Jensen, however, found that 54% of their posttraumatic headache patients who were overusing analgesics and who subsequently underwent detoxification did not improve.[81] This suggests that medication overuse was neither the cause of the headache, nor a factor in its severity, for those patients. Of course, the other 46% did, in fact, have medication overuse headache, which indicates that consideration of this possibility would be prudent. (See Chapter 10.)

In addition to managing pain, it is necessary to address associated problems, such as sleep disorders or mood disorders. It is essential to screen for mood disorders in the chronic headache population (Figures 7-3 and 7-4). Identifying and treating anxiety or depression can diminish the risk of chronicity.[70] Although not specifically studied in the specific populations of whiplash-associated headache or posttraumatic headache, there is class A evidence to support cognitive behavioral therapy and biofeedback in the management of headache disorders.[82-85]

Sleep Questionnaire

Name:_____

Today's date:_____   Your age:_____   Your gender (M/F):_____

a). My ideal amount of sleep is_____ hours (number of hours sleep you need each night in order to feel and function your best)

1. During the weekdays I usually: 2. During the weekends I:

Go to bed at _____ AM or PM (time)   Go to bed at_____ AM or PM (time)

Get up at _____ AM or PM (time)   Get up at _____ AM or PM (time)

Sleep _____ (total hours)   Sleep _____ (total hours)

b). I awaken from sleep with headache: daily_____ sometimes_____ rarely_____ never_____

c). Sleep helps my headache: daily_____ sometimes_____ rarely_____ never_____

d). Oversleeping produces headache: daily_____ sometimes_____ rarely_____ never_____

e). I snore: nightly_____ sometimes_____ rarely_____ never_____

f). After a typical night's sleep, I feel:

refreshed _____ fairly rested _____ somewhat tired_____ very drowsy_____

Figure 7-3   Sleep Questionnaire.

Sleep disorders are a common concomitant of any chronic headache disorder, and whiplash-associated headache and posttraumatic headaches are no exception.[86] Behavioral strategies can be an effective strategy for improving sleep regulation and are preferable to medication as an initial effort[87] (Table 7-2). Individuals with anxiety are particularly prone to post-accident sleep disorders.[86] If not addressed, this may lead to further chronicity. Anxiety can easily be exacerbated by traumatic events. Depression, of course, is classically correlated with sleep difficulties and should be screened as well.

Regardless of specific headache diagnosis, there are patterns of headache that suggest a potential sleep disorder: the "awakening" or morning headache, and chronic daily headache.[88-90] Morning headache is that which occurs during or after sleep. These should lead to further screening of sleep patterns. Taking a sleep history need not be lengthy or arduous. Four key questions can be recalled with the mnemonic REST, which prompts for the **Restorative** nature of the patient's sleep; **Excessive** daytime sleepiness, tiredness, or fatigue; the presence of habitual **Snoring**; and whether **Total** sleep time is sufficient.[91] A sleep diary can be added to a headache diary if these four questions suggest a need for further information. Effective management of sleep disorders is important in the overall management of pain, as there is a reciprocal relationship between sleep quality and pain.[90]

Greater occipital nerve blockade has proven to be useful in blocking the pain of cervicogenic headaches, as well as primary headaches.[92-95] Some patients benefit from upper cervical radiofrequency neurolysis.[96] Careful patient selection can identify those patients who will benefit from invasive procedures.[97]

It is important to set realistic expectations for the patient with chronic headache. There have been no randomized controlled trials of medications for the whiplash-associated headache or posttraumatic headache populations. Even when dealing with better-characterized chronic headache populations, a reduction of 30% in headache days per month is considered an acceptable target for studies of chronic daily headache. A 50% reduction in headache severity and headache frequency is considered a good result in the management of episodic migraine. (Episodic migraine is less than 15 headache days per month.)

TABLE 7-2

Behavioral Treatment for Sleep Disorders

Relaxation training	High physiological, emotional, or cognitive arousal	Progressive relaxation training to reduce physical tension (may be facilitated by EMG or other forms of biofeedback) Autogenic training to establish calm mental state and deter intrusive and arousing thoughts
Cognitive therapy	Racing/obsessive thoughts at bedtime, catastrophizing, ruminative worry about sleep	1. Patients may be asked to self-monitor or solicit beliefs and fears about sleep (or questionnaire). 2. Identify anxiety-provoking insomnia-perpetuating cognitions. 3. Cognitive techniques are taught to challenge dysfunctional beliefs and restructure rational statements that the patient will apply when the dysfunctional thought or emotional state occurs.
Stimulus control	Delayed sleep onset, sleep maintenance	1. Go to bed only when sleepy. 2. If unable to fall asleep 10-20 minutes (without watching clock, 10-20 minutes is equal to repositioning twice to try to fall asleep), leave the bedroom. Return only when sleepy again. 3. Use the bed and bedroom for sleep only. 4. Set alarm and rise daily at a regular time—do not snooze. 5. Do not nap during the day.
Sleep restriction	Excessive time spent in bed not sleeping, fragmented/poor quality sleep	1. Use the sleep diary to determine "time in bed" and "actual sleep time." 2. Restrict "time in bed" to approximately the average number of hours of "actual sleep time" per night. (Prescribe specific bed/wake times) 3. As diary demonstrates, actual sleep time is 85% of time in bed, increase by 15- to 30-minute increments. 4. Keep a fixed wake time, regardless of the actual sleep duration (short nights are expected and increase sleep drive on subsequent night). 5. If sleeping <85% time in bed for 10 days, restrict time in bed further by 15- to 30-minute increments.
Sleep hygiene education	Any above or generally poor sleep habits	1. Avoid daytime naps. 2. Eliminate stimulants (caffeine, nicotine, etc.). 3. Maintain a regular bed/wake schedule 7 days per week. 4. Dark, quiet, comfortable sleep environment. 5. Avoid alcohol. 6. Regular exercise (avoid exercising 5 hours before bed). 7. Use the bed only for sleep and sex (behaviors conducive to sleep).

Adapted from Rains JC, Poceta JS: Headache and sleep disorders: review and clinical implications for headache management, *Headache*; 46(9):1344-1363, 2006; and Rains JC: Chronic headache and potentially modifiable risk factors: screening and behavioral management of sleep disorders, *Headache*; 48(1):32-39, 2008.
EMG, electromyography.

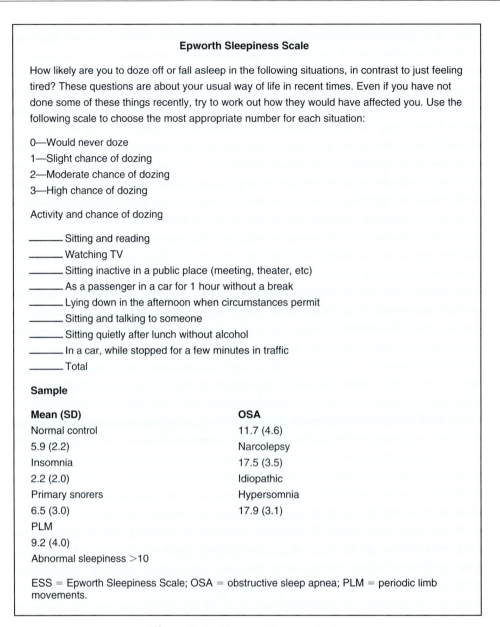

Epworth Sleepiness Scale

How likely are you to doze off or fall asleep in the following situations, in contrast to just feeling tired? These questions are about your usual way of life in recent times. Even if you have not done some of these things recently, try to work out how they would have affected you. Use the following scale to choose the most appropriate number for each situation:

0—Would never doze
1—Slight chance of dozing
2—Moderate chance of dozing
3—High chance of dozing

Activity and chance of dozing

_____ Sitting and reading
_____ Watching TV
_____ Sitting inactive in a public place (meeting, theater, etc)
_____ As a passenger in a car for 1 hour without a break
_____ Lying down in the afternoon when circumstances permit
_____ Sitting and talking to someone
_____ Sitting quietly after lunch without alcohol
_____ In a car, while stopped for a few minutes in traffic
_____ Total

Sample

Mean (SD)	**OSA**
Normal control	11.7 (4.6)
5.9 (2.2)	Narcolepsy
Insomnia	17.5 (3.5)
2.2 (2.0)	Idiopathic
Primary snorers	Hypersomnia
6.5 (3.0)	17.9 (3.1)
PLM	
9.2 (4.0)	
Abnormal sleepiness >10	

ESS = Epworth Sleepiness Scale; OSA = obstructive sleep apnea; PLM = periodic limb movements.

Figure 7-4   Epworth Sleepiness Scale.

SUMMARY

Both the head-injured patient and the whiplash patient may be subject to post-injury headaches. Although the majority of these headaches will be self-limiting, there are some that will become chronic. A high index of suspicion must be maintained to rule out ominous secondary headaches, and judicious work-up of the post-injury headache patient will screen for treatable causes of potentially dangerous conditions.

Although the evidence base is scant for the effective management of chronic whiplash-associated headache and posttraumatic headache populations, there is increasing interest in these patient populations. Evidence garnered from military populations suggests that the majority of posttraumatic headaches are migrainous in character and respond acutely to triptans.

A good history, careful evaluation, and an excellent ongoing therapeutic alliance with the patient will ensure that your care of the post-injury headache patient will be exemplary.

REFERENCES

1. Sterner Y, Gerdle B: Acute and chronic whiplash disorders—a review, *J Rehabil Med* 36:193-210, 2004.
2. Lipton RB, et al: In-office discussions of migraine: results from the American Migraine Communication Study, *J Gen Intern Med* 23(8):1145-1151, 2008.
3. Kosinski M, et al: Development of HIT-6, a paper-based short form for measuring headache impact, *Cephalalgia* 21:334, 2001.
4. Stewart WF, et al: Reliability of the migraine disability assessment score in a population-based sample of headache sufferers, *Cephalalgia* 19:107-114, 1999.
5. Schrader H, et al: Examination of the diagnostic validity of "headache attributed to whiplash injury": a controlled, prospective study, *Eur J Neurol* 13(11):1226-1232, 2006.
6. Burke JP, et al: Whiplash and its effect on the visual system, *Graefes Arch Clin Exp Ophthalmol* 230(4):335-339, 1992.
7. Mosimann UP, et al: Saccadic eye movement disturbances in whiplash patients with persistent complaints, *Brain* 123(4):828-835, 2000.
8. Heritage J, et al: Reducing patients' unmet concerns in primary care: the difference one word can make, *J Gen Intern Med* 22(10):1429-1433, 2007.
9. International Headache Society (IHS): International classification of headache disorders, 2nd ed, *Cephalalgia* 2003.
10. Packard RC: Mild head injury, *Headache Quarterly, Current Treatment, and Research* 4(1):42-52, 1993.
11. Lenaerts ME, Couch JR: Posttraumatic headache, *Curr Treat Options Neurol* 6:507-517, 2004.
12. Couch JR: Chronic daily headache in the posttrauma syndrome: relation to extent of head injury, *Headache* 41:559-564, 2001.
13. Yamaguchi M: Incidence of headache and severity of head injury, *Headache* 32:427-431, 1992.
14. Lenaerts ME: Post-traumatic headache: from classification challenges to biological underpinnings, *Cephalalgia* 28(suppl 1):12-15, 2008.
15. Packard RC: Current concepts in chronic post-traumatic headache, *Curr Pain Headache Rep* 4:19-24, 2005.
16. Sturzenegger M, et al: Presenting symptoms and signs after whiplash injury, *Neurology* 44:688-693, 1994.
17. Pearce JMS: Headaches in the whiplash syndrome, *Spinal Cord* 39(4):228-233, 2001.
18. Radanov BP, Di Stefano G, Augustiny KF: Symptomatic approach to posttraumatic headache and its possible implications for treatment, *Eur Spine J* 10(5):403-407, 2001.
19. Sjaastad O, Fredriksen T, Pfaffenrath V: Cervicogenic headache: Diagnostic criteria, *Headache* 38(6):442-445, 1998.
20. Bevilaqua-Grossi D, et al: Cervical mobility in women with migraine [Internet], *Headache* 49(5):726-731, 2009.
21. Stovner LJ, Obelieniene D: Whiplash headache is transitory worsening of a pre-existing primary headache, *Cephalalgia* 28(suppl 1):28-31, 2008.
22. Obelieniene D, et al: Pain after whiplash: a prospective controlled inception cohort study, *J Neurol Neurosurg Psychiatry* 66(3): 279-283, 1999.
23. Vincent MB: Is a *de novo* whiplash associated pain most commonly cervicogenic headache? *Cephalalgia* 28(suppl 1):32-34, 2008.
24. Esposito CJ, Fanucci PJ, Farman AG: Associations in 425 patients having temporomandibular disorders, *J Ky Med Assoc* 98(5):213-215, 2000.
25. Gatchel RJ, Stowell AW, Buschang P: The relationship among depression, pain, masticatory functioning in temporomandibular disorder patients, *J Orofacial Pain* 20(4):288-296, 2006.
26. Ojima K, et al: Temporomandibular disorder is associated with a serotonin transporter gene polymorphism in the Japanese population, *Biopsychosoc Med* 1:3, 2007.
27. Ishikawa S, et al: Epidural blood patch therapy for chronic whiplash associated disorder, *Anesth Analg* 105:809-814, 2007.
28. Lay C, Newman L: Posttraumatic hemicrania continua, *Headache* 39:275-279, 1999.
29. Turkewitz LJ, et al: Cluster headache following head injury: a case report and review of the literature, *Headache* 32(10):504-506, 1992.
30. VAMC St. Louis University Mental Status (SLUMS) Examination. medschool.slu.edu/agingsuccessfully/pdfsurveys/slumsexam_05.pdf. Accessed July 18, 2009.
31. Tariq SH, et al: Comparison of the Saint Louis University Mental Status Examination and the Mini-Mental State Examination for detecting dementia and mild neurocognitive disorder—a pilot study, *Am J Geriatr Psychiatry* 14(11):900-910, 2006.
32. Folstein MF, Folstein SE: Mini-Mental State Examination, ed 2, (MMSE-2), Lutz, FL, Par Inc. http://www.minimental.com.
33. Folstein MF, Folstein SE, McHugh PR. "Mini-mental state": a practical method for grading the cognitive state of patients for the clinician, *J Psychiatr Res* 12:189-198, 1975.
34. Sharp LK, Lipsky MS: Screening for depression across the lifespan: a review of measures for use in primary care settings, *Am Fam Physician* 66:1001-1008, 1045-1046, 1048, 1051-1052, 2002.
35. Hinse P, Thie A, Lachenmayer L: Dissection of the extracranial vertebral artery: report of four cases

and review of the literature, *J Neurol Neurosurg Psychiatry* 54:863-869, 1991.

36. Prabhakar S, et al: Vertebral artery dissection due to indirect neck trauma: an underrecognised entity, *Neurol India* 49:384, 2001.

37. Mas J-L, et al: Extracranial vertebral artery dissections: a review of 13 cases, *Stroke* 18; 1037-1047, 1987.

38. Reddy K, et al: Carotid artery dissection secondary to seatbelt trauma: case report, *J Trauma* 30(5):630-633, 1990.

39. Duncan MA, et al: Traumatic bilateral internal carotid artery dissection following airbag deployment in a patient with fibromuscular dysplasia, *Br J Anaesth* 85:476-478, 2000.

40. Rubinstein S, et al: A systematic review of the risk factors for cervical artery dissection, *Stroke* 36:1575-1580, 2005.

41. Mainardi F, et al: Spontaneous carotid artery dissection with cluster-like headache, *Cephalalgia* 22:557-559, 2002.

42. Squires B, Gargan MF, Bannister GC: Soft-tissue injuries of the cervical spine: 15-year follow-up, *J Bone Joint Surg* 78:955-957, 1996.

43. Kasch H, Bach FW, Jensen TS: Handicap after acute whiplash injury: a 1-year prospective study of risk factors, *Neurology* 56:1637-1643, 2001.

44. Pearce JMS: Polemics of chronic whiplash injury, *Neurology* 44:1993-1997, 1994.

45. Radanov BP, et al: Factors influencing recovery from headache after common whiplash, *BMJ* 307(6905):652-655, 1993.

46. Ferrari R, Schrader H: The late whiplash syndrome: a biopsychosocial approach, *J Neurol Neurosurg Psychiatry* 70(6):722-726, 2001.

47. Bogduk N, Lambert GA, Duckworth JW: The anatomy and physiology of the vertebral nerve in relation to cervical migraine, *Cephalalgia* 1:11-24, 1981.

48. Barré JA: Sur un syndrome sympathique cervical postérieur et sa cause fréquente, l'arthrite cervicale, *Rev Neurol (Paris)* 1:1246-1248, 1926.

49. Bärtschi-Rochaix W: *Migraine cervicale (das encephale Syndrom nach Halswirbeltrauma)*, Bern, 1949, Huber.

50. Bogduk N: The anatomical basis for cervicogenic headache, *J Manipulative Physiol Ther* 15(1):67-70, 1992.

51. Bogduk N: Anatomy and physiology of headache, *Biomed Pharmacother* 49(10):435-445, 1995.

52. Goadsby PJ, Classey JD: Glutamatergic transmission in the trigeminal nucleus assessed with local blood flow, *Brain Res* 875(1-2):119-124, 2000.

53. Bartsch T: Migraine and the neck: new insights from basic data, *Curr Pain Headache Rep* 4:73-78, 2005.

54. Goadsby PJ, Bartsch T: On the functional neuroanatomy of neck pain, *Cephalalgia* 28(suppl 1):1-7, 2008.

55. Burstein R, et al: Chemical stimulation of the intracranial dura induces enhanced responses to facial stimulation in brain stem trigeminal neurons, *J Neurophysiol* 79(2):964-982, 1998.

56. Bartsch T, Goadsby PJ: Increased responses in trigeminocervical nociceptive neurons to cervical input after stimulation of the dura mater, *Brain* 126(8):1801-1813, 2003.

57. Koltzenburg M: Neural mechanisms of cutaneous nociceptive pain, *Clin J Pain* 16(suppl 3):S131-S138, 2000.

58. Strassman AM, Raymond SA, Burstein R: Sensitization of meningeal sensory neurons and the origin of headaches, *Nature* 384(6609):560-564, 1996.

59. Malick A, Burstein R: Peripheral and central sensitization during migraine, *Funct Neurol* 15(suppl 3):28-35, 2000.

60. Yarnitsky D, et al: 2003 Wolff Award: possible parasympathetic contributions to peripheral and central sensitization during migraine, *Headache* 43(7):704-714, 2003.

61. Welch KA: Contemporary concepts of migraine pathogenesis, *Neurology* 61 (8 suppl 4):S2-S8, 2003.

62. Piovesan EJ, Kowacs PA, Oshinsky ML: Convergence of cervical and trigeminal sensory afferents, *Curr Pain Headache Rep* 2:155-161, 2003.

63. Theeler BJ, Erickson JC: Mild head trauma and chronic headaches in returning US soldiers, *Headache* 49(4):529-534, 2009.

64. Theeler BJ, Mercer R, Erickson, JC: Prevalence and impact of migraine among US Army soldiers deployed in support of Operation Iraqi Freedom, *Headache* 48(6):876-882, 2008.

65. Evans RW: Expert opinion: Posttraumatic headaches among United States soldiers injured in Afghanistan and Iraq, *Headache* 48(8):1216-1225, 2008.

66. Theeler B, Flynn F, Ericson, J: Search engines for the World Wide Web: Post-traumatic headaches after mild head injury in U.S. soldiers returning from Iraq or Afghanistan (AAN Abstract IN6-2.005). Poster presented at the American Academy of Neurology 2009 Annual Meeting, April 25-May 2, 2009. Seattle, WA. http://www.**aan**.com/globals/axon/assets/5305.pdf. Accessed October 9, 2009.

67. Diener HC, et al: Lower cervical disc prolapse may cause cervicogenic headache: prospective study in patients undergoing surgery, *Cephalalgia* 27(9):1050-1054, 2007.

68. Ishikawa S, et al: Epidural blood patch therapy for chronic whiplash associated disorder, *Anesth Analg* 105(3):809-814, 2007.

69. Kongsted A, et al: Acute stress response and recovery after whiplash injuries. A one-year prospective study, *Eur J Pain* 12(4):455-463, 2008.

70. Lenaerts M, Couch J, Couch J: Posttraumatic headache, *Curr Treat Options Neurol* 6(6):507-517, 2004.

71. Lenaerts M: Post-traumatic headache: from classification challenges to biological underpinnings, *Cephalalgia* 28(suppl 1):12-15, 2008.

72. Stewart MJ, et al: Randomized controlled trial of exercise for chronic whiplash associated disorders, *Pain* 128(1-2):59-68, 2007.

73. Ham L, Packard R: A retrospective, follow-up study of biofeedback-assisted relaxation therapy in patients with posttraumatic headache, *Biofeedback Self Regul* 21(2):93-104, 1996.

74. Gurr B, Coetzer BR: The effectiveness of cognitive-behavioural therapy for post-traumatic headaches, *Brain Inj* 19(7):481-491, 2005.

75. Tyler GS, McNeely HE, Dick ML: Treatment of post-traumatic headache with amitriptyline, *Headache* 20(4):213-216, 1980.

76. Weiss HD, Stern BJ, Goldberg J: Post-traumatic migraine: chronic migraine precipitated by minor head or neck trauma, *Headache* 31(7):451-456, 1991.

77. Packard RC: Treatment of chronic daily posttraumatic headache with divalproex sodium, *Headache* 40(9):736-739, 2000.

78. Freund BJ, Schwartz M: Treatment of chronic cervical-associated headache with botulinum toxin A: a pilot study, *Headache* 40(3):231-236, 2000.

79. Loder E, Biondi D: Use of botulinum toxins for chronic headaches: a focused review, *Clin J Pain* 18(suppl 6):S169-S176, 2002.

80. Peloso PM, et al: Medicinal and injection therapies for mechanical neck disorders: a Cochrane systematic review, *J Rheumatol* 33(5):957-967, 2006.

81. Baandrup L, Jensen R: Chronic post-traumatic headache: a clinical analysis in relation to the International Headache Classification 2nd edition, *Cephalalgia* 25(2):132-138, 2005.

82. Cohen M, McArthur D, Rickles W: Comparison of four biofeedback treatments for migraine headache: physiological and headache variables, *Psychosom Med* 42(5):463-480, 1980.

83. Andrasik F, Buse DC, Grazzi L: Behavioral medicine for migraine and medication overuse headache, *Curr Pain Headache Rep* 13(3):241-248, 2009.

84. Buse DC, Andrasik F: Behavioral medicine for migraine, *Neurol Clin* 27(2):445-465, 2009.

85. Andrasik F, Rime C: Can behavioural therapy influence neuromodulation? *Neurol Sci* 28(Suppl 2):S124-S129, 2007.

86. Rao V, et al: Prevalence and types of sleep disturbances acutely after traumatic brain injury, *Brain Inj* 22(5):381-386, 2008.

87. Rains JC: Optimizing circadian cycles and behavioral insomnia treatment in migraine, *Curr Pain Headache Rep* 12(3):213-219, 2008.

88. Rains JC, Poceta JS: Sleep and headache disorders: clinical recommendations for headache management, *Headache* 46(suppl 3):S147-S148, 2006.

89. Rains JC, Poceta JS: Sleep-related headache syndromes, *Semin Neurol* 25(1):69-80, 2005.

90. Moldofsky H: Sleep and pain, *Sleep Med Rev* 5(5):385-396, 2001.

91. Rains JC: Chronic headache and potentially modifiable risk factors: screening and behavioral management of sleep disorders, *Headache* 48(1):32-39, 2008.

92. Naja ZM, et al: Occipital nerve blockade for cervicogenic headache: a double-blind randomized controlled clinical trial, *Pain Pract* 6(2):89-95, 2006.

93. Peres MFP, et al: Greater occipital nerve blockade for cluster headache, *Cephalalgia* 22(7):520-522, 2002.

94. Caputi CA, Firetto V: Therapeutic blockade of greater occipital and supraorbital nerves in migraine patients, *Headache* 37(3):174-179, 1997.

95. Antonaci F, et al: Chronic paroxysmal hemicrania and hemicrania continua: anaesthetic blockades of pericranial nerves, *Funct Neurol* 12(1):11-15, 1997.

96. Govind J, et al: Radiofrequency neurotomy for the treatment of third occipital headache, *J Neurol Neurosurg Psychiatry* 74(1):88-93, 2003.

97. Bogduk N: Role of anesthesiologic blockade in headache management, *Curr Pain Headache Rep* 8(5):399-403, 2004.

Chapter 8

Whiplash-Associated Disorders of Joints and Ligamentous Structures

Meridel I. Gatterman

Trauma from whiplash can cause joint and ligamentous disorders of the cervical spine. When the rapid stretch of the spinal muscles fails to protect the vulnerable cervical articulations, injury and, more commonly, dysfunction occur. Left untreated, these disorders significantly prolong healing time and can result in chronic problems. The residuals of cervical spine injury are most commonly characterized by neck pain, restricted motion, and headaches. In addition, upper extremity symptoms frequently present. Conditions that produce recognizable signs and symptoms are not entities but rather syndromes.[1] This chapter discusses several syndromes related to whiplash-associated disorders of the cervical zygapophyseal joints and associated ligaments.

STABILITY OF THE CERVICAL SPINE AND WHIPLASH INJURY

The wide range of motion of the cervical spine makes stability problematic and predisposes the neck to traumatic injury.[2] When the physiological limits of cervical structures are exceeded, disruption of the soft tissues of the neck occurs. When the muscles of the cervical spine, which offer the first line of defense from whiplash injuries, are unable to compensate for the rapidity of head and torso movement caused by the acceleration forces generated at the time of impact (see Chapter 3), ligamentous structures may be injured along with dysfunction and damage to cervical articulations.

CERVICAL JOINT SPRAIN

Cervical joint sprain is noted when there is ligamentous and capsular damage, which may be evident on functional imaging. (See Chapter 5.) Differentiation of sprain from strain is indicated by the patient's complaints. Muscle strain is indicated with pain on active motion when injured muscles contract. Pain at the end range of movement with passive motion induced by the clinician indicates joint sprain. (See Chapter 4.) Joint sprains are divided into four categories according to severity of the ligamentous damage. A mild sprain is characterized by only a few torn fibers, and the problem quickly resolves in a few days. A moderate sprain exhibits more severe tearing of the fibers, but the ligament remains intact. A severe sprain results in complete tearing of the ligament either from its attachment or within the ligament itself. A sprain or fracture occurs when a fragment of bone (avulsion) is torn from the ligamentous attachment.[3] Functional imaging is necessary to determine the severity of ligamentous damage. (See Chapter 5.)

The inflammatory reaction from a ligamentous sprain can produce scar tissue that is less elastic and

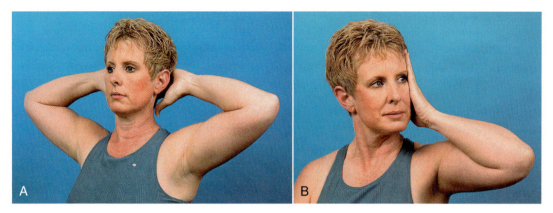

Figure 8-1   **A,** Neck extension against resistance. **B,** Cervical rotation against resistance.

less functional if inflammation persists. Immobilization of joints and/or functional inactivity in mild to moderate cervical joint sprain is not recommended, as it can cause post-traumatic joint stiffness. The patient should be encouraged to move within the normal range of movement while avoiding excess movement. If a cervical collar is recommended, it should not be designed to restrict total movement but used to prevent further injury when riding in an automobile or when the patient complains of extreme fatigue in the cervical region. Isometric neck exercises can be introduced within 2 weeks of injury (Figure 8-1), and patients should be encouraged to return to their normal activities as soon as possible. Repair of injured capsular and ligamentous tissue is slow, taking up to 6 to 8 weeks. During this period, the patient must be careful to avoid overstretching the damaged ligaments, without restricting the joints from their normal range of movement. The Quebec Guidelines for Whiplash Associated Disorders recommend a multimodal approach to management (see Chapter 6) and suggest that the patient be instructed to repeat active cervical movements, within a comfortable range.[4]

WHIPLASH-ASSOCIATED JOINT DYSFUNCTION

Various terms are used to describe joint dysfunction. The term "subluxation" or "fixation" is used by chiropractors, "joint dysfunction" or "somatic dysfunction" by osteopaths, and "spinal stiffness" by physical therapists. Some manual medicine practitioners prefer "joint blockage." The common feature of these terms is that they refer to hypomobility (restricted motion) of the joints. Cervical joint

dysfunction, including subluxation following whiplash, may take the form of simple joint restriction or, more likely, be accompanied by hypermobility in other motion segments. It is critical that hypermobile segments be differentiated from those with restricted motion. It is not rational to introduce forceful manipulation at the level of spinal segmental hypermobility, which can create further damage to sprained articulations. Subluxation has been defined by chiropractors through a rigorous consensus process as *a motion segment in which alignment, movement integrity and or physiological function are altered although joint surfaces remain intact.*[5] Manipulation is not appropriate for all subluxations, and the medical use of the term often refers to an unstable segment (nonmanipulable subluxation) that may require a surgical procedure. It is important to differentiate between restricted joint motion and hypermobile motion segments because the therapeutic approaches to these syndromes are not the same. On a continuum of segmental motion, manipulation is appropriate for articulations with restricted motion, whereas on the other end of the spectrum, hypermobile and unstable segments require a stabilizing approach. Hypermobility has been described as the mobility of a motion segment that is excessive but not so extreme as to be life threatening or require surgery. Instability, on the other hand, is more severe and may require surgery if life threatening or if the patient is exhibiting neurological deficits attributable to the unstable segment.[6] Functional imaging is useful if clinical findings suggest instability. (See Chapter 5.) The biomechanical injuries to joints and ligaments that result from whiplash commonly seen clinically tend to follow characteristic patterns that are recognizable as subluxation syndromes. The torque and lofting of the head produced by the whiplash action tends to produce hypomobility and subluxation of the upper cervical and lower cervical articulations, with hypermobility common at the apex of the curve in the mid cervical region where ligaments are stretched. Radiographically degenerative changes that occur following whiplash injury suggest that the greatest amount of soft tissue injury occurs at the C4-C5, C5-C6 motion segments. Jaeger's report[7] on 11 cervicogenic headache patients related to whiplash noted that tenderness and misalignment around the transverse process of C1 was the most frequent finding. Clinically, blocked movement of spinal motion segments is seen anywhere in the spine with whiplash injuries,[3,8] but upper cervical subluxations[7] are most common followed by restriction at the C7-T1 spinal motion segment, and first costovertebral articulations.[3]

CLINICAL INDICATORS OF CERVICAL SUBLUXATION

Clinical indicators of subluxation outlined by the Medicare Benefit Policy Manual (Box 8-1)[9] include palpatory and radiographic findings. Radiographic and other imaging indicators of subluxation can be found in Chapter 5. Specific palpatory findings along with functional radiographs give the most useful clinical indications of subluxation of the zygapophyseal joints of the spinal motion segments.

BOX **8-1**	**Diagnostic Criteria for Detection of Cervical Subluxation**

Palpation or imaging of the cervical motion segments fulfills two of the following four criteria mentioned, one of which must be A or B:
  A Asymmetry/misalignment on palpation of cervical C0-C1 or C1-C2 or zygapophyseal joint or demonstrable on imaging
  B Movement abnormality on palpation of cervical C0-C1 or C1-C2 or zygapophyseal joint or demonstrable on functional imaging
  C Pain/tenderness on palpation of affected joint
  D Palpable tension/tautness in soft tissue surrounding affected joint

From Medicare Benefit Policy Manual, Chapter 15. Covered medical and other health services. http://www.cms.gov/manuals/Downloads/bp102c15.pdf

PALPATORY FINDINGS INDICATING CERVICAL SUBLUXATION

Static palpation for alignment, tenderness, tone, and texture of the bony and soft tissue structures of the neck provides valuable information in the post-whiplash patient.[10] Palpation for tenderness relies on the patients' pain response and their verbal confirmation that the site is a pain generator. This alone is not a valid indicator for manipulation, as pain and tenderness can be caused by multiple disorders, including sprain or strain, neoplasia, and fractures.

Cervical muscle tone and texture is palpated with the patient supine to promote optimal relaxation in injured structures[10] (Figure 8-2). Palpation is a skill learned only through patience and perseverance. The ability to differentiate abnormal from normal tissue characteristics and aberrant motion is essential for identification of manipulable lesions. The art of manipulation is easier to master than the determination of where and how to perform this procedure,[11] but caution is advised when using long lever procedures because the forces generated can easily cause injury.

Palpation of bony landmarks must take into consideration the possibility of osseous anomalies when assessing symmetry. The least pressure possible provides more information and prevents pain that can induce protective muscle splinting.[11] Surface anatomy and osseous landmarks of the cervical spine are outlined in Table 8-1.

Palpation for flexion, extension, or rotation alignment of C1 in relation to C2 evaluates the C1 transverse process to mandible distance (Figure 8-3). Lateral flexion alignment of the

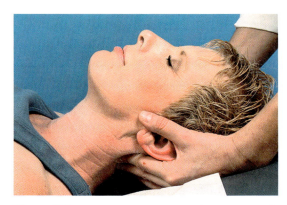

Figure 8-2   Cervical muscle tone and texture are palpated with the patient supine to promote optimal relaxation.

TABLE **8-1**

Surface Anatomy and Osseous Landmarks of the Cervical Spine

Landmark	How to Locate	Clinical Significance
External occipital protuberance (EOP)	Posterior: Midline projection of posterior aspect of skull at junction of head and neck.	A reference landmark for manipulative contact points lateral to EOP used with occipital (C0-C1) subluxations.
C2 spinous process	Posterior: First bony point palpated in midline inferior to EOP.	A reference landmark and contact point for manipulation. Tender with spinal fractures, infections, sprain/strains, neoplasia, and subluxations.
C6 spinous process	Posterior: Easily palpated in cervical flexion; moves (anteriorly) away from palpating finger during cervical extension.	Commonly used as a reference landmark and contact point for manipulation.
C7 spinous process	Posterior: Commonly the most prominent spinous process in this region. (T1 in some individuals). C7 moves on T1 during cervical flexion and extension.	Reference landmark and contact point for manipulation. Tender with spinal fractures, infections, sprain/strain, neoplasia, and subluxations.
Cervical facet joints	Posterior: Palpated 1.5-2 cm lateral to spinous processes.	Tenderness of soft tissue over these areas with common with joint sprain/strain, and subluxations.
C1 transverse process	Lateral: Palpated between mastoid process and angle of the jaw.	Commonly used as a contact point for manipulation. Tender with subluxation, sprain/strain.

Modified from Scaringe JG, Faye LJ: Palpation: the art of manual assessment. In Redwood D, Cleveland C, editors, *Fundamentals of chiropractic*, St Louis, 2003, Mosby, 211-237.

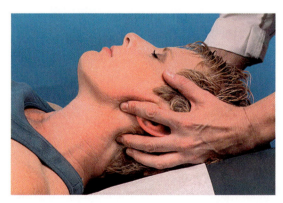

Figure 8-3   Palpation for flexion, extension, or rotation alignment of C1 on C2, evaluation of C1 transverse process to mandible distance.

atlanto-occipital articulation employs the inferior tip of the mastoid to C1 transverse process distance (Figure 8-4). Rotational and lateral flexion alignment at the atlantoaxial articulation can be palpated by comparing the bilateral relationship of the C1 transverse processes to the C2 articular pillars (Figure 8-5). Palpation for the alignment of the spinous processes in the lower cervical spine is conducted with the patient in the sitting position with the head flexed (Figure 8-6).[12]

Palpation for segmental motion includes evaluation of the discrete short-range movements of a joint that are independent of the action of voluntary muscles. This is determined by springing each vertebra in the neutral position (joint play), or at the limit of its passive range of movement (end feel), in addition to segmental range of motion. Joint play in the articulations of the cervical spine can be

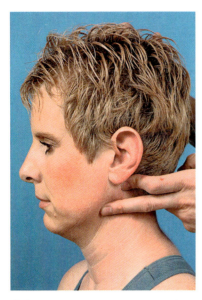

Figure 8-4   Lateral flexion alignment of the atlanto-occipital articulation using the inferior tip of the mastoid to C1 transverse process distance.

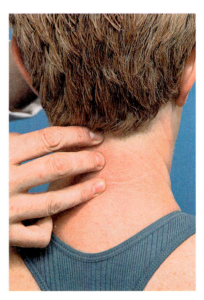

Figure 8-6   Palpation for alignment of the spinous processes in the lower cervical spine.

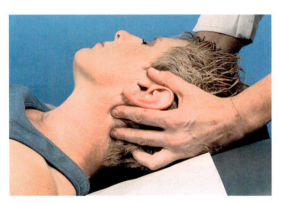

Figure 8-5   Palpation for rotation and lateral flexion alignment of the atlanto-occipital articulation compares the bilateral relationship of the C1 transverse process to the C2 articular pillars.

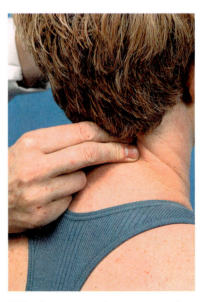

Figure 8-7   Sitting joint play assessment for posterior to anterior glide in the mid cervical spine.

evaluated with the patient seated or in the supine position. In the supine position the patient's head rests on the table, which is more comfortable when the patient is acute. Joint play and posterior-to-anterior glide are assessed in the cervical spine with the patient in the sitting position by bilaterally contacting the posterior joints with the palmar surfaces of the finger and thumb of the contact hand with the patient's forehead supported by the stabilizing hand (Figure 8-7). Each individual motion segment is evaluated for a fluid posterior-to-anterior gliding motion along the horizontal plane. With the patient

in the supine position, joint play and posterior-to-anterior glide are assessed by contacting the posterior joints with the fingertips (Figure 8-8). Lateral-to-medial glide may be assessed by contacting the posterolateral surface of adjacent vertebrae with the index fingers. One hand springs the segment toward the midline as the other hand stabilizes the patient's neck.[12]

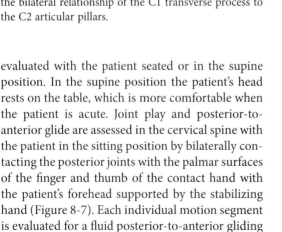

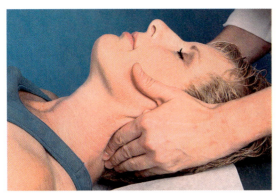

Figure 8-8 Joint play assessment for posterior-to-anterior glide in the mid cervical spine in the supine position.

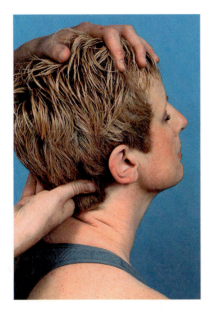

Figure 8-9 Palpation for flexion-extension movement of the right atlanto-occipital articulation.

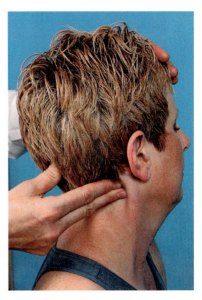

Figure 8-10 Palpation of left rotation at the atlanto-occipital articulation.

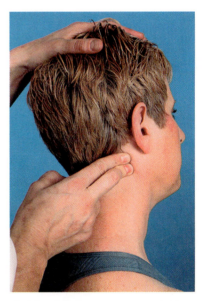

Figure 8-11 Palpation of left lateral flexion at the atlanto-occipital articulation.

Joint play motion should be uniform bilaterally and pain free. Unilateral resistance or a tendency for the spine to rotate away from the midline may indicate a subluxation. A subtle gliding motion with recoil is indicative of normal joint play, and absence of this motion is indicative of joint blockage. A boggy sensation or excessive sponginess indicates possible hypermobility or instability. End feel is assessed by application of pressure at the end of segmental range of motion testing. Atlanto-occipital (C0-C1) flexion and extension are evaluated by placing the tip of the index finger in the space between the mandibular ramus and the anterior tip of the atlas transverse process. This space increases during extension and decreases during flexion (Figure 8-9).[12] There is limited occipital rotation that occurs at the end of cervical rotation. The space between the mandibular ramus and the atlas transverse process will increase on the side opposite rotation and decrease on the side of rotation (Figure 8-10). To assess lateral flexion at the atlanto-occipital articulation, the index finger is placed between the inferior tip of the mastoid process and the atlas transverse process (Figure 8-11). The space

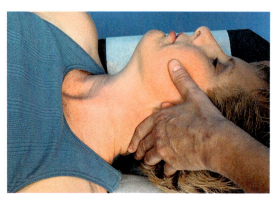

Figure 8-12   Palpation of right rotation at the atlantoaxial articulation.

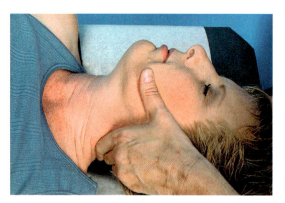

Figure 8-13   Palpation of right rotation at the C3-C4 motion segment with the patient in the supine position.

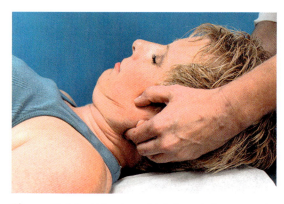

Figure 8-14   Palpation of left lateral flexion in the supine position with a fingertip contact.

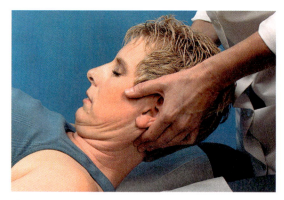

Figure 8-15   Palpation of cervical flexion with the patient in the supine position.

between the mastoid and atlas transverse increases as the head is laterally flexed away from the side of contact.[12]

Segmental range of motion at the atlantoaxial (C1-C2) region is assessed by contacting the posterolateral aspect of the transverse process of the atlas and the axis with the middle and index fingers so that they bridge the C1-C2 intertransverse space. The head is slightly laterally flexed toward the contact, then passively rotated away from the side of contact (Figure 8-12). Separation of the C1-C2 intertransverse space on the side opposite rotation should increase with rotation.[12]

Segmental range of motion in the lower cervical spine from C2 to C7 can be assessed with the patient seated or supine. Contact is established on the posterior surface of the articular pillars with the index finger on the side opposite cervical rotation (Figure 8-13). The superior pillar should move forward in relation to the one below with a stair-stepping effect from the lower to the upper cervical spine on full rotation.

To assess lateral flexion from C2 to C7, the patient is in the supine position. Either a bilateral fingertip or index contact is established over the articular pillars slightly posterior to the mid coronal plane (Figure 8-14). Lateral flexion with a slight inferior inclination is induced, and movement to each side is evaluated. To evaluate flexion and extension, contact is established bilaterally with the fingertips over the posterior articular pillars (Figure 8-15). Posterior inferior gliding of the articular pillars is palpated during extension, with anterior superior gliding palpated on flexion.[12]

Reliability and Validity of Clinical Indicators of Subluxation

Jull, working with others,[13-16] employed diagnostic anesthetic blocks to the facet joints as a gold standard to demonstrate the reliability and validity of motion palpation in the detection of cervical subluxations. These studies have reported on both noncontrolled and controlled trials. Humphrys, Delahaye, and Peterson[17] used anatomically blocked vertebrae as a gold standard to demonstrate the validity of motion palpation. The results of these studies justify the clinical use of motion palpation by trained clinicians in the diagnosis of restricted joint motion in the cervical spine.

Palpation of static segmental misalignment and tenderness can also be useful in the identification of subluxated motion segments in patients suffering from whiplash injuries.[18] (See Table 8-1.) Palpable misalignment of the C1 transverse processes, the C2 spinous process, and the C0-C3 posterior joints are common findings. (See Table 8-1.) This is supported by Jaeger,[7] who noted misalignment around the transverse process of C1 in cervicogenic headache patients following whiplash injury.

SYNDROMES ASSOCIATED WITH SUBLUXATION OF THE CERVICAL ARTICULATIONS

Several syndromes associated with subluxation of the cervical articulations have been identified.[19,20] Subluxation of the joints of the typical and atypical cervical motion segments produces neck pain and tenderness over the involved joints. Pain from subluxated articulations in the cervical region can refer up into the head, producing headache,[19] and down the ipsilateral upper extremity from lower cervical subluxations, creating cervical-brachial syndromes with symptoms characteristic of thoracic outlet syndromes.[19] Dysfunction of the cervical sympathetic ganglion thought to be due to the close relationship to cervical articulations can produce a cervical sympathetic syndrome. Pain referred into the upper thoracic region from the cervical articulations can produce cervicogenic dorsalgia.[19]

WHIPLASH-ASSOCIATED NECK PAIN

The predominant symptom following whiplash injury is neck pain that typically occurs in the posterior region of the neck.[20] The pain may radiate upward to the head and down the shoulder and arms, the thoracic region, and interscapular regions.[21] The onset of symptoms may be delayed up to 12 to 15 hours,[22] reaching peak intensity 48 to 72 hours post-whiplash injury.[4] After 72 hours, a decrease in symptoms can be expected in the majority of cases.[4] The delay in the onset of symptoms is thought to be due to the time required for traumatic edema and hemorrhage to occur in the injured soft tissues.[23] Low back pain may accompany neck pain[21] and is often overlooked initially because of the more severe cervical complaints.[3] Patients should be assessed for subluxation in all regions of the spine following whiplash trauma.[3]

Manipulation and mobilization are effective in the treatment of whiplash-associated neck pain with joint and ligamentous involvement. Table 8-2 summarizes the leading neck pain clinical trials involving spinal manipulation. Forceful manipulation should be delayed for the first 2 to 3 days in patients who have not experienced this form of therapy previously, as they may think that the manipulation has made them worse.[3] The RAND Appropriateness Study: Manipulation and Mobilization of the Cervical Spine suggested that short-term pain relief and enhancement of range of movement in cases of subacute and chronic neck pain can be accomplished by manipulation and mobilization. The study found that literature describing acute neck pain was scant.[24] Another study found that for neck complaints only, the mean improvement in the complaint as shown by the visual analogue scale (where patients rate the level of their pain on a scale of 0 to 10) was slightly better for manipulative rather than physical therapy.[25] A study of 100 subjects with unilateral neck pain with referral into the trapezius muscle found that immediately after the intervention, 85% of the manipulated group and 69% of the mobilized group reported pain improvement. The decreased pain intensity was more than 1.5 times greater in the manipulated group.[26]

WHIPLASH-ASSOCIATED HEADACHE RELATED TO JOINT SUBLUXATION DIAGNOSIS

Because studies of whiplash-associated headache from several diagnostic categories outlined in Chapter 7 have demonstrated response to cervical manipulation (see Table 8-2), this section will discuss these whiplash-associated headaches with the understanding that there are common characteristics in the diagnostic categories reported. The common pathway of the trigeminal complex (see Chapter 7) explains the pathophysiological process that produces the confusion over the three most commonly diagnosed benign, intermittent headache types: cervicogenic, tension type, and migraine without aura. There is considerable overlap in the pattern of symptoms that is characteristic of these three headache diagnoses. (See Chapter 7.) A fourth type of headache, the vertebrogenic headache,[27] has

TABLE **8-2**

Summary of Leading Neck Pain Clinical Trials Involving Spinal Manipulation

Author/Year	Branches	Number of Subjects	Complaint	Outcome	Follow-up
Sloop/1982	Detuned modalities, diazepam, physiotherapy	21 18	Chronic neck pain	Pain. No significant difference. Distinct trend favored manipulation.	3 weeks
Koes/1992	Manipulation and mobilization, massage, exercise, heat modalities, advice	21 13 17	Chronic neck pain	Severity of main complaint, physical functioning, perceived global efficiency.	6 weeks- 12 months
Skargren/1997	Chiropractic manipulation	219	Chronic neck pain	Pain improvement.	6-12 months
Rogers/ 1997	Manipulation/ exercise	10 10	Chronic neck pain	Pain improved 44% for manipulation 41% for exercise 12%.	
Jordon/1998	Manipulation/ physiotherapy Intensive training	40 40 39	Chronic neck pain	Disability. Medication use. All 3 groups showed improvement at end.	4-12 months
van Schalkwyk/ 2000	Rotary manipulation Lateral manipulation	10 10	Acute and chronic neck pain	Pain. Disability. Range of motion. Both groups improved; neither group had benefit over the other.	1 month

been used as a diagnosis for headaches generated by cervical subluxation, and although an accurate term, this diagnosis has largely fallen by the wayside.

The Medicare diagnostic criteria (see Box 8-1) for detecting subluxations that respond to manipulation when combined with the history and functional imaging are helpful in the diagnosis of this headache syndrome. In the absence of a single precise diagnostic category for headaches that respond to manipulation (Table 8-3), response to treatment will confirm that the pain-generating

structures are indeed related to the cervical articulations. Diagnostic blocks have been used to confirm the presence of cervicogenic headaches. In a posttraumatic headache study that compared headache subjects with an age and gender matched control group, at least one segment in the headache group demonstrated marked hypomobility in the upper cervical spine. Much greater joint dysfunction was noted between C0-C3 in the headache group compared with the control group. Jensen, Nielsen, and Vosmer[28] also reported findings of hypomobility in

TABLE **8-3**

Headache Outcomes Research Using Spinal Manipulation

Headache Type	Author/Year	Number of Patients/Arms	Outcomes	Design
Tension	Bitterli/1977	Manipulation/no treatment	Pain.	RCT
Tension	Hoyt/1979	22 (Group 1) Palpation; (Group 2) Palpation plus manipulation; (Group 3) No treatment	Group 2 showed significant improvement in mean headache severity.	
Tension	Droz/1985	332 Manipulation	Pain, 80% success.	RS
Tension	Boline/1995	126 Manipulation/ amitriptyline	Frequency. Total pain. OTC, Global Health. Manipulation group maintained improvement at end of treatment/medication group reverted to baseline.	RCT
Tension	Mootz/1994	11 Manipulation/cold packs	Frequency/duration. Statistically significant decrease.	
Tension	Bove/1998	75 Manipulation/laser	Analgesic use. Frequency/ intensity decreased. All groups improved; no significant distinction between them.	RCT
Tension	Vernon/2009	9 Manipulation/ amitriptyline manipulation/placebo sham/amitriptyline sham/placebo	Frequency/duration. In adjusted analysis, neither the main effects of manipulation nor amitriptyline was statistically significant nor clinically important, but effect of combined treatments was in both respects.	RCT
Cervicogenic	Nilsson/1995	54 Manipulation/ analgesic use	Frequency/intensity. Improvement in manipulation group was statistically significant over analgesic use group.	RCT
Cervicogenic	Whittingham/2001	105 Toggle manipulation/ sham (inactivated Pettibon adjustment)	Sickness impact. Neck Disability Index. Pain drawings and diaries. Manipulation group showed significant improvements in frequency, severity duration, and medication use.	RCT

Continued

TABLE **8-3**

Headache Outcomes Research Using Spinal Manipulation—Cont'd

Headache Type	Author/Year	Number of Patients/Arms	Outcomes	Design
Cervicogenic	Jull/2002	200 Manipulation/exercise/combined	Frequency/intensity/duration. Frequency and intensity improved in both groups and in combined treatment (10% more in latter arm).	RCT
Cervicogenic	Haas/2004	24 Manipulation dose response	Disability. Number of headaches. Significant benefits in pain, disability with higher (9-12) doses.	RCT
Migraine	Parker/1978	85 Mobilization/manipulation DC/manipulation MD	Frequency/intensity/duration. In manipulation group: 28% success, 47% success at 2 years.	RCT
Migraine	Nelson/1998	209 Manipulation/amitriptyline manipulation/amitriptyline and OTC use	Frequency/intensity. All 3 groups improved; post treatment; showed more sustained improvement for manipulation only.	RCT
Migraine	Tuchin/2000	Manipulation/detuned ultrasound	Intensity/duration/disability. Associated symptoms. Medications. Statistically significant improvement in frequency, duration, disability, medication use.	RCT
Posttraumatic	Jensen/1990	19 Manipulation/cold packs	Pain Index/ROM/associated symptoms. Significant improvements in all outcomes in manipulation group.	RCT
Pediatric	Kastner/1995	12 Manipulation		
Pediatric	Anderson/Peacock/1996	5 Manipulation	Chief complaints (frequency, severity) resolved in all cases	Case reports

DC, Doctor of Chiropractic; MD, Medical Doctor; OTC, over-the-counter; RCT, randomized clinical trial; ROM, range of motion.
Modified by Rosner AJ. From Redwood D, Cleveland C, editors, *Fundamentals of chiropractic*, St Louis, 2003, Mosby, pp. 482-483.

a clinical trial of 19 posttraumatic headache patients treated with manipulation.

INCIDENCE OF POST-WHIPLASH HEADACHE

A retrospective study by Radanov, Di Stephano, and Augustiny[29] of 112 patients with post-whiplash headaches reported neck pain was associated with headache in 93% of cases. Most patients reported that headaches only began following the whiplash injury. Of these, 37% were given the label of tension type headache, 27% migraine, and 18% cervicogenic. An additional 18% were unclassified. Two further prospective studies of whiplash-induced headache reported a similar incidence of the three major headache types.

HEADACHE RESPONSE TO MANIPULATION

Headache response to manipulation has been demonstrated utilizing various research designs. Although not specific to post-whiplash headaches, the outcomes of these studies validate the use of manipulation for the treatment of the three main headache types commonly diagnosed post whiplash. (See Table 8-3.) These included randomized controlled trials,[30-38] and case series, retrospective series, or prospective series.[39-42]

POSTERIOR CERVICAL SYMPATHETIC SYNDROME AND THE VERTEBRAL ARTERIES

In 1958, Ruth Jackson[43] reported a number of seemingly bizarre symptoms that appeared to be precipitated by whiplash trauma. The first to describe this syndrome were Barré[44] in 1926 and Liéou[45] in 1928. Symptoms include blurring of vision, dilation of pupil, vertigo, tinnitus, auditory disturbance, and headache. Barré[44] described the headache as mainly suboccipital and the vertigo as mainly precipitated by turning the head and not accompanied by any other vestibular dysfunction. Similar symptoms have been observed in patients injured in motor vehicle accidents.[46] These symptoms were described by Jackson in her classic work on cervical syndrome.[43] She suggested that they are due in part to occlusion of the vertebral arteries. She noted the susceptibility of the vertebral arteries to trauma at the time of neck injuries. Encroachment on the arteries by osteophytes and bony anomalies such as

a ponticulus posticus can become symptomatic when swelling and other components of inflammation result from whiplash-associated injury. In addition, irritation of the vertebral sympathetic plexus surrounding the vertebral artery can produce similar symptoms.[46] Headaches, dizziness, tinnitus, and ocular symptoms following whiplash injuries have been attributed to root sleeve defects at C3-C4, where the C4 nerve root communicates with the superior cervical ganglion of the sympathetic chain through a branch of the postganglionic fibers.[47] Clinically, a subluxation can cause some or all of these signs and symptoms. If extension and rotation produce any of these symptoms, caution is advised against performing manipulation of the neck in an extension and rotation position. This does not preclude manipulation with modification of the position of the cervical spine. An additional test can suggest a vertebral artery syndrome (Figure 8-16). Cervical manipulation of post-whiplash subluxation syndromes may relieve the characteristic signs and symptoms.[48]

Calcification of the atlanto-occipital ligament(s), known as the ponticulus posticus and ponticulus lateralis, may also be a factor that produces symptoms of vertebral artery compromise during extension and rotation.[48] These anomalous ossification centers bridge the vertebral artery sulci, forming bony arches enclosing the foramen arcuate. The complex has been called Kimerle's anomaly and can produce a bony canal that can compromise the vertebral artery as it passes upward into the skull.[48] It has been reported that surgical excision in some cases has relieved symptoms including vertigo, headaches, and nausea.[49] Four of five patients with symptoms of vertebral artery compromise on extension and rotation in a series of 2,000 patients tested showed a ponticulus posticus on radiographic evaluation. Surgical repair of the fifth with a ligated carotid artery had complete remission of symptoms and a negative test after surgical repair.[49] In patients with this anomaly who become symptomatic following whiplash trauma, a trial of more conservative therapy is recommended first. Resolution of the symptoms can occur with time in some cases.

CERVICOGENIC DORSALGIA

Cervicogenic dorsalgia is pain expressed in the thoracic region having its genesis in the cervical spine.[50] The diagnosis of cervicogenic dorsalgia is inadequate for a precise diagnosis, and the cervical

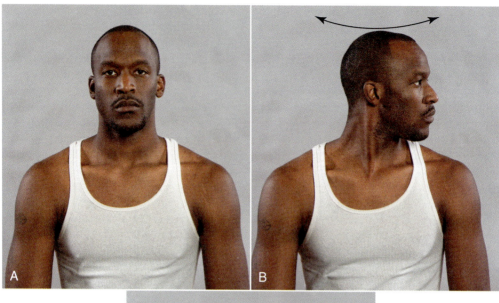

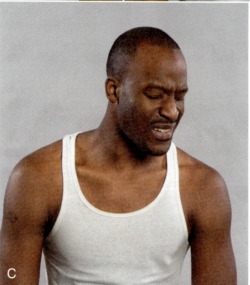

Figure 8-16 **A,** The patient is seated as comfortably and erect as possible following blood pressure and pulse assessment. **B,** The patient rotates the head maximally from side to side. This movement is performed slowly at first and then accelerated until the patient's tolerance is reached. **C,** A vertebral artery syndrome is suggested by vertigo, nystagmus, blurred vision, nausea, or syncope. These symptoms may occur singly or in any combination. The test should be halted if the patient exhibits any of the listed signs.

segment involved must be identified. Although frequently caused by postural stresses, cervicogenic dorsalgia can result from whiplash trauma to the cervical spine. The thoracic pain may be accompanied by neck pain, but this is not always present, making diagnosis more difficult.[51] Palpatory findings of restricted motion in a cervical segment are most definitive, but pain in the thoracic region when the patient actively rotates the head may be the first clue. With treatment including manipulation directed to the involved cervical motion segment, the thoracic pain can be relieved.[51]

CERVICAL-BRACHIAL SYNDROME

Cervical-brachial pain is often referred to as nonspecific arm pain, or neck/arm syndrome. Symptoms may include neck pain, and shoulder, arm, and hand pain in addition to sensory symptoms such as paresthesia, hypoesthesia, hyperesthesia, vasomotor changes and weakness.[52] Barnsley, Lord, and Bogduk[53] reported a frequent occurrence of these symptoms in chronic whiplash patients. This is supported by Sterling, Treleaven, and Jull,[54] who found that approximately 60% of chronic whiplash patients with symptoms longer than 3 months duration also reported the presence of arm pain. Individuals with arm symptoms have been found to be more disabled than those with neck pain only, with an effect on overall health status.[55]

Potential causes of cervical-brachial pain are neurovascular irritation or compression from inflammation, somatic referral from trigger points in injured muscles (see Chapter 6), radiculopathy, and referral from the cervical zygapophyseal joints.[56] The segmental levels that may refer pain from the zygapophyseal joints are C5-C6, C6-C7, and C7-T1.[57] It is critical that all of these pain generators be assessed to prevent long-term upper extremity symptoms in patients suffering from whiplash trauma. Referred pain is more likely to be felt as a deep ache with radicular pain described as sharper, shooting, or lancinating in nature. This is not always definitive, however, and nerve conduction studies are necessary for a more precise diagnosis. Provocation tests (see Chapter 4), in addition to palpatory findings from muscle trigger points that pinpoint referred pain from muscles, and palpation of cervical joint motion, are also useful.[58]

CONSERVATIVE MANAGEMENT OF CERVICAL-BRACHIAL PAIN

Significant and immediate reduction in pain following manual therapy when compared to ultrasound has been reported in the cervical spine.[53] In the lumbar spine, an animal study indicated that the effects of manipulation reduced pain severity and duration in rats with induced dorsal root ganglia inflammation.[59] In addition, electrophysiological and pathological manifestations of inflammation were reduced.[54]

CERVICAL SUBLUXATION SYNDROMES

A subluxation syndrome has been defined as *an aggregate of signs and symptoms that relate to pathophysiological or dysfunction of spinal and pelvic motion segments or to peripheral joints.*[5] Although the signs and symptoms characteristic of subluxation syndromes are not always due to a subluxation, when they are, the condition is commonly responsive to manual and manipulative procedures. Subluxation of the upper cervical complex is a risk factor for headache and localized neck pain. Subluxation of the lower cervical vertebra and the first rib are risk factors for a cervical-brachial syndrome. Victims of whiplash injuries may develop symptoms in the upper extremities from subluxation of the lower cervical spine and first rib that can be considered risk factors for cervical-brachial problems. A careful differential diagnosis that identifies subluxation of this region is necessary as there are a number of sites where dysfunction can cause hand and arm symptoms.

REFERENCES

1. Sjaastad O: Cervicogenic headache: A mini state-of-the-art, *Headache Quarterly, Current Treatment and Research* 8:151, 1997.
2. Adams MA: Biomechanics of the cervical spine. In Gunzburg R, Szpalski M, editors: *Whiplash injuries: current concepts in prevention, diagnosis, and treatment of the cervical whiplash syndrome,* Philadelphia, 1998, Lippincott Williams & Wilkins, pp 13-20.
3. Gatterman MI, Panzer DM: Disorders of the cervical spine. In Gatterman MI, editor: *Chiropractic management of spine-related disorders,* 2nd ed, Baltimore, 2003, Lippincott Williams & Wilkins, pp 229-281.
4. Spitzer WO, et al: Scientific monograph of the Quebec task force on whiplash-associated disorders: redefining "whiplash" and its management, *Spine* 20:S8-S58, 1995.
5. Gatterman MI, Hansen D: Development of chiropractic nomenclature through consensus, *J Manipulative Physiol Ther* 17:302-309, 1994.
6. Peterson CK, Gatterman MI: The nonmanipulable subluxation. In Gatterman MI, editor: *Principles of chiropractic: subluxation,* 2nd ed, St Louis, 2005, Mosby, pp 168-190.
7. Jaeger B: Cervicogenic headache: a relationship to cervical spine dysfunction and myofascial trigger points, *Cephalalgia* (suppl 7):398, 1987.
8. Grice AS: Pathomechanics of the upper cervical spine. In Vernon H, editor: *Upper cervical syndromes,* Baltimore, 1988, Williams & Wilkins, pp 103-112.
9. Medicare Benefit Policy, Chapter 15. Covered medical and other health services. http://www.cms.gov/manuals/Downloads/bp102c15.pdf
10. Bergmann T: Chiropractic technique. In Gatterman MI, editor: *Principles of chiropractic: subluxation,* 2nd ed, St Louis, 2005, Mosby, pp 133-167.

11. Scaringe JG, Faye LJ: Palpation: the art of manual assessment. In Redwood D, Cleveland C, editors: *Fundamentals of chiropractic*, St Louis, 2003, Mosby, pp 211-237.

12. Gatterman MI, Hyland JK: Whiplash. In Gatterman MI, editor: *Principles of chiropractic: subluxation*, 2nd ed, St Louis, 2005, Mosby, pp 429-447.

13. Jull G: Manual diagnosis of C2-3 headache, *Cephalalgia* 5(suppl 5):308-309, 1985.

14. Jull GA: Headaches associated with the cervical spine: a clinical review. In Grieve GP, editor: *Modern manual therapy of the vertebral column*, New York, 1986, Churchill Livingstone, pp 322-329.

15. Jull G, Bogduk N, Marsland A: The accuracy of manual diagnosis for cervical zygapophyseal joint pain syndromes, *Med J Aust* 148:233-236, 1988.

16. Jull G, et al: Interexaminer reliability to detect painful upper cervical zygapophyseal joint dysfunction, *Aust J Physiother* 43:125-129, 1997.

17. Humphrys BK, Delahaye M, Peterson CK: An investigation into the validity of cervical spine motion palpation using subjects with congenital block vertebrae as a "gold standard," *BMC Musculoskelet Disord* 5:19, 2004.

18. Treleavan J, Jull G, Atkinson L: Cervical musculoskeletal dysfunction in post-concussion headache, *Cephalalgia* 14:273-279, 1994.

19. Gatterman MI: Introduction to Part 3. In *Principles of chiropractic: subluxation*, 2nd ed, St Louis, 2005, Mosby, pp 373-375.

20. Jull G, et al: Whiplash associated disorders. In Jull G, et al, editors: *Principles of chiropractic: subluxation*, 2nd ed, St Louis, 2005, Mosby, pp 373-375.

21. Barnsley L, Lord S, Bogduk N: Clinical review: whiplash injury, *Pain* 58:283-307, 1994.

22. Provinciali L, Baroni M: Clinical approaches to whiplash injuries: a review, *Crit Rev Phys Rehabil Med* 11:339-368, 1999.

23. Teasal RW, Shapiro AP: Whiplash injuries. In Giles LGF, Singer KP, editors: Clinical management of cervical spine pain, vol 3, Oxford, 1998, Butterworth Heinemann, pp 71-86.

24. Coulter I, et al: *The appropriateness of spinal manipulation and mobilization of the cervical spine: literature review, indications and ratings by a multidisciplinary expert panel (Monograph no DRU-982-1-CCR)*, Santa Monica, 1995, RAND.

25. Koes BW, et al: A randomized clinical trial of manual therapy and physiotherapy for persistent back and neck complaints: subgroup analysis and relationship between outcome measures, *J Manipulative Physiol Ther* 16:211-219, 1993.

26. Cassidy JD, Lopes AA, Yong-Hing K: The immediate effect of manipulation versus mobilization on pain and range of motion in the cervical spine: a randomized controlled trial, *J Manipulative Physiol Ther* 15(9):570-575, 1992.

27. Vernon HT: Vertebrogenic headache. In Vernon HT, editor: *Upper cervical syndrome: chiropractic diagnosis and management*, Baltimore, 1988, Williams & Wilkins, pp 152-188.

28. Jensen IK, Nielsen FF, Vosmer L: An open study comparing manual therapy with the use of cold packs in the treatment of post-traumatic headache, *Cephalalgia* 10:241-250, 1990.

29. Radanov B, Di Stephano G, Augustiny K: Symptomatic approach to posttraumatic headache and its possible implications for treatment, *Eur Spine J* 10:403-407, 2001.

30. Boline P, et al: Spinal manipulation vs. amitriptyline for the treatment of chronic tension type headaches: a randomized clinical trial, *J Manipulative Physiol Ther* 18:148-154, 1995.

31. Nilsson N: A randomized controlled trial of the effect of spinal manipulation in the treatment of cervicogenic headache, *J Manipulative Physiol Ther* 18:435-440, 1995.

32. Nilsson N, Christensen HW, Hartvigsen J: The effect of spinal manipulation in the treatment of cervicogenic headache, *J Manipulative Physiol Ther* 20:326-330, 1997.

33. Bove G, Nilsson N: Spinal manipulation in the treatment of episodic tension-type headache: a randomized controlled trial, *N Engl J Med* 280:1576-1579, 1998.

34. Parker GB, Tupling H, Pryor DS: A controlled trial of cervical manipulation for migraine, *Aust NZ J Med* 8:589-593, 1978.

35. Parker GB, Pryor DS, Tupling H: Why does migraine improve during a clinical trial? Further results from a trial of cervical manipulation, *Aust NZ J Med* 10:192-198, 1980.

36. Tuchin P, Pollard H, Bonello R: A randomized controlled trial of chiropractic spinal manipulative therapy for migraine, *J Manipulative Physiol Ther* 23:91-95, 2000.

37. Whitingham W: *Randomized placebo controlled clinical trial of efficacy of chiropractic treatment of chronic cervicogenic headaches*. Symposium proceedings, 6th biennial congress, World Federation of Chiropractic. Paris, May 21-26, 2001.

38. Nelson CF, et al: The efficacy of spinal manipulation, amitriptyline and the combination of both therapies in the prophylaxis of migraine headache, *J Manipulative Physiol Ther* 21:511-519, 1998.

39. Mootz RD, et al: Chiropractic treatment of chronic episodic tension-type headache in male subjects: a case series analysis, *J Can Chiropr Assoc* 38:152-159, 1994.

40. Droz JM, Crot F: Occipital headaches: statistical results in the treatment of vertebrogenic headache, *Ann Swiss Chiro Assn* 8:127-136, 1985.

41. Vernon HT: Spinal manipulation and headaches of cervical origin, *J Manipulative Physiol Ther* 12(6):455-468, 1989.

42. Stodolny J, Chmielewski H: Manual therapy in the treatment of patients with cervical migraine, *Man Med* 4:49-51, 1989.

43. Jackson R: *The cervical syndrome*, 4th ed, Springfield, IL, 1977, Charles C Thomas.

44. Barré J: Sur un syndrome sympathique cervical postérieure et sa cause fréquente: l'arthrite cervicale, *Rev Neurol* 45:1246-1248, 1926. In Sandstorm J: Cervical syndrome with vestibular symptoms, *Acta Otolaryngol* 54:207, 1961.

45. Liéou YC: *Syndrome sympathique cervical postérieur et arthrite chronique de la colonne vertébrale cervicale Étude clinique et radiologique.* Thèse de Strasborg 1928. In Sandstorm J, Cervical syndrome with vestibular symptoms, *Acta Otolaryngol* 54:207, 1961.

46. Stewart DY: Current concepts of "Barré syndrome" or the posterior cervical sympathetic syndromes, *Clin Orthop Rel Res* 24:40-48, 1962.

47. Tamura T: Cranial symptoms after cervical injury. Aetiology and treatment of the Barré-Liéou syndrome, *J Bone Joint Surg Br* 71:283-287, 1989.

48. Gatterman MI: Patient safety. In Gatterman MI, editor: *Chiropractic management of spine-related disorders*, 2nd ed, Baltimore, 2003, Lippincott Williams & Wilkins, pp 69-86.

49. Wight S, Osborne N, Breen AC: Incidence of ponticulus posterior of the atlas in migraine and cervicogenic headache, *J Manipulative Physiol Ther* 22:15-20, 1999.

50. Terrett A, Terrett R: Referred posterior thoracic pain of cervical posterior rami origin: a cause of much misdirected treatment, *Chiro J Aust* 3:42-51, 2002.

51. Engel GR, Gatterman MI: Cervicogenic dorsalgia. In Gatterman MI, editor: *Principles of chiropractic: subluxation*, 2nd ed, St Louis, 2005, Mosby, pp 448-456.

52. Cohen M, et al: In search of the pathogenesis of refractory cervicobrachial pain syndrome, *Med J Aust* 156:432-436, 1992.

53. Barnsley L, Lord S, Bogduk N: Clinical review. Whiplash injury, *Pain* 58:283-307, 1994.

54. Sterling M, Treleaven J, Jull G: Responses to a clinical test of mechanical provocation of nerve tissue in whiplash associated disorders, *Man Ther* 7:89-94, 2002.

55. Daffner S, et al: Impact of neck and arm pain on overall health status, *Spine* 28:2030-2035, 2003.

56. Fukui S, et al: Referred pain distribution of the cervical zygapophyseal joints and cervical dorsal rami, *Pain* 68:79-83, 1996.

57. Bogduk N: The neck, *Baillieres Clin Rheumatol* 13:261-285, 1999.

58. Coppieters M, et al: Aberrant protective force generation during neural provocation testing and the effect of treatment in patients with neurogenic cervicobrachial pain, *J Manipulative Physiol Ther* 26:99-106, 2003.

59. Song X-J, et al: Spinal manipulation reduces pain and hyperalgesia after lumbar intervertebral foramen inflammation in the rat, *J Manipulative Ther* 29:5-13, 2006.

Chapter 9

Epidemiology of Whiplash Injuries

Michael T. Haneline

Epidemiology has been defined as "the science concerned with the study of the factors determining and influencing the frequency and distribution of disease, injury, and other health-related events and their causes in a defined human population for the purpose of establishing programs to prevent and control their development and spread."[1] Hence, this chapter will cover the numbers of persons who experience whiplash injuries, mainly in the United States, as well as factors that are thought to influence the risk of becoming injured in a motor vehicle crash (MVC) or of developing chronic symptoms post-injury. Many such factors have been suggested, including the injured person's age, gender, anthropometry, certain pre-existing conditions, position within the vehicle, the vehicle's crashworthiness, and others. Clinicians should be familiar with the significant risk factors in order to formulate more personalized treatment plans and prognoses in whiplash patients.

Epidemiological studies have been used extensively to investigate the whiplash phenomenon, primarily because the condition is not amenable to investigation using randomized controlled trials, which are considered to be the gold standard of clinical research. This is primarily because it would be unethical to expose people to the kinds of forces that are capable of causing injuries involved in MVCs. Thus, whiplash studies typically compare a group of people who have already been involved in MVCs with another group who have not. Researchers either follow the groups forward in time (i.e., cohort studies) or assess various aspects of their medical history retrospectively, before as well as after the time of the crash (i.e., case-control studies).

Studies have been carried out where human volunteers were exposed to whiplash-like forces (i.e., crash tests) similar to what would be expected in a real-life MVC. However, they have always simulated relatively low-speed crashes and rarely resulted in symptoms.[2-4] When symptoms did occur, they have been mild and short-lived. Also, these types of studies have never randomized subjects to groups for comparisons.

Epidemiology is commonly used in the field of public health, which focuses on the study of populations with the purpose of identifying the causes of diseases and conditions. Once the causes are identified, strategies can be developed that are designed to prevent the diseases from occurring. Public health interventions, such as advising people about the best ways to avoid risk factors or how they can integrate protective factors into their lifestyles, can effectively prevent future injuries and illness, as well as enhance the healing process when injury or illness has already occurred. Traffic safety matters, including whiplash, are of interest to public health practitioners, health care providers, as well as local, state, and national governments because of the potential to prevent or reduce the severity of crash-related injuries using these preventive methods.

One aspect of epidemiology involves collecting data from various sources and then analyzing it. However, the data pertaining to the epidemiology of whiplash is at times conflicting—sometimes because of inconsistencies in the way the data were gathered and other times in the way they were analyzed. It is also possible, and not that uncommon, for data collection and analysis to go awry at the same time. These inaccuracies can often be resolved by relying on higher-quality information sources, though even high-quality sources are not always in agreement. In addition to the potential flaws associated with the collection, analysis, and reporting of data, the way data are interpreted is often inconsistent. This chapter will call attention to some of these controversial aspects in relation to whiplash, relying on the highest-quality studies available.

Not only is the way data are collected and interpreted inconsistent in this area of investigation, the term "whiplash" itself is controversial: whereas some researchers use it to describe a mechanism of injury in which the head and neck are forcibly moved beyond the limits of anatomical integrity, others use it to describe the injury that often results. Consequently, the Quebec Task Force on Whiplash-Associated Disorders coined the term "whiplash-associated disorders" (WAD) in 1995 to describe an array of symptoms that have been reported in association with whiplash injuries.[5] According to the Quebec Task Force, WAD symptoms may include neck pain and stiffness, headache, dizziness, tinnitus, memory loss, deafness, dysphagia, upper extremity syndromes (e.g., radicular symptoms and carpal tunnel syndrome), temporomandibular joint disorder, and others.

BASIC EPIDEMIOLOGICAL TERMS

There are some basic terms that are essential to the understanding of the science of epidemiology, a few of which are listed here.

- Association—When two or more attributes are related to each other in such a way that they change predictably together.
- Bias—Anything that causes the conclusions of a study to be systematically different from the truth. Bias may occur in the way data are collected, analyzed, and/or interpreted.
- Case—A person in an epidemiological study who has the disease or condition under investigation. These persons are members of the cases group in a case-control study.
- Case-control study—A type of epidemiological study in which participants are separated into two groups: members of one group have the disease or condition under study (the cases), and those in the other group do not (the controls). The groups are assessed concerning previous exposure to various factors or the presence of certain traits, and then rates of exposure/traits are compared between cases and controls.
- Cause—Refers to a factor that has a direct effect on the occurrence of a disease or condition. The factor could be an intrinsic trait or a behavior of the persons being studied or some event they were exposed to.
- Cohort—A distinct group of people who have something in common, such as being exposed to a common risk factor or being born in the same year.
- Cohort study—A type of epidemiological study that follows one or more cohorts forward in time to determine the incidence of new diseases, conditions, and/or deaths that occur. Typically, one cohort is exposed to a risk factor, while the comparison cohort is not. The rates of the measured outcomes are then compared between the groups to see if members of the exposed cohort are more likely to develop the disease or condition.
- Exposure—An external factor that may have an impact on the health of a person if the person is exposed to that factor.
- Incidence—The number of newly diagnosed cases of a disease within a specified population during a specified time period, which is typically 1 year. The denominator is the population under consideration and the numerator is the number of new cases that develop during the given time period. The incidence rate may be calculated by dividing the number of new cases of a disease in a given time period by the number of persons in the population who are at risk for the disease.
- Odds ratio (OR)—An estimate of the odds of developing a disease given that a person was exposed to a relevant risk factor. It is the odds of being exposed to the risk factor under investigation in the cases divided by the odds of being exposed in the control group, which is calculated from data in case-control studies.

- Prevalence—The number of persons in a population who have a given disease or attribute at a particular point in time (point prevalence) or over a specified period of time (period prevalence). The prevalence rate is calculated by dividing the total number of cases of a disease within a population by the total population.
- Relative risk (RR)—The probability of disease being present in the exposed group, divided by the probability of disease in the unexposed group, which is commonly calculated in cohort studies.
- Risk—The likelihood that a person will experience a given event (e.g., become injured).
- Risk factor—A behavior, environmental exposure, or inherent characteristic of an individual that increases the likelihood of that individual's developing a disease or condition.

FREQUENCY OF WHIPLASH

Incidence

The incidence of whiplash refers to the number of new cases that are diagnosed each year in a given population. Due to the previously mentioned problems with collecting whiplash-related data, estimates of whiplash incidence vary greatly, ranging from 3.4 per 100,000[6] to 800 per 100,000[7] population per year. A Swedish study reported the annual incidence of whiplash in the local catchment area to be 4.2 per 1,000 inhabitants for grade 1 WAD and 3.2 per 1,000 for grade 3.[8] Holm et al[9] reported that the incidence of reported WAD in the Western world is probably at least 300 per 100,000 inhabitants per year. A commonly quoted statistic that refers to the rate of whiplash in the United States is 1,000,000 total cases per year.[10]

The Insurance Institute for Highway Safety (IIHS) reported that approximately 2 million whiplash insurance claims are filed each year in the United States, resulting in more than $8.5 billion in insurance claims.[11] In fact, neck sprains and strains are the most frequent type of injury claim reported to insurance companies in the United States, comprising 25% of all injury-related claim dollars paid out by insurers each year. The institute also reported that about 10% of whiplash injuries result in long-term medical problems. In the Canadian province of Saskatchewan, 83% of traffic injury claims were for whiplash in 1994-1995, resulting in an annual incidence of 677 insurance claims per 100,000 adult population.[12]

In addition to the cases that were included in the IIHS data, there are likely other cases of whiplash that occur but do not give rise to an insurance claim. This is because injured persons may not choose to open a claim (perhaps they do not want their insurance rates raised or they think their injuries are minor) or they are not insured. Thus, the true number of cases per year in the United States is almost certainly higher than 2,000,000, especially when non–traffic related whiplash injuries are factored in.

There are quite a few reasons why the various data sources so often generate different numbers. For instance, the National Accident Sampling System (NASS) provides data on all types of MVCs, including those that result in whiplash injuries. NASS data are collected from police-reported traffic crashes,[13] which is very problematic when trying to obtain an estimate of the actual number of whiplash injuries that occur in the United States. Many MVCs that give rise to whiplash injuries are not reported to police because they do not typically investigate crashes that involve minor vehicle damage, and many whiplash-causing crashes are associated with minor to no vehicle damage. These injured persons "slip through the cracks" and are not included in the NASS database, and this results in an underestimation of the annual number of injuries by possibly hundreds of thousands. Even when police do investigate MVCs that result in whiplash, sometimes symptoms are delayed for hours and days; consequently, these cases are also unreported.

Prevalence

The prevalence of WAD includes the previously mentioned incident cases (i.e., newly injured), but it also includes the total number of people who have persistent symptoms and physical impairments that are not included when only incident cases are counted. It represents the estimated number of persons in a population who manifest WAD symptoms at any given time. Many people experience residual problems for years after a whiplash injury and some never recover. These cases keep mounting in numbers until some of them recover or die. In either case, they are no longer included in calculation of prevalence.

The duration of a disease has an effect on its reported incidence and prevalence. For instance, short-duration diseases like the common cold tend to have a high annual incidence but low prevalence. Because people recover so quickly, not many will have the condition at any one point in time. On the other hand, long-duration diseases like diabetes may have a relatively low annual incidence, yet its prevalence is quite high because the total number of cases keeps accumulating. This principle applies to WAD too, because many affected people experience long-term symptoms. A study from the Netherlands reported that the highest prevalence of MVC-related neck sprain was 28.3 per 100,000 and occurred in those who were in the 25- to 29-year-old age group, with the 40- to 44-year-old group a close second at 27.9 per 100,000.[6] As mentioned earlier, the incidence of WAD in the United States is probably into the millions, and approximately half of those with WAD continue to report neck pain 1 year after their injuries,[14] so its prevalence is undoubtedly very high. In fact, Freeman et al[15] estimated, from a case-control study comprised of 419 chronic neck pain cases and 246 chronic low back pain controls, that about 6.2% of the U.S. population may have chronic neck pain attributable to a whiplash injury.

Chronicity

There is a great deal of controversy and debate surrounding the determination of which risk factors actually contribute to chronic WAD (aka, late whiplash syndrome) and which ones are merely associated by chance. Furthermore, some even question the legitimacy of chronic WAD, considering it to be a psychosocial phenomenon rather than being physically based.[16] As a result of this dichotomy, there has been much debate about this issue in the whiplash-related literature. As stated so well by Dr. Murray Allen, "There are two great puzzles in this world that foster debate among humans. One is the wonder of the universe, the other is whiplash."[17]

A large proportion of persons with chronic neck pain in the United States were initially injured in an MVC. This estimate was based on a case-control study involving 419 cases and 246 control subjects which reported that 45% of those with chronic neck pain considered its origin to have been a prior MVC.[15] On the other hand, a study that was based on a random sample of 6,000 subjects from two counties in Northern Sweden reported that 42% had chronic neck pain and only about 8% of them attributed their condition to a previous whiplash injury.[18]

Most WAD patients recover in time, although many have long-lasting and even permanent pain and impairment. For instance, a cohort of 2,627 persons with whiplash that resulted from an MVC in Canada was followed for up to 7 years.[19] The median time to recovery for the overall group was 32 days, although 12% of the subjects still had symptoms at 6 months. Several risk factors for chronic symptoms were identified in this study, including neck pain on palpation, muscle pain, pain or numbness radiating from the neck to the upper extremities, and headache. Females over 60 years old who had the identified risk factors required a median of 262 days to recover compared with only 17 days for younger males without any risk factors.

Several studies have reported that approximately 50% of WAD patients continue to complain of symptoms 1 year following injury.[20-22] Other studies, however, have found the rate of long-term WAD symptoms to be lower,[8,23-25] and some have reported it as being much lower.[26-28] To complicate the issue further, one study found the prevalence of long-term pain following whiplash injuries to be very close to the same level as the prevalence of chronic neck pain in the general population.[29]

Neck and shoulder pain are commonly reported symptoms of chronic WAD. Symptoms involving other bodily regions and overall health have been reported as well, including headache, back pain, jaw pain, fatigue, dizziness, paraesthesiae, nausea, sleep disturbances, and ill health.[30,31] Depression has also been reported following whiplash injuries. In one study, 42.3% of 5,211 subjects who did not have pre-injury mental health problems reported depressive symptoms within 6 weeks of the injury.[32] Furthermore, the symptoms were recurrent or persistent in almost 40% of the cases. Berglund et al[30] concluded that whiplash injuries due to rear-impact MVCs have a substantial impact on health complaints, even a long time after the injury.

A systematic review and meta-analysis involving 38 cohort studies that followed subjects with acute whiplash reported that recovery rates were extremely variable across studies.[33] Most subjects recovered within 3 months after the injury, and recovery rates leveled off after 3 months had elapsed. The review's authors suggested that data concerning prognostic factors thought to be associated with a poor recovery were difficult to interpret because of the dissimilar ways studies assessed associations, differences in their methods of reporting data, as well as differences in the outcome measures that were used.

WHIPLASH RISK FACTORS

Risk Factors for Developing WAD

Numerous studies have assessed the influence of a variety of risk factors on the probability of developing WAD subsequent to an MVC. Example risk factors include position of the occupant within the vehicle, head position (e.g., rotated), female gender, head-to-neck ratio, prior neck injury, use of safety belts, and crash severity. The results of these studies have been conflicting for the most part, but a few WAD risk factors have emerged as being important.

The underlying mechanism of whiplash is best explained by distortion of the neck that results from sudden movement of the head in relation to the torso. Thus, automobile head restraints and reactive seat backs are designed to minimize the difference between the rates of acceleration of the head compared with the torso. If there is very little or no movement of the head relative to the torso, the neck will probably not be injured, even in severe crashes that result in a lot of vehicle damage. In fact, studies have reported that the incidence of whiplash is surprisingly low in high-energy crashes, as well as in crashes where occupants sustain multiple traumas.[34,35]

A recent systematic review[9] that included studies pertaining to the determinants of developing WAD following MVC found several relevant factors, including the occupant's seat position (i.e., being a front-seat versus a rear-seat passenger) and the direction of collision impact. The authors found preliminary evidence suggesting that head restraints and/or car seats that limit head extension have a preventive effect on reporting WAD, although this relationship was mainly evident in females. Being a younger person and/or female seemed to be associated with filing claims or seeking care for WAD, although the evidence was not consistent. Preliminary evidence presented in one of the studies included in the review reported that the elimination of insurance payments for pain and suffering were associated with a lower incidence of WAD injury claims.

Holm et al[36] conducted a study in Sweden wherein questionnaires were mailed to 1,187 persons who reported WAD after an MVC and filed an insurance claim for injuries. The questionnaire asked about prior health, details about the collision, and symptoms after the collision. The following factors were reported to be significantly associated

with severe initial neck pain intensity: low educational level (OR 2.8), being sole adult in the family (OR 1.6), prior neck pain (OR 2.9), prior headache (2.2), prior poor general health (OR 2.6), and exposure to rollover MVC (OR 1.9). The authors concluded that sociodemographic and economic status, pre-injury health status, and collision-related factors were associated with the degree of participants' initial neck pain intensity.

Several factors, including job style, severity of injury, and social class, were also found to have an impact on the time taken off work following whiplash injuries.[37] The data for this study were extracted from the files of 800 medicolegal cases in a private orthopedics practice. The mean time off work corresponded to the severity of injury: 10.6 days for minor injuries, 12.1 days for moderate, 13.8 days severe, and 24.9 days very severe. Heavy manual workers were off work an average of 20.5 days, 15.7 days light manual, 13.9 days for drivers, 9.2 days secretarial, and 12.8 days sedentary. Analysis for each social class showed that professionals were off 7.0 days, 16.1 days for skilled nonmanual workers, and 34.2 days skilled manual, and 11.5 days unskilled manual. Approximately 31% of the 800 cases took no time off work, about 52% returned to work after only 4 days off, and 90% returned to work after 30 days off. Only 4.9% were still off work after 12 weeks.

Sturzenegger et al interviewed a sample of 137 consecutive WAD patients soon after their MVC and found three attributes of crash mechanisms that were associated with more severe symptoms. These included occupant unpreparedness, a rear-end collision vector, and rotated or inclined head position at the time of impact.[38]

Some studies have suggested that the introduction of automobile safety belts has increased the incidence and/or severity of whiplash injuries,[39-41] although others have not found an association.[6,38] A recent best evidence synthesis did not find a relationship between the use or type of safety belt and the prognosis for recovery from WAD.[14] A report from the early 1990s indicated that there was a progressive increase in the number of whiplash patients seen in emergency departments in the United Kingdom since 1982 when safety belt laws were established,[42] but the authors suggested that the increase was not necessarily due to the introduction of seatbelts. Thus, the evidence seems to point away from safety belts having an impact on the incidence of whiplash injuries. Their use should always be encouraged, however, because they have been shown to significantly reduce the risk of serious injury and death in MVCs.[43,44]

Risk Factors for Developing Chronic WAD

Risk factors for developing chronic symptoms following whiplash include some of the same that increase the risk of being injured in the first place. A number of risk factors have been investigated that were initially thought to increase the chance of developing chronic WAD symptoms (e.g., advancing age, female gender, neck pain on palpation, pain or numbness radiating from the neck to the upper extremities, headache, pretraumatic neck pain, low educational level, and position of the occupant at impact). However, the findings of most studies pointing to a positive association are not robust, are sometimes conflicting, and many are of poor methodological quality.[45] Ultimately, only a few risk factors have emerged as being significant. Table 9-1 provides a list of commonly reported risk factors for developing chronic whiplash.

A best evidence synthesis was recently conducted by Carroll et al[14] on the prognostic factors for chronic neck pain after WAD. Articles were judged for relevance and quality to ensure that the best evidence was included. The authors considered 47 related studies, finding that higher initial pain level, more symptoms, and greater initial disability were predictive of a slower recovery. Collision-related factors, such as direction of the collision and type of head restraint, were not prognostic. They concluded that recovery from WAD appeared to be multifactorial, as more than one contributing risk factor is typically present when a group of WAD patients is studied.

A meta-analysis that included 14 cohort studies covering a total of 2,933 whiplash patients reported that high neck pain intensity (defined as a pain score that was 5 or greater on the 11-point numeric rating scale) 3 weeks after injury was the best predictor of chronic pain. The odds ratio for this risk factor was 5.34, meaning the likelihood was increased more than fivefold when it was present.[46] Other significant risk factors included greater than nine total complaints, the presence of headache, low education level, WAD grade 2 or 3, no seatbelt use, past history of neck pain, and female gender. The age of subjects, collision factors, and employment status were not found to be predictive. For ease of understanding, these authors segregated WAD risk factors into four categories: (1) patient demographics, (2) collision

TABLE 9-1

Some of the Reported Risk Factors for Developing Chronic Whiplash

Category	Risk Factor
Patient demographics	• Advancing age • Female gender • Low educational level • Having dependents • Not being employed full-time • Presence of a compensation claim • Early intensive health care following injury • Expectation for recovery
Collision parameters	• Position of the occupants at impact • Being a passenger • Rear impact collision • Collision with a moving object • Head-on or perpendicular collision • Seatbelt use • Improper head restraint • Type of vehicle • Car equipped with a towbar
Previous history	• Headache • Neck pain • Widespread body pain • Head trauma
Presenting symptoms	• High neck pain intensity • High neck disability • Neck pain on palpation • Symptoms of radicular irritation • Muscle pain • Unspecified pain • Headache • Emotional or psychological distress • WAD symptoms • Higher WAD grades • Sleep disturbances • Reduced speed of information processing • Nervousness • Depression

WAD, whiplash-associated disorder.

parameters, (3) previous history, and (4) presenting symptoms.[47]

A cohort study reported that several sociodemographic factors were associated with a longer recovery from WAD, including older age, female sex, having dependents, and not being employed full-time.[48] Each one of these factors decreased the recovery rate by 14% to 16%.

Another cohort study administered questionnaires to a group of 765 WAD patients at 3, 6, and 12 months post-injury. Twenty-seven percent of the cohort complained of symptoms at each evaluation.[49] The authors suggested that the most useful predictors of persistent neck pain following an MVC included psychological distress, precollision symptoms of widespread body pain, WAD symptoms, and high initial neck disability. The type of vehicle (i.e., truck, bus, or car) was the only collision-related factor that influenced the likelihood of the patients developing chronic symptoms.

Pobereskin[22] followed a group of 503 whiplash patients for 12 months, finding that age and prior history of neck pain were the most important predictors of early neck pain, and the patients' initial neck pain visual analogue scale (VAS) score and the presence of a compensation claim were the most important predictors of pain at 1 year. The researchers also investigated measures of impact severity to determine what influence they had on outcomes and found the influence to be weak.

Initial symptoms of radicular irritation and high neck pain intensity were associated with poor improvement reported at all examinations in a group of 117 whiplash patients who were examined initially and then followed up at 3, 6 and 12 months.[25] In addition to the degree of injury severity, poor recovery was also associated with a prior history of head trauma and headache, as well as the presence of sleep disturbances, reduced speed of information processing, and nervousness soon after the injury. Psychosocial factors at any follow-up examination were not predictive of poor recovery. In another paper that involved this same group of whiplash patients,[50] the authors pointed out that even though patients commonly suffered from psychological symptoms and cognitive impairment, improvement of these symptoms was associated with recovery from their somatic symptoms. The authors suggested these data support the viewpoint that psychological and cognitive problems in whiplash patients are principally related to their somatic symptoms.

Prior neck pain and a high degree of emotional distress after the MVC were found to be independently associated with an increased risk of developing chronic neck pain in a series of 186 acute whiplash patients who were seen in an emergency room.[51] Patients were followed for 1 year and evaluated at 1, 3, 6, 12 weeks and 1 year after the MVC. Significant neck pain was still present in 18% of the patients at 1 year. Chronic neck pain was associated with patient-specific characteristics in this study, rather than with physical signs of injury or the follow-up regimen that was employed.

Another study that followed whiplash patients referred from hospital emergency departments or primary care providers included 740 subjects.[52] The study's objectives were to determine if post-collision ratings of pain and psychological distress that were experienced before the collision were associated with reduced work capability and neck pain at follow-up 12 months after the injury. The authors concluded that unspecified pain (in contrast to specified neck pain) prior to the collision was associated with poor recovery and negatively affected work capacity. Also, a high level of psychological distress before the collision was associated with considerable neck pain at follow-up. No association was found between the level of pre-collision neck pain or severity of the MVC and a poor outcome.

A Canadian study that analyzed data obtained from the databases of a provincial universal automobile insurance plan and police crash records reported several sociodemographic factors as being independently associated with a slower recovery from whiplash, including female gender, older age, having dependents, and not having full-time employment. The authors also identified several crash-related factors that were associated with a slower recovery, including occupancy in a truck or bus, being a passenger in the vehicle, colliding with a moving object, and being in a head-on or perpendicular collision.[28]

An injured person's expectation for recovery was found to be an important prognosticator of their level of disability 6 months after a whiplash injury.[53] Symptom severity and mental symptoms were controlled for in this study, yet those who stated that they were "less likely to make a full recovery" were more likely to have a high level of disability than those who stated that they were "very likely to make a full recovery." The odds ratio for this association was fairly strong at 4.2. The authors also noted a dose response relationship, where the more positive the injured person was about making a full recovery, the more likely they were to have a low level of disability at follow-up.

Based on an analysis of the records of a cohort of 1,693 patients who experienced a whiplash injury, Côté et al[54] reported that early intensive health care following whiplash leads to poor recovery. In this study, the intensity of care patients received during the first 30 days after the collision was negatively associated with their rate of recovery; that is, the more care they received, the more delayed was their recovery and vice versa. The authors opined as to the reasons recovery was delayed in those who received early aggressive care: "Because patient pressure is a known predictor of physician behavior, doctors may use treatments, schedule follow-up visits, and refer patients when not medically needed. This in turn may lead to adverse outcomes and even prolong recovery by legitimizing patients' fears and creating unnecessary anxiety."[54] They also felt that early aggressive clinical care delays recovery by promoting the use of passive coping strategies that reinforce the patients' beliefs that whiplash injuries often lead to disability.

The conclusions of the Côté et al study, as well as another one published in 2005[55] that used very similar methodology, has been criticized by practitioners and researchers from across health care disciplines. For instance, Freeman et al[56] pointed out numerous limitations of the study, emphasizing the fact that whiplash patients who have more severe injuries are likely to be treated more frequently at the beginning of care and take longer to recover from their injuries.

Therefore, they thought the authors' conclusion that treatment for a painful injury prolongs the duration of the injury was not supported by the study's data. This argument seems more rational than the notion that early treatment could actually contribute to a delayed recovery.

SOCIETAL IMPACT

Musculoskeletal conditions are the leading cause of disability in the United States and are responsible for more that one half of all chronic disorders in people greater than 50 years of age in developed countries.[57] The direct and indirect costs associated with all bone and joint health in the United States were estimated to be $849 billion in 2004, which represented about 7.7% of the gross domestic product. MVCs are a major source of musculoskeletal injuries, being responsible for about 11% of

visits to hospital emergency rooms for treatment of nonfatal unintentional injuries.

About one half of persons involved in MVCs reported an associated sprain or strain injury, and when considering musculoskeletal sprain or strain injuries in general, MVCs were the most common cause.[57b]

Whiplash injuries have an enormous socioeconomic impact, with the average whiplash injury related to a rear-impact collision in the United States costing approximately $9,994 in 2002 dollars. This includes $6,843 in economic costs and $3,151 in costs related to quality-of-life impacts. From these data, the total annual cost of rear-impact whiplash injuries in the United States has been estimated to be approximately $2.7 billion.[58] In addition to the monetary costs of treatment and lost productivity, there are also psychological, cognitive, and emotional aspects of whiplash that should be considered in order to determine the total impact the condition has on society.[59]

Given the enormous costs of whiplash, government agencies and the automotive and insurance industries have attempted to minimize the occurrence and severity of whiplash injuries. However, their efforts have not proven to be effective. In fact, the incidence of whiplash has actually increased over the past 30 years.[9] For instance, a study by Holm et al[60] reported that the amount of medical impairment due to WAD increased between 1989 and 1994 in Sweden, from 16% to 28% respectively. The authors also identified some predictor variables in this study that were associated with reduced or complete work disability, including being over 40 years old, a medical impairment judgment of 15% or more, and having low professional status.

A WHIPLASH CULTURE

Some studies have pointed to a difference in the likelihood of developing chronic symptoms following whiplash that hinges on the country from which the data were gathered. For instance, a prospective cohort study originating in Greece reported that all 180 members of their cohort of whiplash victims returned to their pre-injury state of health within 6 months after injury and no cases of chronic disability occurred.[61] Another report originated from data collected in Lithuania[62] and was derived from a cohort of 202 whiplash victims. Although 35% of the injured cohort noticed initial neck pain and headaches, this was not significantly different from a group of matched controls who were randomly selected from the general population. Furthermore, none of the subjects had disabling or persistent symptoms as a result of the MVC. Another study involving patients from Germany reported findings that were similar to those emanating from Greece and Lithuania.[63]

The findings of these studies have served to advance the concept that the likelihood of developing chronic symptoms following a whiplash injury is largely dependent on the cultural expectations of the population and have prompted Ferrari and his colleagues[64] to opine, "The late whiplash syndrome, if it exists at all in these countries, is uncommon." Ferrari et al[64,65] have proposed a biopsychosocial model to explain the discrepancies that can be found in the epidemiology of the late whiplash syndrome between different countries. This model presumes that symptoms are not merely the result of a somatic expression of anxiety or other psychological disorder, but psychosocial factors in those countries with a whiplash culture in which the occurrence of the late whiplash syndrome is common. The biopsychosocial model was inspired partly by data derived from studies that highlighted the differences in rates of chronic whiplash between various countries (e.g., Lithuania and Greece versus the United States and Great Britain) and partly by studies that point out how people have certain expectations about their symptoms, that is, that an acute whiplash injury may cause chronic symptoms and disability. The outcome of these cultural differences, as well as the potential for patients' expectations to hamper their recovery, results in modified illness behaviors of some whiplash patients, making them susceptible to long-term problems.[64]

In countries that have a whiplash culture, in which the population generally accepts chronic whiplash as being a real condition, a substantial proportion of persons with whiplash develop chronic symptoms. In contrast, in countries without a whiplash culture, in which the population does not generally accept chronic whiplash as being a real condition, very few people develop chronic WAD symptoms.[65,66] However, Carroll et al[14] indicated that the reported differences in rates of recovery following whiplash between countries is not well understood. The authors listed a number of reasons that could be responsible for the reported differences in recovery rates, including societal beliefs and attitudes. Nevertheless, they thought other factors may be responsible, including methodological issues of the studies, differences in the

context in which the injuries occurred, and differences in compensation policies.

An earlier writing on the topic noted the difference between the rates of chronic whiplash symptoms between Singapore, a region where taking on the sick role following this type of injury is not generally accepted, and Western countries like Australia, where whiplash injuries are legitimized.[67] The authors thought this observation supported generalizations about the development of chronic whiplash syndrome as a social illness that is different across various cultures. However, this study was criticized because it represented "little more than anecdotal evidence from interviews of selected Singaporean doctors compared with data from Australia."[68]

The concept of a whiplash culture is also based on the "symptom expectation" theory, wherein persons in some countries are more likely to envision long-term symptoms following a whiplash injury as compared to those from other countries. This theory stems from one study that queried naïve subjects from a country with a "whiplash culture" about what kinds of symptoms would be expected by patients who had experienced whiplash.[69] What the subjects expected was very similar to what actually has been reported by whiplash victims in the literature. No comparisons were made with other countries that lack a "whiplash culture." Thus, it is not really known what, if any, differences actually exist between the countries on this issue. Ferrari and Lang also cited another study to support the symptom expectation theory that dealt with symptoms a group of subjects would expect to occur 6 months after a mild head injury,[70] but any comparison with whiplash is speculative. Based on these studies, however, Ferrari[71] noted, "In North America there is overwhelming information regarding the potential for chronic pain after whiplash injury." And because North Americans are so well-informed, they expect to develop chronic WAD.

The previously mentioned Greek[61] and Lithuanian[62] studies have been criticized by a number of researchers. For instance, Merskey[72] noted that the Norwegian Centre for Health Technology Assessment, a group established by the Department of Health and Social Affairs for Norway, questioned the validity of the Lithuanian study. The Norwegian report indicated that more than 4,000 persons would be needed in each group to reach an 80% probability of finding a statistically significant difference. Moreover, Barnsley[68] pointed out that none of the studies that are commonly used to highlight the differences between the reported rates of chronic whiplash symptoms in countries having or not having whiplash cultures has adequate statistical power to show a real difference, even if one existed.

The notion that residents of North America and many European countries are inclined to expect chronic symptoms and disability following whiplash injuries is debatable. For instance, Aubrey et al[69] found that there were misconceptions among laypersons about whiplash and head injuries. They administered questionnaires to a group of 43 subjects that covered their knowledge of the physical and cognitive consequences of whiplash and head injuries. Most subjects incorrectly thought that high crash speeds would be required to produce the common physical complaints of acute WAD. The subjects were also mistaken about their understanding of post-injury cognitive symptoms. Their knowledge about the physical symptoms of whiplash, however, was consistent with what is found in the whiplash literature. The authors concluded that it was unlikely that patients with persistent complaints following whiplash injuries derive their symptoms from common knowledge about the condition's sequelae.

The work of Ferrari and his colleagues and the concept that the rates of chronic whiplash vary between countries because of cultural conditioning has also been criticized as not providing a balanced perspective of the whiplash literature. As noted by Barnsley,[68] "They fiercely interrogate research that does not support their view, yet uncritically embrace literature favoring their preconceptions." However, in spite of the criticisms of the work of Ferrari and his colleagues on the reality of whiplash cultures, certain aspects may actually have merit. Perhaps there are real differences between residents of countries without whiplash cultures and North Americans as a result of their litigious disposition. Another possible reason may be the large number of bigger vehicles (i.e., trucks and SUVs) that are preferred by so many Americans, which may contribute to the severity of injuries and the consequential greater number of late whiplash syndromes found in the United States. Finally, although there is no supporting evidence, citizens of countries with a whiplash culture may be less tolerant of pain as compared with their more stoic counterparts in non–whiplash culture countries.

In the end, there are still many unanswered questions about the basis of chronic WAD. Its occurrence is almost certainly not solely related to

biopsychosocial issues, yet it is surely not entirely physical. There is doubtless a tissue injury component in the majority of chronic WAD victims that is aggravated in those who are susceptible to various biopsychosocial factors.

PREVENTION

From an epidemiological perspective, prevention of whiplash injuries involves primary, secondary, and tertiary strategies. Thus, injury prevention can be targeted at three levels: Primary prevention involves preventing the injury from occurring in the first place or, if the event does occur, reducing the extent of the injuries. For instance, enforcing laws that prevent people from driving while under the influence of drugs or alcohol can avert a rear-impact collision. Secondary prevention involves the prompt and appropriate management of a person's injuries. For example, a community that makes certain adequate emergency response facilities are in place. Tertiary prevention is directed at improving the final outcome of a person's injuries. An example would be adequately trained physicians who know the best practices for managing WAD patients.

Primary Prevention

Efforts to prevent whiplash injuries have involved various automobile design tactics aimed at reducing the rate of acceleration of the head that results when the torso is abruptly shifted during an MVC, for example, head restraints that minimize the distance between the back of the head (i.e., backset) and ensure that the level of the head restraint is high enough, including active head restraints.[73] Several studies have shown that the presence of a highly rated and appropriately fitted head restraint is an important primary whiplash prevention strategy that is especially important for females.[74,75] Chapline et al[76] recommended that vehicle occupants should adjust their head restraints, if possible, behind the head's centers of gravity with the back of the head as close as possible to the head restraint (Figure 9-1).

Farmer et al[74] used insurance claims data to compare neck injury rates for drivers of cars that were struck from the rear based on IIHS head restraint ratings. The authors reported that drivers sustained 24% fewer neck injuries when they were in cars with "good" rated seats, compared to cars with "poor" rated seats.[74] The same authors conducted another study using similar methodology,

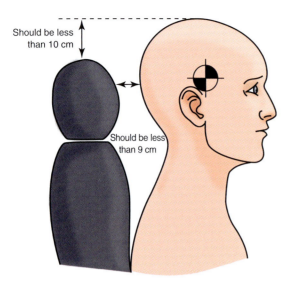

Figure 9-1   The distance between the back of the head and the head restraint should be as small as possible, and the head restraint should be directly behind the head's center of gravity.

but this time they investigated the rates of neck injuries in rear-end crashes for vehicles with and without redesigned head restraints, redesigned seats, or both.[75] They reported that newer head restraints with improved geometric fit significantly reduced the risk of whiplash injury among female drivers, although they did not appear to protect male drivers. However, the risk was reduced in both males and females by about 43% when they looked at the data on new seat designs that incorporate active head restraints that move upward and closer to the occupants' heads in a rear-impact collision.

Some have suggested that energy-absorbing bumpers may prevent whiplash, although this assumption is probably wrong, as there is evidence pointing to their ineffectiveness.[77] Enforcement of driving laws may also be effective at preventing whiplash (e.g., sobriety checkpoints and banning cell phone use while driving).

Secondary and Tertiary Prevention

A number of different treatments for WAD have been studied,[78-92] although, when considering non-surgical methods, no one type of therapy has emerged as being clearly superior.[93] A recent best evidence synthesis of noninvasive treatments for neck pain reported that educational videos, mobilization, and exercises appeared to be more advantageous than usual care or physical modalities for

WAD patients.[94] The authors also suggested that, for patients with common neck pain, manual therapy (including cervical manipulation) plus exercise was more effective than alternative strategies. Other reviews have been in agreement with these findings,[95,96] although most of the included studies focused on acute whiplash. Accordingly, there is little evidence available to support the effectiveness of any particular therapy for chronic whiplash.[23,97]

On the other hand, a study by Suissa et al[98] compared outcomes of two groups of whiplash patients, with injured persons in one group receiving a managed treatment approach, referred to as the Whiplash Management Model (WMM), and the other group (the reference group) receiving typical medical care. The WMM consisted of initial and ongoing care by a family physician, who referred patients for physical therapy and provided home exercises. Patients continued with this care only if their conditions improved; if no improvement was observed, they were referred to an occupational therapist for assessment. A physician and a psychologist would also evaluate the patient at this point to confirm the diagnosis and/or assess for obstacles to healing. Interdisciplinary rehabilitation might be initiated on the recommendation of these evaluations. This model seemed to work well, with the rate of ending insurance compensation being much higher in the WMM group than the reference group (RR: 3.2; 95% CI 2.8-3.6). The average cost per patient was also much lower in the WMM group.

CONCLUSION

Whiplash injuries are common in modern society and represent a major cause of both acute and chronic neck pain. Considerable costs result from WAD-related neck pain which permeate society at many levels (e.g., monetary costs, lost productivity, and emotional distress). There are few concrete answers as to which risk factors truly contribute to the incidence of whiplash injuries, which treatments are effective, and which prevention strategies should be adopted.

The most current systematic reviews on whiplash injuries have identified only a few variables that are helpful in predicting the occurrence of acute WAD or the chances of injured persons developing chronic pain. Whether the occupant was a front seat versus rear seat passenger and the direction of collision impact were the main predictors of sustaining an acute whiplash injury. Nonetheless, telling people to avoid riding in the rear seat when they are a passenger in an automobile is probably not a reasonable prevention strategy.

There is some evidence pointing to better-fitting head restraints as being helpful in the prevention of whiplash injuries in females and that active head restraints noticeably protect both females and males. Thus, counseling patients on the proper adjustment of their head restraints (see Figure 9-1) and pointing out which vehicles they should consider purchasing in order to protect their necks during an MVC (i.e., active and/or those IIHS-rated good) would be effective primary prevention strategies.

Higher initial pain levels, the presence of more symptoms, and greater initial disability are probably the best predictors of a slow recovery. Hence, practitioners should consider these factors as they prepare treatment plans and prognoses for their WAD patients. The evidence in support of a whiplash culture is very weak and in some cases improperly extrapolated. The reported difference in the rates of recovery from WAD between countries, which is the basis of the concept of a whiplash culture, is not well understood and may be caused by a number of other factors.

There is no strong evidence supporting any particular therapy for neck pain associated with chronic WAD. However, manual therapy (i.e., cervical mobilization and/or manipulation), together with exercise, appears to be the most effective noninvasive treatments for patients with acute WAD-related neck pain. Interdisciplinary evaluation and care by appropriate specialists may be of benefit when patients do not respond to treatment within a reasonable length of time.

REFERENCES

1. Dorland's illustrated medical dictionary, 30th ed, Philadelphia, 2003, Saunders, pp xxvii.
2. Szabo TJ, et al: *Human occupant kinematic response to low speed rear-end impacts.* SAE Tech Paper no. 940532, 23-35, 1994.
3. Brault JR, Siegmund GP, Wheeler JB: Cervical muscle response during whiplash: evidence of a lengthening muscle contraction, *Clin Biomech (Bristol, Avon)* 15(6):426-435, 2000.
4. McConnell WE, et al: Human head and neck kinematics after low velocity rear-end impacts—Understanding "whiplash." SAE Tech Paper no. 952724, November 1, 1995. In 39th Stapp Car Crash Conference, Society of Automotive Engineers, San Diego, California, 1995.
5. Spitzer WO, et al: Scientific monograph of the Quebec Task Force on Whiplash-Associated Disorders: redefining "whiplash" and its management, *Spine* 20(suppl 8):S1S-S73, 1995.
6. Versteegen GJ, et al: Neck sprain in patients injured in car accidents: a retrospective study covering the period 1970-1994, *Eur Spine J* 7(3):195-200, 1998.
7. Cassidy JD, et al: Effect of eliminating compensation for pain and suffering on the outcome of insurance claims for whiplash injury, *N Engl J Med* 342(16):1179-1186, 2000.
8. Sterner Y, et al: The incidence of whiplash trauma and the effects of different factors on recovery, *J Spinal Disord Tech* 16(2):195-199, 2003.
9. Holm LW, et al: The burden and determinants of neck pain in whiplash-associated disorders after traffic collisions: results of the Bone and Joint Decade 2000-2010 Task Force on Neck Pain and Its Associated Disorders, *Spine* 33(suppl 4): S52-S59, 2008.
10. Evans RW: Some observations on whiplash injuries, *Neurol Clin* 10(4):975-997, 1992.
11. Insurance Institute for Highway Safety (IIHS): *New crash tests of SUVs: Nissan Murano is top safety pick; 3 SUVs are marginal or poor for protection in side crashes (news release)*, Arlington, VA, 2008, Insurance Institute for Highway Safety, February 22, 5.
12. Côté P, et al: The association between neck pain intensity, physical functioning, depressive symptomatology and time-to-claim-closure after whiplash, *J Clin Epidemiol* 54(3):275-286, 2001.
13. National Accident Sampling System (NASS): Washington, DC, 2008, U.S. Department of Transportation.
14. Carroll LJ, et al: Course and prognostic factors for neck pain in whiplash-associated disorders (WAD): results of the Bone and Joint Decade 2000-2010 Task Force on Neck Pain and Its Associated Disorders, *Spine* 33(suppl 4):S83-S92, 2008.
15. Freeman MD, et al: Chronic neck pain and whiplash: a case-control study of the relationship between acute whiplash injuries and chronic neck pain, *Pain Res Manag* 11(2):79-83, 2006.
16. Ferrari R, et al: The best approach to the problem of whiplash? One ticket to Lithuania, please, *Clin Exp Rheumatol* 17(3):321-326, 1999.
17. Allen M: *Musculoskeletal pain emanating from the head and neck: current concepts in diagnosis, management, and cost containment*, New York, 1996, Haworth Medical Press, pp xiv, 1.
18. Guez M, et al: The prevalence of neck pain: a population-based study from northern Sweden, *Acta Orthop Scand* 73(4):455-459, 2002.
19. Suissa S, Harder S, Veilleux M: The relation between initial symptoms and signs and the prognosis of whiplash, *Eur Spine J* 10(1):44-49, 2001.

20. Buitenhuis J, Spanjer J, Fidler V: Recovery from acute whiplash: the role of coping styles, *Spine* 28(9):896-901, 2003.
21. Mayou R, Bryant B: Outcome of "whiplash" neck injury, *Injury* 27(9):617-623, 1996.
22. Pobereskin LH: Whiplash following rear end collisions: a prospective cohort study, *J Neurol Neurosurg Psychiatry* 76(8):1146-1151, 2005.
23. Cassidy JD, et al: Does multidisciplinary rehabilitation benefit whiplash recovery? Results of a population-based incidence cohort study, *Spine* 32(1):126-131, 2007.
24. Herrström P, Lannerbro-Geijer G, Högstedt B: Whiplash injuries from car accidents in a Swedish middle-sized town during 1993-95, *Scand J Prim Health Care* 18(3):154-158, 2000.
25. Radanov BP, et al: Relationship between early somatic, radiological, cognitive and psychosocial findings and outcome during a one-year follow-up in 117 patients suffering from common whiplash, *Br J Rheumatol* 33(5):442-448, 1994.
26. Schrader H, et al: Natural evolution of late whiplash syndrome outside the medicolegal context, *Lancet* 347(9010):1207-1211, 1996.
27. Obelieniene D, et al: Pain after whiplash: a prospective controlled inception cohort study, *J Neurol Neurosurg Psychiatry* 66(3):279-283, 1999.
28. Harder S, Veilleux M, Suissa S: The effect of socio-demographic and crash-related factors on the prognosis of whiplash, *J Clin Epidemiol* 51(5):377-384, 1998.
29. Bovim G, Schrader H, Sand T: Neck pain in the general population, *Spine* 19(12):1307-1309, 1994.
30. Berglund A, et al: The association between exposure to a rear-end collision and future health complaints, *J Clin Epidemiol* 54(8):851-856, 2001.
31. Ferrari R, et al: A re-examination of the whiplash associated disorders (WAD) as a systemic illness, *Ann Rheum Dis* 64(9):1337-1342, 2005.
32. Carroll LJ, Cassidy JD, Côté P: Frequency, timing, and course of depressive symptomatology after whiplash, *Spine* 31(16):E551-E556, 2006.
33. Kamper SJ, et al: Course and prognostic factors of whiplash: a systematic review and meta-analysis, *Pain* 138(3):617-629, 2008.
34. Malik H, Lovell M: Soft tissue neck symptoms following high-energy road traffic accidents, *Spine* 29(15):E315-E317, 2004.
35. Giannoudis PV, Mehta SS, Tsiridis E: Incidence and outcome of whiplash injury after multiple trauma, *Spine* 32(7):776-781, 2007.
36. Holm LW, et al: Factors influencing neck pain intensity in whiplash-associated disorders in Sweden, *Clin J Pain* 23(7):591-597, 2007.
37. Hagan KS, Naqui SZ, Lovell ME: Relationship between occupation, social class and time taken off work following a whiplash injury, *Ann R Coll Surg Engl* 89(6):624-626, 2007.
38. Sturzenegger M, et al: Presenting symptoms and signs after whiplash injury: the influence of accident mechanisms, *Neurology* 44(4):688-693, 1994.
39. Crouch R, et al: Whiplash associated disorder: incidence and natural history over the first month for patients presenting to a UK emergency department, *Emerg Med J* 23(2):114-118, 2006.
40. Thomas J: Road traffic accidents before and after seatbelt legislation—study in a district general hospital, *J R Soc Med* 83(2):79-81, 1990.
41. Bourbeau R, et al: Neck injuries among belted and unbelted occupants of the front seat of cars, *J Trauma* 35(5):794-799, 1993.
42. Galasko CS, et al: Neck sprains after road traffic accidents: a modern epidemic, *Injury* 24(3):155-157, 1993.
43. Zhu M, et al: Association of rear seat safety belt use with death in a traffic crash: a matched cohort study, *Inj Prev* 13(3):183-185, 2007.
44. Schlundt D, Warren R, Miller S: Reducing unintentional injuries on the nation's highways: a literature review, *J Health Care Poor Underserved* 15(1):76-98, 2004.
45. Williamson E, et al: A systematic literature review of psychological factors and the development of late whiplash syndrome, *Pain* 135(1-2):20-30, 2008.
46. Walton D, et al: Risk factors for persistent problems after whiplash: a meta-analysis. In *World Congress on Neck Pain*, Los Angeles, CA, January 20-22, 2008.
47. Walton DM, et al: Risk factors for persistent problems following whiplash injury: results of a systematic review and meta-analysis, *J Orthop Sports Phys Ther* 39(5):334-350, 2008.
48. Suissa S: Risk factors of poor prognosis after whiplash injury, *Pain Res Manag* 8(2):69-75, 2003.
49. Atherton K, et al: Predictors of persistent neck pain after whiplash injury, *Emerg Med J* 23(3):195-201, 2006.
50. Radanov BP, et al: Common whiplash: psychosomatic or somatopsychic? *J Neurol Neurosurg Psychiatry* 57(4):486-490, 1994.
51. Kivioja J, Jensen I, Lindgren U: Neither the WAD-classification nor the Quebec Task Force follow-up regimen seems to be important for the outcome after a whiplash injury. A prospective study on 186 consecutive patients, *Eur Spine J* 17(7):930-935, 2008.
52. Carstensen TB, et al: Post-trauma ratings of pre-collision pain and psychological distress predict poor outcome following acute whiplash trauma: A 12-month follow-up study, *Pain* 139(2): 248-259, 2008.
53. Holm LW, et al: Expectations for recovery important in the prognosis of whiplash injuries, *PLoS Med* 5(5):e105, 2008.

54. Côté P, et al: Early aggressive care and delayed recovery from whiplash: isolated finding or reproducible result? *Arthritis Rheum* 57(5):861-868, 2007.

55. Côté P, et al: Initial patterns of clinical care and recovery from whiplash injuries: a population-based cohort study, *Arch Intern Med* 165(19):2257-2263, 2005.

56. Freeman MD, et al: Greater injury leads to more treatment for whiplash: no surprises here, *Arch Intern Med* 166(11):1238-1239, 2006, author reply 1239-1240.

57. Watkins-Castillo SI, project coord: *Burden of musculoskeletal diseases in the United States: Prevalence, societal and economic cost*, Rosemont, IL, 2008, American Association of Orthopaedic Surgeons, pp ix.

57b. Ibid, 127-128.

58. Request to list in the compendium of candidate global technical regulations (compendium of candidates). The United States of America Federal Motor Vehicle Safety Standard (FMVSS) No. 202—Head restraints, in No. WP.29-135-17. UN Economic and Social Council: World Forum for Harmonization of Vehicle Regulations (WP.29), 139th session, 2005, p. 6.

59. Gargan M: Psychological aspects of whiplash injuries, *J Bone Joint Surg Br* 88-B(Suppl 1):12, 2006.

60. Holm L, et al: Impairment and work disability due to whiplash injury following traffic collisions. An analysis of insurance material from the Swedish Road Traffic Injury Commission, *Scand J Public Health* 27(2):116-123, 1999.

61. Partheni M, et al: A prospective cohort study of the outcome of acute whiplash injury in Greece, *Clin Exp Rheumatol* 18(1):67-70, 2000.

62. Schrader H, Obelieniene D: Natural evolution of late whiplash syndrome outside the medicolegal context, *Lancet* 347(9010):1207-1211, 1996.

63. Bonk AD, et al: Prospective, randomized, controlled study of activity versus collar, and the natural history for whiplash injury, in Germany, *J Musculoskel Pain* 8(1/2):123-132, 2000.

64. Ferrari R, et al: Laypersons' expectation of the sequelae of whiplash injury. A cross-cultural comparative study between Canada and Lithuania, *Med Sci Monit* 8(11):CR728-CR734, 2002.

65. Ferrari R, Lang C: A cross-cultural comparison between Canada and Germany of symptom expectation for whiplash injury, *J Spinal Disord Tech* 18(1):92-97, 2005.

66. Ferrari R: *The whiplash encyclopedia: the facts and myths of whiplash*, ed 2, Sudbury, MA, 2006, Jones & Bartlett, pp xxxviii, 3.

67. Balla JI: The late whiplash syndrome: a study of an illness in Australia and Singapore, *Cult Med Psychiatry* 6(2):191-210, 1982.

68. Barnsley L: Epidemiology of whiplash, *Ann Rheum Dis* 59(5):394, 2000; author reply 395-396.

69. Aubrey JB, Dobbs AR, Rule BG: Laypersons' knowledge about the sequelae of minor head injury and whiplash, *J Neurol Neurosurg Psychiatry* 52(7):842-846, 1989.

70. Mittenberg W, et al: Symptoms following mild head injury: expectation as aetiology, *J Neurol Neurosurg Psychiatry* 55(3):200-204, 1992.

71. Ferrari R: Prevention of chronic pain after whiplash, *Emerg Med J* 19(6):526-530, 2002.

72. Merskey H: Social influences on the concept of fibromyalgia, *CNS Spectr* 13(3 Suppl 5):18-21, 2008.

73. Voo L, et al: *Performance of seats with active head restraints in rear impacts (Paper No. 07-0041)*. In 20th International Technical Conference on the Enhanced Safety of Vehicles, Washington, DC, 2007, National Highway Traffic Safety Administration.

74. Farmer CM, Wells JK, Werner JV: Relationship of head restraint positioning to driver neck injury in rear-end crashes, *Accid Anal Prev* 31(6):719-728, 1999.

75. Farmer CM, Wells JK, Lund AK: Effects of head restraint and seat redesign on neck injury risk in rear-end crashes, *Traffic Inj Prev* 4(2):83-90, 2003.

76. Chapline JF, et al: Neck pain and head restraint position relative to the driver's head in rear-end collisions, *Accid Anal Prev* 32(2):287-297, 2000.

77. Kornhauser M: *Delta-V thresholds for cervical spine injury*. SAE Tech Paper No. 960093, 1-13, 1996.

78. Padberg M, de Bruijn SF, Tavy DL: Neck pain in chronic whiplash syndrome treated with botulinum toxin. A double-blind, placebo-controlled clinical trial, *J Neurol* 254(3):290-295, 2007.

79. Vikne J, et al: A randomized study of new sling exercise treatment vs traditional physiotherapy for patients with chronic whiplash-associated disorders with unsettled compensation claims, *J Rehabil Med* 39(3):252-259, 2007.

80. Soderlund A, Lindberg P: Cognitive behavioural components in physiotherapy management of chronic whiplash associated disorders (WAD)—a randomised group study, *G Ital Med Lav Ergon* 29(1 Suppl A):A5-A11, 2007.

81. Kongsted A, et al: Neck collar, "act-as-usual" or active mobilization for whiplash injury? A randomized parallel-group trial, *Spine* 32(6):618-626, 2007.

82. Lemming D, et al: Managing chronic whiplash associated pain with a combination of low-dose opioid (remifentanil) and NMDA-antagonist (ketamine), *Eur J Pain* 11(7):719-732, 2007.

83. Scholten-Peeters GG, et al: Education by general practitioners or education and exercises by physiotherapists for patients with whiplash-associated disorders? A randomized clinical trial, *Spine* 31(7):723-731, 2006.

84. Aigner N, et al: Adjuvant laser acupuncture in the treatment of whiplash injuries: a prospective, randomized placebo-controlled trial, *Wien Klin Wochenschr* 118(3-4):95-99, 2006.

85. Ferrari R, et al: Simple educational intervention to improve the recovery from acute whiplash: results of a randomized, controlled trial, *Acad Emerg Med* 12(8):699-706, 2005.

86. Schnabel M, et al: Randomised, controlled outcome study of active mobilisation compared with collar therapy for whiplash injury, *Emerg Med J* 21(3):306-310, 2004.

87. Rosenfeld M, et al: Active intervention in patients with whiplash-associated disorders improves long-term prognosis: a randomized controlled clinical trial, *Spine* 28(22):2491-2498, 2003.

88. Byrn C, et al: Subcutaneous sterile water injections for chronic neck and shoulder pain following whiplash injuries, *Lancet* 341(8843):449-452, 1993.

89. Foley-Nolan D, et al: Low energy high frequency pulsed electromagnetic therapy for acute whiplash injuries. A double blind randomized controlled study, *Scand J Rehabil Med* 24(1):51-59, 1992.

90. Mealy K, Brennan H, Fenelon GC: Early mobilization of acute whiplash injuries, *Br Med J (Clin Res Ed)* 292(6521):656-657, 1986.

91. Olson VL: Whiplash-associated chronic headache treated with home cervical traction, *Phys Ther* 77(4):417-424, 1997.

92. Stewart MJ, et al: Randomized controlled trial of exercise for chronic whiplash-associated disorders, *Pain* 128(1-2):59-68, 2007.

93. van der Velde G, et al: Identifying the best treatment among common nonsurgical neck pain treatments: a decision analysis, *Spine* 33(suppl 4):S184-S191, 2008.

94. Hurwitz EL, et al: Treatment of neck pain: noninvasive interventions: results of the Bone and Joint Decade 2000-2010 Task Force on Neck Pain and Its Associated Disorders, *Spine* 33(suppl 4):S123-S152, 2008.

95. Gross AR, et al: Conservative management of mechanical neck disorders: a systematic review, *J Rheumatol* 34(5):1083-1102, 2007.

96. Gross AR, et al: Manipulation and mobilisation for mechanical neck disorders. *Cochrane Database Syst Rev* (1):CD004249, 2004.

97. Verhagen AP, et al: Conservative treatments for whiplash. *Cochrane Database Syst Rev* (2):CD003338, 2007.

98. Suissa S, et al: Assessing a whiplash management model: a population-based non-randomized intervention study, *J Rheumatol* 33(3):581-587, 2006.

Chapter 10

The Safety and Effectiveness of Common Treatments for Whiplash

William J. Lauretti

JUDGING SAFETY AND EFFECTIVENESS: AN EVIDENCE-BASED APPROACH

In the past, management of whiplash-associated disorders (WADs) was based upon traditional treatment approaches, opinions of experts, and simple common sense. However, the safety and effectiveness of many of these common approaches had little if any formal evidence basis. Even though we are increasingly entering the era of evidence-based medicine, much of whiplash treatment continues to be based upon the individual practitioner's personal experience and opinions.

In light of the large burden that modern societies bear from the financial and productivity costs of whiplash-associated disorders, it's no wonder that there is increasing pressure to apply a more consistent evidence-based approach toward the treatment of these common, expensive, and often debilitating conditions.

Recent research has helped clarify the evidence for (or against) the safety and effectiveness of a variety of treatments commonly used for WADs. Two recent comprehensive literature reviews in particular have helped to define the current state-of-the-art of whiplash treatment: the Quebec Task Force on Whiplash-Associated Disorders and the

Bone and Joint Decade Task Force on Neck Pain and Its Associated Disorders.

THE QUEBEC TASK FORCE ON WHIPLASH-ASSOCIATED DISORDERS

One of the first comprehensive studies comparing the safety and effectiveness of a variety of common treatments for whiplash was performed by the Quebec Task Force. This multidisciplinary task force consisted of leading researchers and clinicians from North America and Europe and was sponsored by the public auto insurer in Quebec, Canada. The Quebec Task Force submitted a report on whiplash-associated disorders in 1995, which made specific recommendations on prevention, diagnosis, and treatment of WAD. The task force's monograph, titled *Redefining "Whiplash" and Its Management,* was published in the April 15, 1995, issue of *Spine.*[1] An update was published in January 2001.[2]

Among the task force's conclusions were that joint manipulation and mobilization were recommended to improve range of motion and reduce pain, and as part of a management strategy based on early return to function and activities, as opposed to rest or use of a cervical collar. It was also concluded that certain prescription medications might be beneficial, whereas surgery is rarely indicated in simple WAD cases. Notably, the task force's comprehensive literature review found that the "vast literature on the subject of whiplash" (over 10,000 titles were reviewed) was generally of poor scientific quality.

THE BONE AND JOINT DECADE TASK FORCE

The United Nations has declared the decade of 2000-2010 as the Bone and Joint Decade (BJD). The goal of this multinational, multi-specialty organization is to improve the health-related quality of life for people with musculoskeletal disorders throughout the world. One major project that was undertaken by the BJD was the creation of a Task Force on Neck Pain and Its Associated Disorders. This task force published its major findings in a 250-page supplement to the journal *Spine* in 2008,[3] and this document was republished as a supplement in the *Journal of Manipulative and Physiological Therapeutics* in February 2009. Included in these publications was a comprehensive review of noninvasive interventions for the treatment of neck pain by Hurwitz et al.[4] Because this task force's report, particularly the Hurwitz et al review, is the most comprehensive and best researched summary of the risks and evidence of various commonly utilized treatments for whiplash that has been published to date, the results of these reviews will be heavily incorporated in the remainder of this chapter.

COMPARING SAFETY AND EFFECTIVENESS OF COMMON THERAPIES

Common Pharmaceutical Treatments

Nonsteroidal Anti-Inflammatory Drugs (NSAIDs)

The most common conventional first-line treatment for most musculoskeletal pain syndromes is nonsteroidal anti-inflammatory drugs (NSAIDs). These are a broad class of prescription and over-the-counter drugs that include common aspirin, ibuprofen, naproxen, and similar drugs. NSAIDs are generally considered safe and are among the most prescribed drugs in the United States. NSAIDs also account for millions of dollars in annual sales of over-the-counter formulations.

Although they are generally considered safe, NSAID use has been associated with a variety of serious adverse effects, including bleeding and ulcers in the stomach and intestine, stroke, kidney problems (including kidney failure), life-threatening allergic reactions, and liver failure.[5]

One study published in *The New England Journal of Medicine*[6] estimated that at least 103,000 patients are hospitalized per year in the United States for serious gastrointestinal complications due to NSAID use. At an estimated cost of $15,000 to $20,000 per hospitalization, the annual direct costs of such complications exceed $2 billion. These authors also estimated that 16,500 NSAID-related deaths occur every year in the United States. This figure is similar to the annual number of deaths from AIDS and is considerably greater than the number of deaths from multiple myeloma, asthma, cervical cancer, or Hodgkin's disease. If deaths from gastrointestinal toxic effects of NSAIDs were tabulated separately in the National Vital Statistics reports, these effects would constitute the 15th most common cause of death in the United States.

Complications from NSAID use apparently do not result only from chronic, long-term use. One double-blind trial found that 6 of 32 healthy volunteers developed a gastric ulcer that was visible on endoscopic examination after only 1 week's treatment with naproxen (at a commonly prescribed dose of 500 mg twice daily).[7]

Although less common than gastrointestinal complications, kidney disease is also an infrequent but potentially serious complication from NSAIDs. One study[8] found NSAID use was associated with a fourfold increase in hospitalization for acute renal failure, a risk that was dose-dependent and occurred especially in the first month of NSAID therapy.

Simple Analgesics

Simple analgesics such as paracetamol (acetaminophen) are commonly seen as being the safest and most conservative pharmaceutical treatment for WAD. In recommended doses, paracetamol (available under a number of trade names, such as Tylenol and Anacin-3), does not irritate the lining of the stomach or affect blood coagulation as much as NSAIDs. Although generally safe at recommended doses, acute overdoses (above 1,000 mg per single dose and above 4,000 mg per day for adults, above 2,000 mg per day if drinking alcohol) of paracetamol can cause potentially fatal liver damage; in rare individuals, a normal dose can do the same. Alcohol consumption significantly heightens the risk.

Paracetamol toxicity is the leading cause of acute liver failure in the Western world and far exceeds all other causes of acute liver failure in the United States.[9] Paracetamol is the largest cause of drug overdoses in the United States, chiefly because of the relatively narrow range between therapeutic dose and toxic dose.[10] This problem is heightened by the widespread use of paracetamol together with NSAIDs and opioid analgesics in combination with pain-management drugs. Paracetamol is also used in many over-the-counter medications marketed for relief of cold and flu symptoms, migraine headache symptoms, menstrual symptoms, and other conditions.

Other Drugs

Skeletal muscle relaxant drugs, including benzodiazepines such as diazepam (Valium), are often used for treatment of acute or subacute WAD. Side effects most commonly reported were drowsiness, fatigue, muscle weakness, and ataxia. Other, less common side effects include confusion, depression, vertigo, constipation, blurred vision, hypotension, and amnesia.[11]

Other drugs that are sometimes used for treatment of WAD, such as corticosteroids and opioid analgesics, have a wide range of significant and potentially serious adverse effects. Opioid analgesics in particular have a significant risk of abuse and/or illicit use. However, these drugs have little evidence supporting their use for WAD or relief of nonspecific neck pain.

EVIDENCE FOR PHARMACOLOGICAL THERAPIES

Despite the widespread use of pharmacological therapies in WAD, the evidence supporting nearly all drugs commonly used for post-whiplash pain is scanty. Hurwitz et al,[4] in their BJD review, commented, "We were unable to identify any studies that evaluated the effectiveness of commonly used analgesic medications including acetaminophen, nonsteroidal anti-inflammatory drugs (NSAIDs), and narcotics, or studies of muscle relaxants and antidepressant medications in WAD. Medications were components of the 'usual care' protocols in several studies, however." There was a similar paucity of studies looking at common medications for patients with "nonspecific" neck pain (i.e., neck pain without history of whiplash).

CONSERVATIVE PHYSICAL TREATMENTS

Manual Therapies: Mobilization/Manipulation

Based on the evidence reviewed, Hurwitz et al[4] concluded that mobilization was "likely helpful" for acute WAD, whereas they concluded that for manipulation there was "not enough evidence to make a determination."

However, for nonspecific neck pain (i.e., neck pain without a history of whiplash), they found 17 studies looking at various types of manual therapies and found that there was overall positive evidence for both mobilization and manipulation, particularly when combined with exercise. This led them to include mobilization, manipulation, and other manual therapies among the "likely helpful" treatments for nonspecific neck pain. However, they also found one randomized controlled trial (RCT)[12] that reported that manipulation was associated with an increased risk of minor adverse reactions in patients with mostly subacute or chronic neck pain when compared with mobilization.

Reported complications from manipulation include sprains or strains, rib fractures, posttreatment soreness, and exacerbation of symptoms. Although these milder adverse reactions are far more common than the major complications of manipulation, they tend to be self-limiting and relatively benign in nature. In a prospective, clinic-based survey of 4,712 treatments on 1,058 new patients by 102 Norwegian chiropractors, Senstad, Leboeuf-Yde, and Borchgrevink[13] found that 55% of patients reported at least one "unpleasant reaction" during the course of a maximum of six visits. The most common were local discomfort (53%), headache (12%), tiredness (11%), or radiating discomfort (10%) (Figure 10-1). Reactions were mild or moderate in 85% of patients, and 74% of reactions had disappeared within 24 hours. There were no reports of serious complications in this study.

There is a fairly widespread impression among some health professionals that chiropractic-style manipulation of the cervical spine can result in dissection of the vertebral artery and lead to stroke of the posterior cerebral circulation.[14] Although recent evidence[15] suggests there may be some association between a recent visit to a chiropractor for treatment of a cervical-related complaint and a subsequent stroke, the same study found a similar association between a recent visit to a primary care

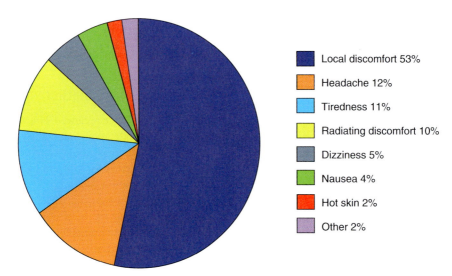

Figure 10-1   Types of complications from spinal manipulation.

physician and stroke. This study suggests any association between these phenomena is due to patients with undiagnosed vertebral artery dissection seeking clinical care for headache and neck pain associated with the evolving dissection (whether that care is from a primary care physician or a chiropractor) before the dissection evolves into a stroke. The study concludes that there is likely no causal relationship between the chiropractic visit and stroke (see Box 10-1).

Immobilization (Cervical Collar)

Immobilization by cervical collar (whether soft, firm, or rigid) has long been one of the mainstays of conventional conservative care for whiplash injuries, so much so that it has almost become a cliché. Increasingly, evidence suggests that the use of an immobilizing collar does little good and, if used for a prolonged period of time, may do more harm than good.

The Hurwitz et al review notes, "There is consistent evidence from 2 RCTs and one nonrandomized study that soft or rigid collars alone or in combination with other treatments were not associated with greater pain or disability reduction in the short- or long-term (up to 1 year) in persons with acute WAD when compared with advice to rest, exercises, and mobilization, and usual or no care."[4]

In spite of this evidence, many practitioners still routinely recommend prolonged use of an immobilizing cervical collar following a whiplash injury. The website of the National Institute of Neurological Disorders and Stroke notes, "Treatment for individuals with whiplash may include pain medications, nonsteroidal anti-inflammatory drugs, antidepressants, muscle relaxants, and a cervical collar (usually worn for 2 to 3 weeks)."[16]

Possible complications due to immobilization (particularly prolonged immobilization) theoretically include immobilization-induced degeneration and osteopenia, and muscular atrophy.

Although the short-term use of a soft collar may give a patient some pain relief and reassurance, long-term use may result in psychological dependency and fear-avoidance of normal neck motion and may promote iatrogenic disability.

Physical Modalities

Commonly used physical modalities for treating whiplash include traction, therapeutic ultrasound, transcutaneous electrical nerve stimulation (TENS), and various other types of therapeutic electrical stimulation (examples include high volt stimulation, low volt stimulation, interferential stimulation, and electrical stimulation using a variety of waveforms). All of these modalities have well-established contraindications and, when used appropriately, appear to have very rare complications. However, the evidence for the effectiveness of all these passive therapeutic modalities for WAD is scanty. For example, the effectiveness of electrotherapies in the treatment of acute neck pain was found lacking in a recent Cochrane review.[17]

BOX **10-1**   **Is Cervical Manipulation Safe?**

Cervical Manipulation: Safety Controversies

Critics of cervical manipulation have often focused on the perceived risk of severe complications from upper cervical manipulation; specifically, the possibility of dissection of the vertebral basilar artery (VBA) subsequently leading to a stroke of the brain stem circulation. By all accounts, this is an extraordinarily rare occurrence. However, it is potentially very serious, possibly resulting in permanent disability, death, or the "locked-in syndrome," in which the patient remains awake and aware but permanently paralyzed from the neck down.

Pathology of Cervical Arterial Dissection and Stroke

Trauma to the neck, either significant or trivial, may create stress to the vertebral artery, most likely between atlas and axis or atlas and occiput. This may cause a VBA dissection—a partial tearing of the inner artery wall (the intima). This dissection can cause turbulence in the blood flow, which can cause the formation of a hematoma or thrombus in the wall of the artery.

This hematoma can evolve in several different ways, affecting the ultimate outcome:

1. The hematoma may seal off, and if it is small, it may only minimally affect cerebral circulation, remaining essentially asymptomatic.
2. The hematoma may expand to occlude the vertebral artery completely, possibly leading to infarction of the brain stem or cerebellum (stroke); the symptoms might also be minimal if the contralateral vertebral artery compensates.
3. The hematoma may disrupt blood flow and form emboli; these emboli may travel into the smaller caliber arteries and arterioles distally, leading to transient ischemia or a completed stroke if there is significant infarction of brain tissue.
4. A subadventitial dissection may rupture further through the middle layer of the artery (the adventitia), resulting in subarachnoid hemorrhage.

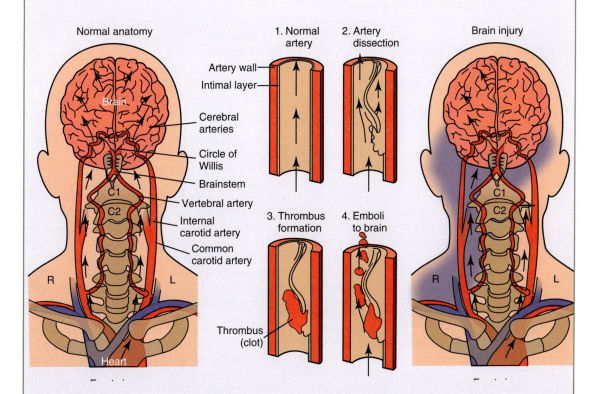

Normal anatomy — Brain, C1, C2, R, L, Heart

1. Normal artery — Artery wall, Intimal layer
2. Artery dissection
Cerebral arteries
Circle of Willis
Brainstem
Vertebral artery
Internal carotid artery
Common carotid artery
3. Thrombus formation — Thrombus (clot)
4. Emboli to brain
Brain injury — C1, C2, R, L

Vertebral basilar dissections are very rare phenomena and have been associated with trivial stresses to the cervical spine from normal activities such as swimming, yoga, stargazing, and overhead work.[20] Even common activities such as talking on the telephone, sexual intercourse, and sleep have been associated with VBA dissections. "Beauty Parlor Stroke," caused by cervical hyperextension over a sink while washing the hair, is also well documented.

Most cases of VBA dissection are spontaneous, with no apparent precipitating event or trauma. Conversely, VBA dissections are rare even in cases where severe cervical trauma is sustained, such as in catastrophic motor vehicle accidents. In other words, a "normal"

Continued

| BOX 10-1 | **Is Cervical Manipulation Safe?—cont'd** |

vertebral artery seems to be a robust structure that is not damaged even under significant trauma; however, an "abnormal" vertebral artery can apparently sustain catastrophic damage from trivial stress.

What are some of the indications that a patient might have an "abnormal" vertebral artery? Several inheritable connective tissue disorders have been associated with an increased risk of dissection of the vertebral artery and other cervical and cranial arteries.[21] These include the following:

- The vascular type of Ehlers-Danlos syndrome (also known as EDS Type IV): an inheritable disorder characterized by weakened linings of the walls of blood vessels and the intestine. Unlike better-known types of EDS (sometimes referred to as the "rubber-man disease"), Type IV EDS is associated with minimal skin and joint hyperextensibility but is associated with a notable tendency toward easy bruising. Affected individuals have an increased risk of spontaneous arterial or intestinal rupture, with a peak incidence in the third or fourth decade of life. A skin biopsy can diagnose this condition.
- Marfan's syndrome: a generalized disorder of connective tissue with skeletal, ocular, and cardiovascular manifestations. Characteristically, the affected person is tall and thin with long extremities, with an arm span greater than the height. They often have long, thin, and hyperextensible fingers. These individuals commonly have a marked spinal kyphosis and deformities of the sternum like pectus excavatum ("funnel chest") or pectus carinatum ("pigeon breast").
- Osteogenesis imperfecta (OI) Type I: a generalized inheritable disorder of the connective tissue. This is the most common and mildest type of OI and is associated with abnormal fragility of the skeleton, easy bruising, loose joints, and low muscle tone. Affected individuals have a tendency toward spinal curvature, often have a triangular-shaped face, and the whites of the eyes (sclera) may have a blue, purple, or gray tint.

Other history that may be associated with an increased risk of VBA dissection includes elevated serum homocysteine levels and a history of migraine headaches.

If a patient is in the process of an evolving VBA dissection, there may be no specific neurological signs or symptoms unless a large thrombus completely occludes the vertebral artery or an embolus that has been shed from the dissection has blocked the blood supply to a portion of the brain. One potential early warning sign is sudden onset of pain in the side of the neck, on the side of the head, or in the occipital region. These symptoms may be particularly significant if they are different from any pain the patient has had before, or in the absence of other exam findings supporting a musculoskeletal pain source. This suggests the pain might be referred pain from an evolving arterial dissection before an ischemic stroke has occurred. However, these early signs of a VBA dissection may be very subtle and difficult or impossible to differentiate from common musculoskeletal causes of neck pain and cervicogenic headache.

Although the signs and symptoms of an evolving VBA dissection are often difficult to differentiate from common cases of benign neck pain or headache, if an embolus breaks off the dissected wall of the artery and disrupts cerebral blood flow, the patient may present with RED FLAGS suggesting a possible ischemic event of the VBA circulation. These include the following:

- "The worst headache ever" or a headache unlike any other
- Severe dizziness or vertigo; nausea or vomiting
- Drop attacks or fainting
- Double vision, nystagmus, or other visual disturbances
- Difficulty swallowing or speaking
- Unsteadiness of gait
- Loss of sensation or movement on one side of the body

The Problem of Dizziness

A patient complaining of dizziness presents a particular diagnostic challenge. The dizziness or vertigo may have its origin in a musculoskeletal lesion of the cervical spine (such as vertebral dysfunction/subluxation or myofascial pain syndrome). If this is the case, a cervical adjustment may be the treatment of choice.[22]

However, the dizziness or vertigo might be an early sign of vertebral basilar ischemia, in which case a neck adjustment might precipitate a full stroke. There is no simple and reliable method to differentiate between these conditions. Determine whether neck rotation and extension aggravate the dizziness (which suggests a vascular cause), whether any other of the "Red Flags" are present, or whether cervical manipulations have aggravated the symptoms in the past. The presence of any of these factors may suggest a vascular cause and a contraindication to cervical manipulation.

When in doubt, a prudent course is to treat the neck with other nonmanipulative conservative methods such as soft tissue massage, physiological therapeutics, or nonforce manual techniques. If the dizziness shows some improvement under this course of care, it suggests a musculoskeletal, nonvascular etiology, and it might be appropriate to consider adding gentle osseous cervical adjustments to the treatment plan.

BOX **10-1**   **Is Cervical Manipulation Safe?—cont'd**

The Question of Causation

One original research project sponsored by the Bone and Joint Decade Task Force on Neck Pain and Its Associated Disorders looked at the relationship between a past history of chiropractic neck treatment and subsequent stroke of the VBA system.[15] This population-based case-control and case-crossover study retrospectively looked at data for hospitalization and diagnostic coding for all hospitals in the Canadian Provence of Ontario from 1993 to 2002. They identified diagnostic codes that were associated with VBA stroke and found 818 individuals who appeared to have had VBA strokes in the 9 years studied (reflecting 109,020,875 person-years of observation). For case-controls, they then randomly selected four age- and sex-matched controls from the registry of all health card numbers in Ontario for each case of VBA stroke found.

To determine whether or not there was an association between chiropractic care and subsequent VBA stroke, the researchers then used provincial insurance records to extract all reimbursed ambulatory encounters with either chiropractors or primary care physicians for both the stroke patients and their controls in the year before the date of the stroke.

The results of this study found that, although there was an association between visiting a chiropractor and having a VBA stroke, there was a similar (and in some patient groups, a greater) association between visiting a primary care physician and having a VBA stroke. The study concluded that any observed association between a VBA stroke and a patient's visit to either a chiropractor or a family physician was likely due to patients with an undiagnosed vertebral artery dissection seeking care for neck pain or headache before their stroke, rather than the stroke being directly caused by any treatment performed.

The results of this study emphasized the importance of developing the ability to differentiate a patient presenting with neck pain or headache as the result of an evolving vertebral basilar dissection and stroke, as opposed to the garden-variety neck pain patient. This differentiation is often difficult and is based on subtle signs. This illustrates how critical it is that all practitioners, whether they practice manipulation or not, screen for issues in the history and exam that suggest that any cervical-related symptoms are from an occult and potentially serious cause.

NONCONSERVATIVE INTERVENTIONS

Botulinum Toxin A Injection

The Hurwitz et al BJD review[4] concluded that muscular injections of botulinum toxin A (BOTOX) was found to be ineffective and harmful in WAD, based upon a single acceptable double-blind, placebo-controlled RCT[18] that looked at its use versus placebo in the treatment of people with disabling neck pain of at least 3 months duration. The study found similar decreases in mean neck pain and disability scores and increases in trigger point pressure thresholds in both groups over 16 weeks post-treatment; however, adverse reactions were much more frequent in the botulinum toxin A group.

SURGICAL INTERVENTIONS

Another review[19] performed by the Bone and Joint Decade Task Force on Neck Pain and Its Associated Disorders found that "the current evidence does not support the use of anterior cervical fusion or cervical disc arthroplasty for neck pain without radiculopathy or serious underlying pathology." In addition, it was found that potentially serious complications after open surgical procedures performed on the cervical spine occurred in approximately 4% of patients. Minor complications after open surgical procedures on the cervical spine (such as dysphagia, hoarseness, and donor site pain) were found to be frequent, but they usually resolved with time.

The review found that serious adverse events associated with less-invasive surgical procedures such as cervical foraminal or epidural injections were relatively uncommon (<1%). However, these procedures led to relatively frequent minor adverse events (5%-20%).

CONCLUSIONS

Although researchers have expended much effort to identify the best treatments for neck pain, and the reviewers of the BJD have contributed a major accomplishment by systematically reviewing the evidence, one can't help but feel unsatisfied and even frustrated with the overall results. The only definitive conclusion that can be drawn from the studies done to date is that the science supporting most clinical interventions for neck pain is

TABLE **10-1**

"Red Flags"* for Neck Pain Patients

Sign or Symptom	Condition to Be Ruled Out
History of a significant trauma, such as a fall or significant auto accident	Possible traumatic fracture
History of osteoporosis, corticosteroid use, or endocrine disease; age over 50	Possible pathological fracture or severe osteoporosis
Recent unexplained weight loss or malaise; history of cancer or other serious disease	Possible pathological fracture or metastatic disease
History of recent bacterial infection (e.g., urinary tract infection); intravenous drug use or immune suppression from steroid use, transplant, or HIV infection; recent fever over 100° F	Possible spinal infection or meningitis
Nonmechanical pain pattern: constant, progressive pain unrelated to movement with no relief from rest, or severe pain at night	Possible metastatic disease or referred pain from organ pathology
Severe or progressive weakness or numbness in the arms, particularly if it extends past the elbow	Possible disc herniation with true radiculopathy
Neck pain that causes shooting pains into the arms or legs, and/or an extremely rigid neck during forward flexion	Possible cervical disc herniation or meningitis
Headache or neck pain accompanied by numbness, weakness, dizziness, nausea, or vomiting	Possible CVA, intracranial bleed, or CNS tumor
Headache or neck pain accompanied by confusion, visual disturbances, difficulties in speech or swallowing, or alteration in consciousness	Possible CVA, vertebral basilar insufficiency, intracranial bleed, or CNS tumor
Severe or progressive headache, or a sudden onset of "the worst headache ever."	Possible CVA, vertebral basilar insufficiency, intracranial bleed, or CNS tumor

*A patient presenting with one or more Red Flags may require further diagnostic studies to rule out potentially serious pathology. The presence of any of these Red Flags is not necessarily a contraindication to conservative care; it simply suggests the need for further diagnostic investigation before any conservative care is initiated.
CNS, central nervous system; CVA, cerebrovascular accident.

incomplete and often conflicting, particularly when it comes to managing neck pain that is the result of whiplash. The authors of the Hurwitz et al review apparently share this opinion, concluding, "Despite an explosion of the neck-pain literature including several methodologically sound studies in the past decade, there remains limited or conflicting evidence for most of the therapies commonly given to WAD patients."[4]

Despite the ambiguity, some general conclusions can be drawn from the evidence. First, one is struck with the impression that, in general, many of the **more invasive** procedures have **less evidence** supporting their use compared to many **less invasive** procedures. For example, the authors of the Hurwitz et al review found that of the 30 systematic reviews identified and accepted as scientifically admissible, 24 involved noninvasive interventions.

Whereas the evidence for many commonly used treatments in acute WAD is variable and less than conclusive, the current state of evidence is almost completely silent on what to do with patients who don't recover in the acute stage and become chronic. The Hurwitz et al[4] review noted, "Because of conflicting evidence and few high-quality studies, no firm conclusions could be drawn about the most effective noninvasive interventions for patients with chronic WAD." This near absence of evidence is especially troublesome because these chronic and nonresponsive cases tend to account for the most costly toll of whiplash, both financially and in terms of patient suffering.

RECOMMENDATIONS

Because there is no current consensus on the best whiplash treatment, and because even a comprehensive review like the one performed by Hurwitz et al failed to find "overwhelming evidence" to suggest that there is one clearly better treatment option, practitioners and patients are faced with a variety of choices for management of WAD. Because of the scientific "toss-up" noted in the Hurwitz review, other elements, such as patients' preferences for treatment and their attitudes toward risk, should play an important role in deciding the best treatment.

Based on the best evidence available, a scientifically valid and patient-centered approach to managing whiplash-associated disorders should incorporate the following principles:

- Screen for "Red Flags" in the patient's history and presentation (Table 10-1).
- In the absence of Red Flags, it is unlikely that further extensive diagnostic testing will yield any clinically useful information.
- Treatment should focus on avoiding iatrogenic disability; WAD patients should be reassured and should be given advice to keep active and avoid unnecessary work absences.
- It is important that practitioners do not invalidate the effect that pain can have on a patient's life; however, pain and disability should not be the focus of treatment. Instead, the restoration of function and independence should be the focus.
- The patient should be given a choice among the treatments that have been shown to be effective and safe, and the patient's personal preference for selecting treatment should be respected.

Generally, an approach emphasizing effective patient education and early return to normal activity levels, together with short-term active therapy including exercise instruction and manual therapies, appears to be the most scientifically valid approach. This contrasts with traditional approaches that often encouraged rest, immobilization, and passive therapies such as pharmaceutical interventions (sometimes including powerful drugs) and extensive use of passive physical modalities.

The care for WAD that has the most evidence of effectiveness is clearly an approach that is conservative and noninvasive. Because of this, it is care that can be provided by a wide variety of licensed health providers, including general practice medical physicians, osteopathic physicians, physical therapists, and doctors of chiropractic. In other words, when seeking quality care for whiplash, a provider's license and credentials are less important than his or her dedication to a conservative, evidence-based, and patient-centered philosophy.

REFERENCES

1. Spitzer WO, et al: Scientific monograph of the Quebec Task Force on Whiplash-Associated Disorders: redefining "whiplash" and its management, *Spine* 20(suppl 8):S1-S73, 1995.
2. Côté P, et al: A systematic review of the prognosis of acute whiplash and a new conceptual framework to synthesize the literature, *Spine* 26(19):E445-E558, 2001.
3. Haldeman S, et al: The Bone and Joint Decade 2000-2010 Task Force on Neck Pain and Its Associated Disorders: executive summary, *Spine* 33(suppl 4):S5-S7, 2008.
4. Hurwitz EL, et al: Treatment of neck pain: noninvasive interventions: results of the Bone and Joint Decade 2000-2010 Task Force on Neck Pain and Its Associated Disorders, *Spine* 33(suppl 4):S123-S152, 2008.
5. FDA medication guide for non-steroidal anti-inflammatory drugs (NSAIDs), http://www.fda.gov/downloads/Drugs/DrugSafety/ucm088657.pdf. Accessed November 23, 2010.
6. Wolfe MM, Lichtenstein DR, Singh G: Gastrointestinal toxicity of nonsteroidal antiinflammatory drugs, *New Engl J Med* 340(24):1888-1889, 1999.
7. Simon LS, et al: Preliminary study of the safety and efficacy of SC-58635, a novel cyclooxygenase 2 inhibitor, *Arthritis Rheum* 41:1591-1602, 1998.
8. Pérez Gutthann S, et al: Nonsteroidal anti-inflammatory drugs and the risk of hospitalization for acute renal failure, *Arch Intern Med* 156:2433-2439, 1996.
9. Larson AM, et al: Acetaminophen-induced acute liver failure: results of a United States multicenter, prospective study, *Hepatology* 42(6):1364-1372, 2005.

10. Joint Meeting of the Drug Safety and Risk Management Advisory Committee with the Anesthetic and Life Support Drugs Advisory Committee and the Nonprescription Drugs Advisory Committee. Meeting announcement, June 29-30, 2009. http://www.fda.gov/AdvisoryCommittees/Calendar/ucm143083.htm. Accessed November 23, 2010.

11. Data sheet for VALIUM brand of diazepam tablets. http://www.accessdata.fda.gov/drugsatfda_docs/label/2008/013263s083lbl.pdf. Accessed November 23, 2010.

12. Hurwitz E, et al: A randomized trial of chiropractic manipulation and mobilization for patients with neck pain: clinical outcomes from the UCLA neck-pain study, *Am J Public Health* 10:1634-1641, 2002.

13. Senstad O, Leboeuf-Yde C, Borchgrevink C: Frequency and characteristics of side effects of spinal manipulative therapy, *Spine* 22(4):435-440, 1997.

14. Ernst E: Spinal manipulation: its safety is uncertain, *CMAJ* 166:40, 2002.

15. Cassidy JD, et al: Risk of vertebrobasilar stroke and chiropractic care: results of a population-based case control and case crossover study, *Spine* 33(suppl):S176-S183, 2008.

16. National Institute of Neurological Disorders and Stroke: NINDS whiplash information page, http://www.ninds.nih.gov/disorders/whiplash/whiplash.htm. Accessed November 23, 2010.

17. Kroeling P, et al: A Cochrane review of electrotherapy for mechanical neck disorders, *Spine* 20:E641-E648, 2005.

18. Wheeler AH, Goolkasian P, Gretz SS: Botulinum toxin A for the treatment of chronic neck pain, *Pain* 94:255-260, 2001.

19. Carragee EJ, et al: Treatment of neck pain injections and surgical interventions: results of the Bone and Joint Decade 2000-2010 Task Force on Neck Pain and Its Associated Disorders, *Spine* 33(suppl 4):S153-S169, 2008.

20. Okawara S, Nibblelink D: Vertebral artery occlusion following hyperextension and rotation of the head, *Stroke* 5(5):640-642, 1974.

21. Schievink WI: The treatment of spontaneous carotid and vertebral artery dissections, *Curr Opin Cardiol* 15(5):316-321, 2000.

22. Fitz-Ritson D: Assessment of cervicogenic vertigo, *J Manip Physiol Ther* 14(3):193-198, 1991.

Chapter 11

Prognosis of Whiplash-Associated Disorders

Meridel I. Gatterman

There is little doubt that soft tissue injuries of the cervical spine can leave persisting symptoms.[1] Jackson[2] discussed posttraumatic chronic cases in patients whose symptoms persisted well beyond the anticipated time. She noted that because of the tendency to dismiss these patients with a psychological diagnosis that they will "be relieved of worry and anxiety knowing that they have explainable reasons for their symptoms." Hohl,[3] in 1974, reported that lasting symptoms are intermittent neck ache, stiffness, and headaches often with interscapular and upper extremity pain and numbness. These findings are consistent with a more recent study by Squires, Gargan, and Banister.[1] They noted that in the patients that they studied, symptoms did not improve after settlement of litigation. This too, is consistent with the published literature of Balla and Moraitis in 1970[4] and Mendelson in 1982.[5] Parmar and Raymakers[6] found that whereas most patients reach their final state after 2 years, a small percentage improves with time.

Holm[8] stated that in the early management of persons with whiplash-associated disorders, it is important to consider psychological status, expectations for recovery, and social circumstances in addition to the biomedical components of the injury. These factors must all be considered in the prognosis of patients with whiplash trauma. The natural course of recovery and the prognosis for whiplash-associated disorders are controversial. Some claim that such injury and its prognosis are solely determined by the physical injury.[9-11] Others are critical of this point of view, stating that psychosocial factors are relevant.[1,8] Some factors are known to contribute to a poor prognosis.

PROGNOSTIC FACTORS

Despite observations of bias with regard to the prognosis of whiplash victims in the literature,[8,12] there is reasonable agreement on several factors affecting prognosis.[8] These factors include severity of the injury,[3,13] position of the head at the time of impact,[8,13,17] gender,[8,14-16] and age.[1,13-15] Holm[8] also includes psychosocial factors that contribute to poor prognosis, such as lower education, passive coping strategies, poor mental health, and low pain tolerance. Despite various possible explanations for the differences in the course of recovery after whiplash injury, the magnitude of the importance of a patient's prognosis is individual, and management must be patient centered to achieve optimal results.

Severity of Injury

Severity of injury can produce an unfavorable prognosis if extensive soft tissue damage occurs. The presence of fracture or dislocation need not be present for the patient to experience ongoing pathology or dysfunction. In a study of patients with complaints of headache, 27% were symptomatic 6 months post-accident, and another study found that 42% of their cohort were symptomatic an average of 2 years post-accident. Squires et al[1] found that 70% of the patients in a 15-year follow-up study continued to complain of symptoms referable to the accident 15 years later. These ranged from mild to severe. This is much higher than the 27% that remained symptomatic in a 2-year post-injury study that reported the prognostic significance of the initial severity of injury.[13]

Instability must be ruled out in late whiplash symptoms. Instability cannot be diagnosed by static tests.[18] A boggy sensation with no abrupt end feel on palpation is suggestive of instability, and dynamic imaging (see Chapter 5) is required for confirmation. In a case series, reported that when these patients were investigated with functional magnetic imaging (see Chapter 5), dramatic findings were obtained.[18] Imaging showed capsule tears and instability of the lateral atlantoaxial joint, and scar tissue around the odontoid process with cord impingement upon rotation of the head. This pathology was consistent with the patient's complaints and the abnormalities confirmed at surgery. The patients' symptoms were previously dismissed as psychogenic, and the possibility of pathology was ignored. Bogduk notes that the psychogenic model of whiplash-associated disorders, although attractive and convenient, is neither reliable nor valid.[18]

Position of Head at Time of Impact

Sideways position of the head at the time of impact tends to produce more severe injury and a poorer prognosis.[8,13,17] If the head is turned sideways at the time of impact, as when looking in the rearview mirror, the force of the impact must be resisted by the unilateral anterior strap muscles on the side facing forward. Damage to these muscles not only produces neck pain but also headache (see Chapters 5, 6, and 7) and upper extremity symptoms on the same side (see Chapter 6). Persistent neck and upper extremity pain can significantly produce a poorer prognosis. Pain maps in a 1996 follow-up study[1] reinforce the view of Hohl[3] that radiating pain is associated with more severe disability. Unilateral involvement of facet joints should also be considered in these cases. (See Chapter 8.) Bogduk and Marsland[19] noted the distribution of pain

conforms more closely to radiation from the facet joints rather than dermatomes.

Gender

A number of authors have found that pain and disability did not vary with gender.[17,21,22] A poorer prognosis for whiplash-associated disorders in females has been explained in terms of both biological and social factors.[8,20] Krafft et al[16] indicate that women run a higher risk of sustaining a whiplash injury when involved in a car crash. This may be due to their lighter frames, less-protective musculature, and their tendency to drive smaller vehicles compared with males. Croft[23] notes that although females may be more at risk of acute injury, they are roughly equal with males for the likelihood of developing late whiplash. Squires et al[1] reported that women and older patients had a worse outcome after 15 years.

Age

There appears to be more agreement that age is a prognostic factor for a worse outcome than gender.[1,17,20,24-25] Elderly patients in the long term tend to have more symptoms (pain, among others) compared with younger patients.[17,25] Age has been found to significantly predict the outcome of disability, with high age corresponding to high ratings of disability.[24]

PSYCHOLOGICAL AND PSYCHOSOCIAL FACTORS THAT DELAY RECOVERY

Holm[8] states that when reviewing the literature on prognosis after whiplash injury, it becomes evident that biomedical, psychological, and social factors play a role and also interact. Bogduk[26] notes that review of the literature reveals a considerable amount of biomechanical and experimental data that substantiates a diverse organic basis for patient's symptoms and that the symptoms of whiplash injury are poorly understood or misrepresented as due to neurosis. Too often, patients' complaints have been dismissed as psychogenic and unrelated to the trauma of whiplash injury.[2,18] In the current multidimensional model of musculoskeletal pain and patient-centered care, psychological and psychosocial factors must be considered as having a role in the perpetuation of symptoms from whiplash trauma. However, the relationship between pain and disability, physical impairment, and psychosocial variables is complex and not fully understood.[27] Clinicians should maintain an open mind with respect to potential interrelationships between these variables.[28] There has been a paucity of investigations of pain and disability related to the cervical spine compared to that of low back pain.[28] Extrapolation from findings of studies of low back pain may not be valid. Recent evidence demonstrates that the development and perpetuation of neck pain probably involves psychological factors unique to this condition.[29-31] In an earlier study, evidence of psychological disturbance was found in approximately half of the patients in the 15-year follow-up study by Squires et al.[1] In a 1992 study, Gargan, Bannister, and Main[7] found that patients who were psychologically normal at the time of injury developed abnormal psychological profiles if symptoms persisted for 3 months. Wallis, Lord, and Bogduk[32] demonstrated that psychological distress resolved following pain relief using zygapophyseal joint blocks in patients with chronic whiplash-associated disorders. This suggests that ongoing psychological distress may be dependent upon symptom persistence.

Posttraumatic stress symptoms, when misdiagnosed or inappropriately treated, can significantly delay recovery from whiplash injury.[31,33] Symptoms may include intrusive thoughts and/or images of the crash, avoidance behavior such as avoiding driving or avoidance through substance abuse, and hyperarousal such as panic attacks, hypervigilance, and sleep disturbance.[28] The presence of posttraumatic stress symptoms is associated with greater levels of pain and disability, more severe whiplash complaints, and poor functional recovery from the injury.[17,33] Whiplash injury differs from other causes of neck injury in that it is precipitated by the trauma of a vehicle crash. Post-accident, those with a whiplash diagnosis such as neck pain are likely to have a posttraumatic stress disorder at 12 months compared to those who did not report neck pain.[34] A diagnosis of moderate posttraumatic stress disorder in patients suffering from whiplash-associated disorder has been found to be a strong predictor of poor outcome.[35,36]

Educational background has been found to be a factor in the prognosis of whiplash injuries.[8] Those with a low educational level appear to be more vulnerable to daily hassles and stress following whiplash injury.[37] Chronic patients with whiplash-associated disorders appear to be more vulnerable and react with more distress than healthy people to all kinds of stressors. Stress responses probably play

an important role in the maintenance or deterioration of whiplash-associated complaints. In the early management of patients with whiplash-associated disorders, it is important to consider psychological status, expectations for recovery, and social circumstances, in addition to the biomedical components of the injury.

Since Engel[38] proposed the biopsychosocial model in 1977, an alternative to the biomedical model of illness or disease has been studied. As opposed to the biomedical model, the biopsychosocial model emphasizes interactions among the various aspects of pathology, psychology, and behavioral adaptations in clinicians' attitudes, in patients, and in the society. A biopsychosocial model, coupled with a patient-centered paradigm,[39] appears to be the most appropriate concept for understanding the clinical course of whiplash-associated disorders. Holm,[8] building on and modifying Gallagher's diagnostic matrix, adapted this matrix to whiplash-associated disorders (Table 11-1). This biopsychosocial net presents factors that should be considered in the prognosis of patients suffering from whiplash-associated disorders. The biopsychosocial model that considers an effect of cultural expectation, cultural factors that generate symptom amplification and attribution, as well as the possibility that physical and psychological causes coexist, seems more helpful.[40]

Given that meta-analysis tends to mix apples and oranges, not to mention pomegranates and pineapples, a recent study evaluated the prognostic literature regarding risk factors for persistent problems following whiplash injury.[41] The study concluded that evidence for prognosis and intervention are difficult to interpret because of differences in inception times, outcomes used, and heterogeneity. Nonetheless the study concluded that the following nine factors are significant predictors of prognosis following whiplash injury: no postsecondary education, female gender, history of previous neck pain, presence of neck pain at baseline, greater intensity of neck pain, presence of headache, catastrophizing, a whiplash-associated disorder grading of 2-3 (more severe injury), and no seat belt at time of collision. It was noted that neck pain intensity, headache, whiplash-associated disorders grade, and postsecondary education were robust to publication bias. The authors recommended that risk factors should be routinely assessed during history taking and considered when establishing a prognosis for recovery. They noted that clinicians should also remember that "lack of evidence" is not

TABLE **11-1**			
Possible Factors in the Prognosis of Whiplash-Associated Disorders			
	Predisposition	**Precipitation**	**Perpetuation**
Physical	Age, gender Previous pain condition, pathology, or degenerative condition	Tissue damage (nerves, blood vessels, muscles, ligaments, joints) Inflammatory response	Tissue damage Other concurrent injuries Neurophysical disturbance (central sensitization) Disturbed immune response
Psychological	Age, gender, education Vulnerable personality Low pain threshold Pretraumatic stress Pretraumatic mental disorder Prior abuse	Severity of injury of significant others or other parties Posttraumatic stress Guilt or anger	Depressive mood, anxiety, cognition, guilt or anger, illness attribution, coping and pain behavior, perceived helplessness, uncertain or decreased recovery expectations Other concurrent injuries
Social	Abusive or traumatic relationship with health care system or insurance system Illness or social dysfunction in other family members Economic stress Media information (prior knowledge)	Severity and direction of collision impact Car design Comfort and social support at work and at home Health care management Paramedical management	Social support: family network and reinforcement of dependency Job-related factors: unemployment, high physical and mental strain Deficiency of health care: poor coordination, iatrogenic effects, Insurance system: financial incentives, slow and lengthy process, prior knowledge

Modified from Holm L: *Epidemiological aspects on pain in whiplash associated disorders*, Stockholm, Sweden, 2007, Karolinska Institute.

synonymous with "evidence against" a point that is especially relevant when considering the absence of hard physical signs as significant predictors in their review.[41]

The late whiplash syndrome is not merely psychosomatic. With appropriate management, the prognosis of whiplash-associated disorders is generally favorable.[18] Neck pain is present in almost all symptomatic subjects, and neck injury can be a trigger for widespread pain.[8] One important aspect of the course of whiplash-associated disorders is whether the neck injury is a trigger for subsequent widespread pain. (See "Central Sensitization," Chapter 6.) When pain persists or other symptoms don't resolve within 3 months, patients generally require more sophisticated management.[18] Functional imaging, including functional magnetic imaging, is necessary to determine movement abnormalities. (See Chapter 5.) "Whiplash can have lesions"[18] that cannot be diagnosed using static

tests; it requires dynamic testing.[18] Severity of injury is complicated by pre-existing conditions, including previous injury and congenital anomalies. Structural variations, degenerative changes, or inflammatory processes can affect both healing ability and the damage sustained during accidents.[20] Narrowing of the spinal canal places the patient at greater risk of suffering neurological deficits when a whiplash injury occurs. It is rational that some late whiplash symptoms associated with zygapophyseal joint dysfunction can be prevented if the patient is initially evaluated for motion segment dysfunction (subluxation).[42,43] (See Chapter 8.) This is suggested by the pain mapping of patients with persistent symptoms and facet joint blocks.[19,26,32]

IN THE PATIENT'S INTEREST

Patient-centered care that focuses on the individual patient's recovery can in many cases prevent long-term effects of whiplash trauma and lead to a more favorable prognosis.

There is reasonable argument, however, for the presence of pathoanatomical lesions in at least some of the injured people,[44] and these should not be dismissed with a psychological diagnosis without appropriate investigations.[18] The essence of patient-centered care is that patients are individuals with individual responses to any injury and especially in those with whiplash-associated disorders.[2] Those that seek to control the cost of management of whiplash-associated disorders should not approach patients solely with population-based recommendations.[45]

Failure to respond to treatment in 12 weeks begs for a complete reassessment.[46] Over-treatment is not only costly but in some cases can be harmful and delay recovery. Failure to respond to treatment may be caused by incorrect diagnosis, inappropriate treatment, incompatibility between doctor and patient, secondary gain (patient receives benefit from pain behavior), and co-existing conditions.[46] It is the responsibility of the patient-centered doctor to take a complete history, perform an appropriate physical examination and any specialized diagnostic procedure that is clinically indicated, assess the patient's general health status, and formulate a diagnosis before providing appropriate care. When indicated, consultation with continuity in the co-management or referral to other health care providers may be necessary. Above all, the patient-centered health care provider must develop a partnership that actively engages the patient in his or her recovery.[47] These steps may lead to a more favorable prognosis, avoiding needless suffering and excessive cost.

REFERENCES

1. Squires B, Gargan MF, Bannister GC: Soft-tissue injuries of the cervical spine: 15-year follow-up, *J Bone Joint Surg* 78B(6):955-957, 1996.
2. Jackson R: *The cervical syndrome*, 4th ed, Springfield, IL, 1977, Charles C Thomas, pp 334.
3. Hohl M: Soft tissue injuries in automobile injuries of the neck in automobile accidents, *J Bone Joint Surg* 56-A:1675-1682, 1974.
4. Balla JI, Moraitis S: Knights in armour: a follow-up study of injuries after legal settlement, *Med J Aust* 2:355-361, 1970.
5. Mendelson G: Not "cured by verdict": effect of legal settlement on compensation claimants, *Med J Aust* 2:132-134, 1982.
6. Parmar HV, Raymakers R: Neck injuries from rear impact road traffic accidents: prognosis in persons seeking compensation, *Injury* 24:75-78, 1993.
7. Gargan MF, Bannister GC, Main CJ: *Behavioural response to whiplash injury.* Paper presented at the British Cervical Spine Society. Bowness-on-Windermere, UK, November 7, 1992.
8. Holm L: *Epidemiological aspects on pain in whiplash associated disorders*, Stockholm, Sweden, 2007, Karolinska Institute.
9. Ferrari R: *The whiplash encyclopedia: the facts and myths of whiplash*, Gaithersburg, MA, 1999, Aspen Pub.
10. Partheni M, et al: A prospective cohort study of the outcome of acute whiplash injury in Greece, *Clin Exp Rheumatol* 18(1):67-70, 2000.
11. Ferrari R, et al: Laypersons' expectation of the sequelae of whiplash injury. A cross-cultural comparative study between Canada and Lithuania, *Med Sci Monit* 8(11):CR728-CR734, 2002.
12. Freeman M, et al: A review and methodologic critique of the literature refuting whiplash syndrome, *Spine* 24(1):86-98, 1999.
13. Radanov BP, Sturzenegger M, Stefano G: Factors influencing recovery from headache after common whiplash, *Br Med J* 307:652-655, 1993.
14. Bannister G, Gargan M: Prognosis of whiplash injuries: a review of the literature, *Spine State of Art* 7:557-569, 1993.
15. Dolinis J: Risk factors for "whiplash" in drivers: a cohort study of rear-end traffic crashes, *Injury* 28(3):173-179, 1997.
16. Krafft M, et al: Soft tissue injury of the cervical spine in rear-end car collisions, *J Traffic Med* 25(3-4):89-96, 1997.
17. Radanov BP, Sturzenegger M, Stefano GD: Long term outcome after whiplash injury: a 2-year follow-up considering features of injury mechanism and somatic, radiologic, and psychosocial findings, *Medicine* 74(5):281-297, 1995.
18. Bogduk N: Whiplash can have lesions, *Pain Res Manag* 11(3):155, 2006.
19. Bogduk N, Marsland A: The cervical zygapophyseal joints as a source of pain, *Spine* 13:610-617, 1988.
20. Foreman SM, Hooper PD: Factors affecting long-term outcome. In Foreman SM, Croft AC, editors: *Whiplash injuries: the cervical acceleration/deceleration syndrome*, ed 3, Baltimore, 2002, Lippincott Williams & Wilkins, pp 499-520.
21. Deans GT, et al: Neck sprain—a major cause of disability following car accidents, *Injury* 18:10-12, 1987.
22. Soderlund A, Lindberg P: Long-term functional and psychological problems in whiplash associated disorders, *Int J Rehabil Res* 22(2):1-7, 1999.
23. Croft AC: Soft tissue injury: long and short-term effects. In Foreman SM, Croft AC, editors: *Whiplash injuries: the cervical acceleration/*

deceleration syndrome, 3rd ed, Baltimore, 2002, Lippincott Williams & Wilkins, pp 334-428.

24. Kyhlback M, Thierfelder T, Soderland A: Prognostic factors in whiplash-associated disorders, *Int J Rehabil Res* 25:181-187, 2002.

25. Gargan MF: Banister GC: Long-term prognosis of soft-tissue injuries of the neck, *J Bone Joint Surg* 72B(5):901-903, 1990.

26. Bogduk N: The anatomy and pathophysiology of whiplash, *Clin Biomech* 1:92-101, 1986.

27. Linton S: Psychological risk factors for neck and back pain. In Nachemson A, Jonsson E, editors: *Neck and back pain. The scientific causes, diagnosis and treatment*. Philadelphia, 2000, Lippincott Williams & Wilkins, pp 57-78.

28. Jull G, et al: *Whiplash, headache and neck pain. Research-based directions for physical therapies*, New York, 2008, Churchill Livingstone.

29. Peebles J, McWilliams L, MacLennan R: A comparison of Symptom Checklist 90-Revised profiles from patients with chronic pain from whiplash with other musculoskeletal conditions, *Spine* 26:766-770, 2001.

30. Wenzel H, Haug T, Mykletun A: A population study of anxiety and depression among persons who report whiplash traumas, *J Psychosom Res* 53:831-835, 2002.

31. Sterling M, et al: The development of psychological changes following whiplash injury, *Pain* 106:481-489, 2003.

32. Wallis B, Lord S, Bogduk N: Resolution of psychological distress of whiplash patients following treatment by radiofrequency neurotomy: a randomized, double-blind, placebo controlled trial, *Pain* 73:15-22, 1997.

33. Buitenhuis J, et al: Relationship between posttraumatic stress disorder symptoms and the course of whiplash complaints, *J Psychosom Res* 61:681-689, 2006.

34. Freidenberg B, et al: Posttraumatic stress disorder and whiplash after motor vehicle accidents. In Young G, Kane A, Nickolson K, editors: *Psychological knowledge in court*, New York, 2006, Springer, pp 215-224.

35. Sterling M, et al: Physical and psychological factors predict outcome following whiplash injury, *Pain* 114:141-148, 2005.

36. Sterling M, Jull G, Kenardy J: Physical and psychological predictors of outcome following whiplash injury maintain predictive capacity at long term follow-up, *Pain* 122:102-108, 2006.

37. Blokhorst MG, et al: Daily hassles and stress vulnerability in patients with a whiplash-associated disorder, *Int J Rehabil Res* 25:173-179, 2002.

38. Engel GL: The need for a new medical model: a challenge for biomedicine, *Science* 196(4286):129-136, 1977.

39. Gatterman MI: A patient-centered paradigm: A model for chiropractic education and research, *J Altern Complement Med* 1:371-386, 1995.

40. Ferrari R, Shrader H: The late whiplash syndrome: a biopsychosocial approach, *J Neurol Neurosurg Psychiatry* 70:722-726, 2001.

41. Walton DM, et al: Risk factors for persistent problems following whiplash injury: results of a systematic review and meta-analysis, *J Orthop Sports Phys Ther* 39:334-350, 2009.

42. Peterson C, Gatterman MI: The nonmanipulable subluxation. In Gatterman MI, editor: *Principles of chiropractic: subluxation*, 2nd ed, St Louis, 2005, Mosby, pp 168-190.

43. Jull G, Bogduk N, Marsland A: The accuracy of manual diagnosis for cervical zygapophyseal joint pain syndromes, *Med J Aust* 148:233-236, 1988.

44. Bogduk N: Point of view, *Spine* 27:1940-1941, 2002.

45. Cassidy JD, Cote P: Is it time for a population health approach to neck pain? *J Manipulative Physiol Ther* 31:442-446, 2008.

46. Jaquet PE: *An introduction to clinical chiropractic*, Geneva, Switzerland, 1994, Grounauer.

47. Hawk C, Dusio ME: A survey of 492 U.S. chiropractors on primary care and prevention related issues, *J Manipulative Physiol Ther* 18:57-64, 1995.

Credits

Figures 2-1, 2-2, 2-19, 2-20, 2-21, 2-22, 2-23, 2-24, 2-25, 2-26, 2-27, 2-29, 2-30, 2-31, 2-32, 2-33, 2-34, 2-35, 6-1, 6-3, 6-5, 6-7, 6-9, 6-11, 6-13, 6-17, 6-19, 6-21, 6-23: Modified from Muscolino JE: *The muscular system: the skeletal muscles of the human body*, St Louis, 2010, Mosby.

Figures 2-3A-C, 2-4A-C, 2-6A-B, 2-10, 2-12, 2-13, 2-14, 2-15, 2-16, 2-17, 2-18, 2-28, 2-40: From Cramer GD, Darby SA: *Basic and clinical anatomy of the spine, spinal cord, and ANS*, 2nd ed, St Louis, 2005, Mosby.

Figures 2-8, 2-9, 2-36, 2-37, 2-38, 2-39: Modified from Cramer GD, Darby SA: *Basic and clinical anatomy of the spine, spinal cord, and ANS*, 2nd ed, St Louis, 2005, Mosby.

Figures 2-5A-D, 4-1: Gatterman, ML: *Chiropractic management of spine related disorders*, 2nd edition, Philadelphia, 2004, Lippincott, Williams & Wilkins.

Figure 2-11: Modified from Yu S, Sether L, Haughton VM: Facet joint menisci of the cerviczl spine: correlative MR imaging and cryomicrotomy study, *Radiology* 164:79–82, 1987.

Figures 4-2A-C, 4-3A-B, 4-4A-B, 4-5A-C, 4-6, 4-7A-B, 4-8A-D, 4-9, 4-10, 4-11, 4-12, 4-13A-C, 4-14A-B, 4-15A-D, 4-16, 4-18A-C, 8-16A-C: Evans, RC: *Orthopaedic illustrated physical assessment*, 3rd edition, St Louis, 2009, Mosby.

Figure 4-17: Jull G, Sterling M, Falla D, Treleavan J, O'Leary S: *Whiplash, headache and neck pain: research-based directions for physical therapies*, New York, 2008, Churchill Livingstonem, p. 138.

Figures 5-1, 5-2, 5-3: Courtesy of Dr. Lisa Hoffman.

Figure 5-5: Images courtesy of Cliff Tao, DC, DACBR and Dio Kim, DC, Lac, Anaheim, CA.

Figure 5-6: Images courtesy of Los Angeles College of Chiropractic.

Figures 5-7, 5-8, 5-9: Images courtesy of Siker Medical Imaging, Portland, OR.

Figure 7-1: http://www.headquartersmigraine.com/about.htm.

Figure 7-2: From Stewart WF, Lipton RB, Kolodner K et al: Reliability of the migraine disability, assessment score in a population-based sample of headache sufferers, *Cephalatgia* 19(2):107-114, 1999.

Index

Page numbers followed by f indicate figures; t, tables;
b, boxes.